Modern Management of Spinal Deformities

Modern Management of Spinal Deformities

Edited by Joe Morrison

STATES
ACADEMIC PRESS
www.statesacademicpress.com

States Academic Press,
109 South 5th Street,
Brooklyn, NY 11249, USA

Visit us on the World Wide Web at:
www.statesacademicpress.com

ISBN: 978-1-63989-361-4

Cataloging-in-Publication Data

Modern management of spinal deformities / edited by Joe Morrison.
p. cm.
Includes bibliographical references and index.
ISBN 978-1-63989-361-4
1. Spine--Diseases. 2. Spine--Abnormalities. 3. Spine--Diseases--Treatment.
4. Spine--Abnormalities--Treatment. I. Morrison, Joe.
RD768 .M63 2022
617.560 59--dc23

Table of Contents

Preface

This book has been a concerted effort by a group of academicians, researchers and scientists, who have contributed their research works for the realization of the book. This book has materialized in the wake of emerging advancements and innovations in this field. Therefore, the need of the hour was to compile all the required researches and disseminate the knowledge to a broad spectrum of people comprising of students, researchers and specialists of the field.

Spinal deformities refer to the conditions of impairment of the backbone. These encompass various diseases associated with the spine such as spinal muscular atrophy, kyphosis, dorsalgia, ankylosing spondylitis, spina bifida, lumbar spinal stenosis, osteoporosis, spinal tumors and cauda equine syndrome. Spinal diseases also encompass the diseases of cervical spine which are diseases of the vertebrae of the neck. Cervical spine is very flexible; because of this it is very likely for a person to damage that area over a long period of time. Some common diseases of cervical spine include cervical stenosis, cervical disc herniation and degenerative disc diseases. Neck pain is caused when spinal canal loses its gap and gets thinner. This book is a compilation of chapters that discuss the most vital concepts and modern management of spinal deformities. It presents researches and studies performed by experts across the globe. This book will serve as a reference to a broad spectrum of readers.

At the end of the preface, I would like to thank the authors for their brilliant chapters and the publisher for guiding us all-through the making of the book till its final stage. Also, I would like to thank my family for providing the support and encouragement throughout my academic career and research projects.

Editor

1

The Quantified Indices for Compensatory Patterns for Low Back Pain and Outcome Measures

Paul S. Sung and Pamela Danial

Abstract

The quantification of balance stability is valuable to a number of populations, including older adults with low back pain (LBP). Investigations into postural stability and one-leg standing should be performed to integrate balance performance using kinematic and kinetic indices. The comparison of postural control between older adults with LBP and healthy older adults might contribute to a further understanding of postural adaptations, especially when considering visual condition. The one-leg standing test would highlight the differences in kinematic and kinetic stabilities between groups. Because the eyes-closed condition results in significantly decreased spinal stability, the normalized kinematic and kinetic indices could be utilized to compare postural integration as well as proprioceptive responses. Older adults with LBP demonstrated higher lumbar spine stability in the eyes-open condition, which might be due to a possible pain avoiding strategy from the standing limb. Clinicians need to consider both kinetic and kinematic indices and visual condition when addressing lumbar spine stability. Quantified indices for compensatory patterns might provide further understanding of optimal injury prevention and rehabilitation strategies for individuals with LBP.

Keywords: low back pain, balance, kinetic, kinematic, biomechanics, postural control

1. Introduction

Low back pain (LBP) is an ailment that impacts work performance and affects up to 80% of the United States population at some point in an individual's, making it one of the most prevalent musculoskeletal conditions causing physical disability [1, 2]. LBP is a major factor in escalating health-care costs with a point prevalence of approximately 12%, a 1-month prevalence of 23%, and a 1-year prevalence of 38% [3]. One study reported that between 24 and 80% of older adults with LBP experienced recurrent episodes within 1 year [3]. As the most commonly encountered medical condition in older adults, LBP poses an even greater challenge in the health care of this population as compared to their younger counterparts.

This chapter proposes biomechanical assessments of spinal function by which to evaluate LBP. The development of a valid and reliable tool for evaluating older adults with LBP is necessary to provide a link between LBP and balance deficits. It might be helpful for clinicians to consider the potential characteristics of kinematic data, such as range of motion, velocity, and acceleration as well as kinetic data, such as ground reaction force (GRF) changes, during the one-leg standing test. This combined approach could provide a better understanding of postural stability and ground reaction forces for integrating motor control and biomechanics. Specifically, an understanding of the compensatory patterns between normalized kinematic and kinetic stability indices for spinal regions, while considering visual condition may reveal possible pain avoiding strategies from the standing limb. These would be important findings since a lack of coordination and altered postural strategy has the potential to cause musculoskeletal injuries. Individual variations between older adults might lead to different compensatory responses and should be elucidated to establish fall prevention strategies. Several studies reported that an analysis of the one-leg standing test via a motion capture system could be used to determine balance strategies in older adults with LBP [4–8]. However, a comprehensive tool for quantifying kinematic and kinetic changes during one-leg standing is still needed to enhance evidence-based practice, prevent fall injuries, and identify factors affecting proprioception and posture.

An evidence-based, quantitative approach may enhance quality of care for older adults with LBP and aid in preventing injury. Furthermore, the development of potential interventions as a result of this quantitative approach could favorably alter motor control, which plays a key clinical role in terms of musculoskeletal and neurological functioning of older adults with LBP.

2. Comprehensive balance parameters

Evidence-based intervention has stressed the importance of establishing a strong link between treatments and outcomes to both researchers and clinicians. Various studies have suggested that exercise programs are effective in the treatment of LBP [9–12]; however, most researchers fail to provide evidence favoring one exercise over another. Contradicting results might be related to poor sensitivity of the instruments, an unmatched research design, small sample sizes, and/or the lack of a valid and reliable index for standardization.

It is necessary to provide sensitive kinetic and kinematic indices for quantitative evaluation of altered postural coordination in older adults with recurrent LBP. Kinetic and kinematic data regarding spinal dysfunction and coordination may provide clinical insight into motor control and identify patterns of compensatory movements in older adults with recurrent LBP [13, 14]. Several studies have measured kinematic changes of the dominant thigh and pelvis to identify variations in balance sway compensation strategies as well as spinal alignment and core stability between older adults with LBP and control subjects [13, 15]. Another study reported that because active limb movements might be associated with early lumbopelvic motion, increased frequency of these movements may contribute to increased lumbar region tissue stress, potentially leading to LBP symptoms [16] since altered movements are known to decrease muscular force-generating capabilities [17, 18]. These outcome studies considered the morphological and functional implications in the neuro-musculoskeletal system.

The one-leg standing test was developed in order to investigate dynamic postural steadiness (**Figure 1**). Clinicians often use the one-leg standing test to assess movement performance and to observe biomechanical deficits. It provides a sensitive analysis of postural stability, considering 40% of human gait movement occurs during one-leg stance [19, 20]. The one-leg standing test examines the ability of the subject to perform spinal load transfers and to optimize pelvic girdle stability while also detecting relative innominate bone motion [21]. A kinematic analysis of the body regions and the kinetic analysis from the force plate during the one-leg standing test could be useful in enhancing the understanding of the role of core spine activity during the test. As shown in **Figure 1**, the core spine model is a reference model for trunk motion used in motion analysis. It compares specific three-dimensional kinematic data to the motion of the lumbar spine [13]. This measure of integrated spinal stability might allow for the development of motor control strategies in older adults with LBP since reaction forces from the platform reflect oscillations in forces about the foot needed to maintain balance [7, 14, 20].

The kinetic and kinematic changes in three-dimensional trunk motion could also be compared to reflect standing balance contributions to postural control [7]. A lack of coordination of the

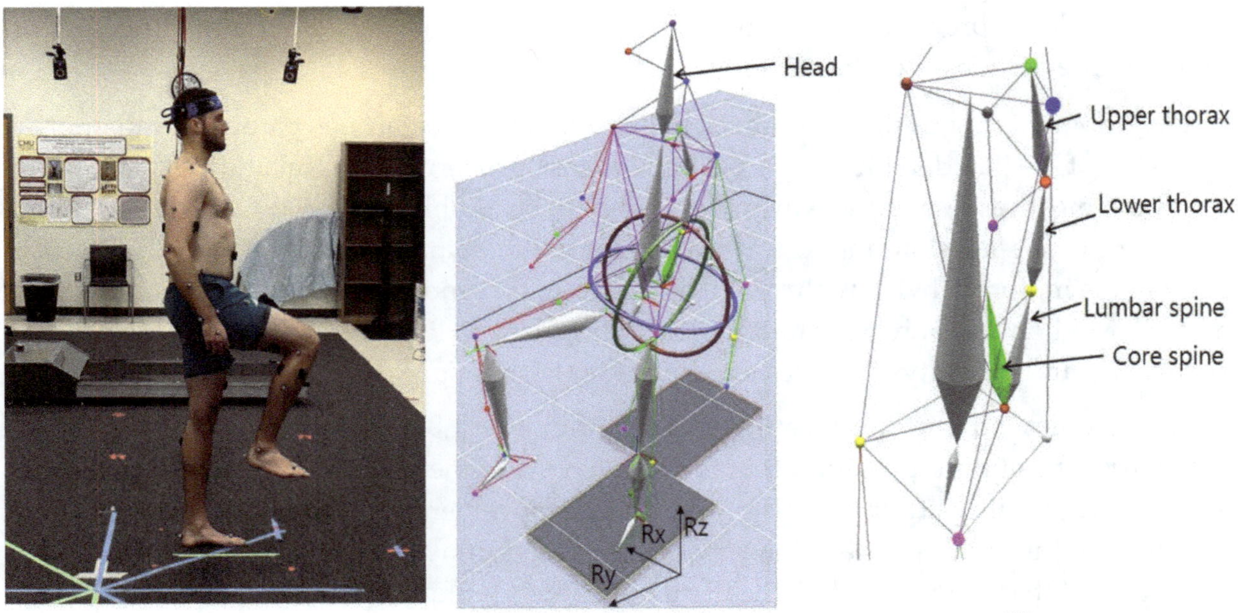

(A) (B) (C)

Figure 1. One-leg standing balance test (A). The subject was asked to stand on a single leg with the contralateral hip and knee flexed 90° for 30 s. During the test, the subject maintained postural stability while kinetic and kinematic data were collected. In order to quantify the data, each segment was calculated as the amount of rotational displacement side-to-side (Rx), back-and-forth (Ry), and up-and-down (Rz) away from a mean value (B). The core spine model was utilized as a reference to compare specific three-dimensional spine motions including the lumbar spine and the lower and upper thoracic spines (C).

lumbar spine may cause musculoskeletal injuries, and altered coordination of the postural reaction might lead to compensatory responses to prevent injuries [14, 22, 23]. Quantifying postural compensation may lead to a better understanding of spinal movement patterns due to a fear of falling in order to clarify the relationship between kinematic and kinetic changes in older adults with recurrent LBP.

The normalized kinematic index of the lumbar spine was calculated based on the three-dimensional rotation angle (*Rxyz*) and relative standing index between control and recurrent LBP groups. The ratio between standing duration and requested duration could be compared with the corresponding older adults' *Rxyz* values. The analysis time window excluded the initial transition time (5 s) from standing with bilateral legs to maintaining single, dominant leg standing.

3. Postural deficits and integrated balance performance

Fear of falling is a major health concern among older adults and has even been reported in those who have no history of falls [24, 25]. The presence of fear of falling was defined as "low perceived self-efficacy at avoiding falls during essential, nonhazardous activities of daily living" [26]. Fear of falling risk drastically increases with age and is known to affect quality of life in older adults, especially for women who fear that falling contains potentially serious outcomes [27–29]. These studies indicated that fear of falling in older women is a common and persistent complaint that is caused mainly by impairments of balance and mobility. The results for balance problems or fear of falling imply that early intervention might be important in the prevention and rehabilitation of balance deficits.

The development of sensitive tools that can quantify loss of balance is paramount to improving quality of life in older adults. It is essential to perform biomechanical and functional analyses of the most representative kinematic and kinetic variables obtained from specific tasks, including the one-leg standing test. Since the control of spinal function might include excitability in the motor pathway with fearful aspects of pain syndromes, the combined kinematic analysis based on spinal regions and kinetic indices from a force plate may provide comprehensive postural integrity strategies to reduce the risk of injury.

Previous studies support the idea that older adults with LBP have reduced proprioceptive sensation on position-reposition accuracy and have a higher prevalence of balance deficits [30–32]. Several other studies focusing on typical movement patterns in older adults with LBP identified increased postural sway and decreased lumbar spine motion [33, 34]. It has been reported that individuals with LBP demonstrate significantly decreased postural stability during one-leg standing and other clinical balance tests [7, 8, 14]. However, the results of these studies lacked an understanding of three-dimensional dynamic variables over time during one-leg standing. Further, most clinical outcome studies are still not convincing in their measurements, and implications of functional activity need to be further investigated [35, 36]. For example, center of pressure (COP) displacement may provide useful information in quantifying standing postural stability as well as predicting dynamic balance [37]. However, the COP provides limited information, as it is only a two-dimensional quantity.

Before one can quantify balance deficits, however, one must first understand their origins and the factors that directly or indirectly impact them. The assessment and classification of balance deficits due to spinal disorders have been carried out in different ways. Patients have been classified according to the injured or painful structure using imaging techniques (i.e., magnetic resonance imaging, computed tomography, and myelography). However, a pathologic-anatomic diagnosis is established in only 10–15% of all patients with disorders of the lumbar region [1]. Additionally, there is great variation in the reported prevalence of balance deficits in older adults, which is associated with multiple factors, including poor health characteristics [38, 39]. Gender, age, body mass index (BMI), time since initial pain onset, and quality of life warrant further investigation for a complete understanding of the role of these factors in providing comprehensive tools to prevent fall injuries. Therefore, valid and reliable measurement tools for balance deficits that account for physiological and socioeconomic factors would be important for clinicians to develop rehabilitation and injury prevention strategies.

The quantification of balance deficits based on three-dimensional kinematic and kinetic indices is valuable to a number of populations, including older adults with LBP. It is generally accepted that individuals with LBP possess altered postural control as well as less-refined proprioception [15, 40, 41]. Previous research has shown that control groups demonstrated significantly longer standing duration in the eyes-open condition [7, 13]. Due to decreased proprioception, the pain-avoiding strategies implemented by the LBP group may be more evident. When proprioception is limited, the differences in standing duration may explain the proprioceptive capability between groups [42]. The normalized kinematic index could be utilized to compare postural integration based on visual input as well as proprioceptive responses. This compensatory pattern needs to be further investigated for optimal injury prevention and the development of effective rehabilitation programs.

Studies have also reported poor coordination of balance performance in individuals with LBP; however, there is a lack of understanding about the individual kinetic and kinematic characteristics of trunk motion in older adults with balance deficits. Recent studies have been performed to evaluate the role of core stability in older adults with LBP [43–45], as kinematic changes of the trunk are compensated for by postural alignment and core spine stability [13, 15]. Further, a comprehensive investigation to determine postural steadiness might be helpful to understand the control of postural segments, including the trunk, pelvis, and lower extremities, during one-leg standing. The ability to adjust postural steadiness as a function of these regions is critical for activities of daily life, as increased balance sway was related not only to spinal motion but also to dynamic functional capacity in older adults with LBP [46]. Therefore, a change in postural steadiness might be related to an increase in kinetic stability [7], which reduces dynamic functional capacity in the trunk, pelvis, and lower extremities.

Older adults with LBP demonstrated differences in lumbar spine stability, possibly due to a pain avoidance strategy and compensation from the standing limb [7]. However, it is not clear how the kinematic chain reaction might change for whole body control mechanisms during one-leg standing. Therefore, the normalized kinematic stability index of the body regions (thorax, pelvis, and bilateral thighs, shanks, and feet) and one-leg standing duration might contribute to an integrated understanding of postural steadiness in older adults with LBP.

Several studies have used the one-leg standing test to investigate postural control using different outcome variables [7, 13, 47]. The one-leg standing test can be divided into two phases: the dynamic phase and the static phase. The dynamic phase is defined as a rapid decrease of force variability during the first 5 seconds (s) of the test. The static phase is defined as the maintenance of a certain level of force variability. One study, which investigated the first 5 s of a 25 s duration test (dynamic phase), concluded that the first few seconds of the one-leg standing test pose the greatest challenge to postural steadiness [48]. They concluded that if participants were unable to perform one-leg standing for at least 5 s, they were at an increased risk for injurious falls. Other studies have investigated the static phase. High variability during the first 5 s of the static phase of the one-leg standing test was reported, which could potentially be caused by muscular or postural adjustments [7, 14]. Based on these findings, it might be possible to analyze the first 5 s increments of the static and dynamic phases of postural stability to discover different aspects of sensorimotor function that older adults with LBP use to enhance pain-avoiding strategies.

It has been reported that impaired back muscle function may lead to an inability to adopt postural control strategies focused on increasing strength and self-efficacy in older adults with LBP [49, 50]. These studies suggested that impaired back muscle function may lead to an adaptation of postural control strategies with the primary purpose of preventing pain and decreasing mobility of the painful region. By contrast, longer one-leg standing duration in the control group can be explained by enhanced motor learning due to greater ability to perform functional activities and implement more functional postural control strategies.

Other studies supported the reorganization of trunk muscle representation at the motor cortex in individuals with recurrent LBP [51, 52]. Their results suggest that this reorganization is associated with deficits in postural control, which persist after the training effect takes place as LBP becomes chronic or recurrent. Eventually, these learned strategies become automatic defense mechanisms to prevent pain and further injury [15, 52].

4. Kinetic and kinematic indices

The stability index was developed with two parameters—relative standing time and relative standstill time [14]. The relative standing time was defined as a ratio between the successful standing time and the requested standing time. The successful standing time was measured as the total standing time before the subject failed to maintain stability, allowing the non-dominant, lifted limb to touch the force plate. The relative standstill time was defined as a ratio between the sum of standstill time and successful standing time. The standstill time was the summation of the temporal segments, where the three-dimensional rotation of the tested axis was below threshold (5°).

In **Figure 2**, the distribution of the normalized standing time was plotted with the corresponding relative kinematic index for the core spine model between the control group and the recurrent LBP group. The data obtained from five subjects were selected as examples

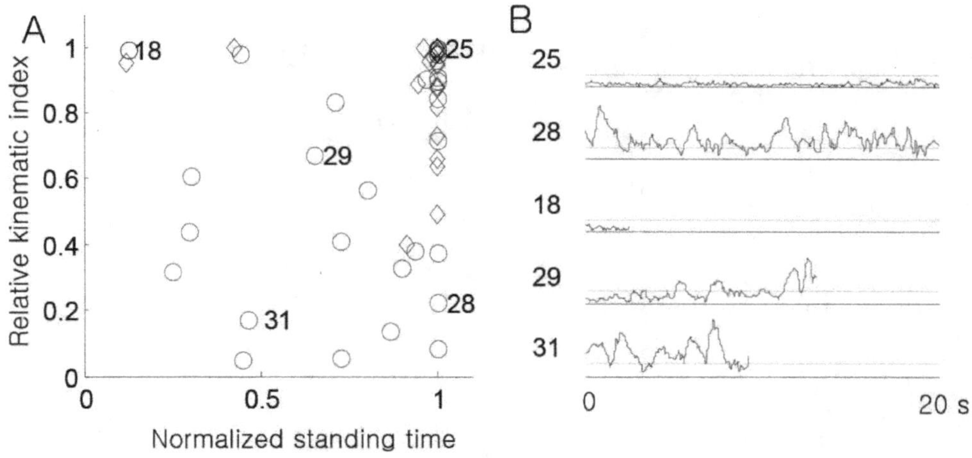

Figure 2. A: Distribution of normalized standing time (x-axis) and relative kinematic index (y-axis) of body regions and corresponding three-dimensional angle (Rxyz) from control group (diamond) and LBP group (open dot). B: Examples of Rxyz traces from A. Subject 25 had stable and long duration, while subject 28 had unstable long duration. Subject 18 had short duration with stable balance and subject 31 had relatively short duration with unstable balance. Subject 29 had longer duration and more stable balance than subject 31. Threshold (dot) and baseline (solid) are plotted for each trace.

of the normalized standing time, and the relative kinematic index was compared with the corresponding subjects' *Rxyz* values. The analysis time window excluded the initial transition time (5 s) from the test [14].

Therefore, the rotational angular displacements were more important than translations during the test. The operational definitions for the terms utilized in this study are included as follows:

- Normalized kinematic index from spinal regions: The rotational angles of the specific spinal regions (core spine model, lumbar spine, lower thorax, and upper thorax) were calculated between two adjacent joints in three dimensions and then combined to quantify the normalized kinematic stability index. As shown in **Figure 3**, the angular displacement of the lumbar spine was calculated from the average, and then, temporal summation of the data was used to calculate the normalized kinematic index for each spinal region.
- Normalized kinetic index from force plate: The older adults stood upright on the non-dominant leg for 20 s on a force plate surface with the dominant hip and knee flexed to approximately 90°, first with their eyes open and then with their eyes closed. The summation of ground reaction forces was computed in the same way as the kinematic index, with the average value subtracted to have each force plane average. Therefore, the normalized kinematic and kinetic changes for postural stability were compared for the balance test under different visual conditions. The kinematic and kinetic data were normalized so that various individual differences might be fairly compared between groups. For reliability, the intra-class correlations were calculated to determine the force plate measures taken. The intra-class correlation coefficients of type (3, 1) were used to determine the degree of test-retest reliability, ranged from 0.85 to 0.98, and were interpreted as excellent according to Shrout and Fleiss [53].

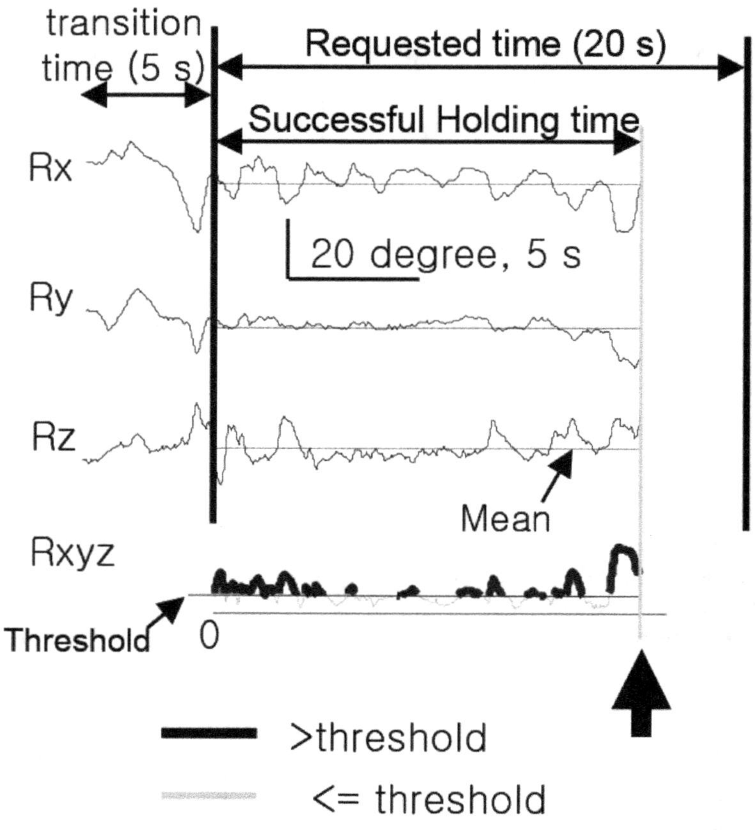

$$Rxyz = \sqrt{(R_x - R_{x\_mean})^2 + (R_y - R_{y\_mean})^2 + (R_z - R_{z\_mean})^2}$$

Figure 3. The rotation angle of the core spine computed from kinematic markers. For computing stability index, initial transition time (5 s) was excluded. Out of 25 s requested holding time, successful holding time (duration) was measured as the total duration until subject fail to stand on one leg (large arrow). The kinematic stability was measured as the square root sum of axial angle subtracted from its own mean value during successful holding time (see equation).

- The dynamic postural steadiness index (DPSI): The DPSI (4) was based on the kinetic data, which was calculated for three principal directions and was reported as a sensitive measure index. The DPSI is a composite of the medio-lateral steadiness index (MLSI; 1), anterior-posterior steadiness index (APSI; 2), and vertical steadiness index (VSI; 3), which are mean square deviations assessing fluctuations around a zero point, rather than standard deviations assessing fluctuations around a group mean. The stabilization time was also determined as an objective postural control measure by using three indices of analysis based on the resultant GRF. The MLSI and APSI assessed the fluctuations from a zero point along the frontal and sagittal planes of the force plate, respectively. The VSI assessed fluctuation of the subject's body weight to normalize the vertical scores for standardization of the vertical GRF along the transverse plane of the force plate. This measure allowed comparison of individuals with different body weights (mass).

$$\text{MLSI} = \sqrt{\left[\frac{\Sigma (0 - x)^2}{\text{number of data points}}\right]} \tag{1}$$

$$\text{APSI} = \sqrt{\left[\frac{\Sigma(0-y)^2}{\text{number of data points}}\right]} \quad (2)$$

$$\text{VSI} = \sqrt{\left[\frac{\Sigma(\text{body weight}-z)^2}{\text{number of data points}}\right]} \quad (3)$$

$$\text{DPSI} = \sqrt{\left[\frac{\Sigma(0-x)^2+\Sigma(0-y)^2+\Sigma(\text{body weight}-z)^2}{\text{number of data points}}\right]} \quad (4)$$

The outcome measures included one-leg standing time, DPSI (composite of MLSI, APSI, and VSI), and stabilization times. In this way, postural stability might be quantified during the one-leg standing test with the underlying premise that dynamic postural stability depends on lower limb kinematics.

5. Applications for the balance indices

The normalized kinematic stability index for specific portions of the body was compared with the kinetic stability index from the force plate.

As shown in **Figure 4**, a threshold was determined as 10 Newtons for the normalized kinetic stability. Although the value might not be the optimal quantity, the results would not be significantly different if neighboring values were selected.

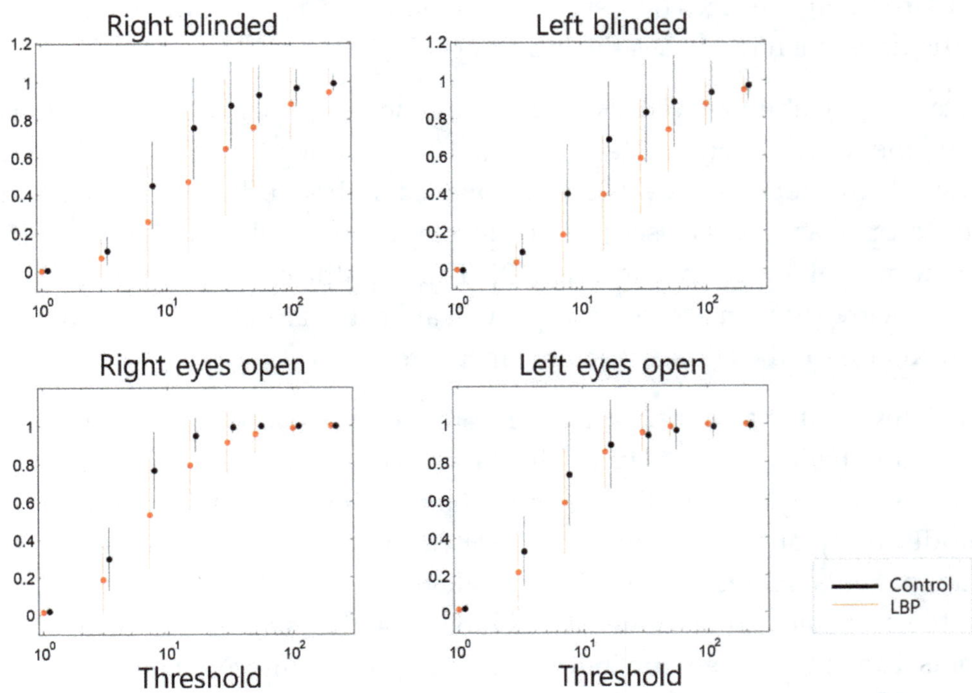

Figure 4. The change of threshold on normalized kinetic stability for the force platform between groups based on visual input. A threshold of approximately 10 Newtons could separate the LBP group from the control group.

A recent review article indicated that there are no evidence-based guidelines currently available to assess spinal instability [54, 55]. Their summary indicated that both spinal stability and mobility concepts represent a new frontier in the study of the painful degenerative spine. The development of new rehabilitation strategies for LBP based on information regarding the kinematic and kinetic stability indices could help restore the normal function of spinal segments and protect the adjacent segments. Previous studies also reported that postural steadiness, including trunk coordination, is a foundational necessity to prevent early mechanical deterioration of the entire body [8, 14, 56]. Postural steadiness has been used to characterize the dynamics of the postural control system associated with maintaining balance [57]. However, the compensatory function of postural steadiness needs to be implemented within the whole body to prevent recurrence of pain and further injuries.

6. Clinical implications

It is important to investigate the effects of an intervention in terms of its musculoskeletal or neurological link with the cardiovascular and integumentary systems during human motion. Although some therapeutic interventions have demonstrated benefits, researchers have not quantified or characterized the results yielded by specific non-surgical interventions [9–12].

The one-leg standing test could be utilized to quantitatively assess postural steadiness in a static position and to investigate various balance disorders in older adults with LBP. The test has been utilized in clinical settings, in which patients perform the test with their eyes open, standing unassisted on one leg. The test is timed in seconds from the time one foot is lifted off the floor to the time when it touches the ground [7, 58].

Other balance and gait abilities were assessed using the Berg Balance Scale [59], the functional reach test [60], the timed up and go test [61], the 10-m walking test [62], and the timed single leg stance test [8]. The performance values established in this study help make the single-limb stance test (eyes open and eyes closed) a reliable, readily available, and easy to perform "bedside" examination tool for balance testing [63]. The quantified performance scores based on the age and the degree of pain across a sample will aid clinicians in understanding the specific level of performance for the clinical outcome measures.

Therefore, it is evident that nonsurgical spine research, as well as other fields of clinical research, should enhance the quality of clinical efforts and develop effective interventions for individuals suffering from LBP. It is important to develop a sensitive tool for evaluating baseline disability and the effectiveness (or detriment) of clinical treatment strategies for individual patients. However, the COP provides limited information on body reactions. Conversely, the combined three-dimensional kinetic analyses from GRF with specific sensitive thresholds, as well as kinematic index analyses, provide more accurate and meaningful data, which could allow for the development of new and more effective intervention strategies for treating LBP [14].

7. Conclusion

The quantification of balance deficits based on kinematic and kinetic indices is valuable to a number of populations, including older adults with LBP. The comparison of postural control based on the normalized kinematic and kinetic stabilities during the one-leg standing test might contribute to a further understanding of postural adaptations that occur as a result of chronic LBP. The compensatory pattern need to be investigated to allow for optimal injury prevention and the development of effective rehabilitation programs.

Acknowledgements

This work was supported by Herbert H. and Grace A. Dow College of Health Professions at Central Michigan University (ION 42041-15647 and FRCE 48151).

Author details

Paul S. Sung* and Pamela Danial

*Address all correspondence to: drpsung@gmail.com

Department of Physical Therapy, Central Michigan University, MI, USA

References

[1] Woolf AD, Pfleger B. Burden of major musculoskeletal conditions. Bulletin of the World Health Organization. 2003;**81**(9):646-656

[2] Manchikanti L, et al., Epidemiology of low back pain in adults. Neuromodulation, 2014; **17 Suppl 2**:3-10

[3] Hoy D, et al. The Epidemiology of low back pain. Best Practice & Research Clinical Rheumatology. 2011;**24**(6):769-781

[4] Sung PS. The ground reaction force thresholds for detecting postural stability in participants with and without flat foot. Journal of Biomechanics. 2016;**49**(1):60-65

[5] Sung PS, Danial P, Lee DC. Comparison of the different kinematic patterns during lateral bending between subjects with and without recurrent low back pain. Clinical Biomechanics (Bristol, Avon). 2016;**38**:50-55

[6] Sung PS, Ham YW. Comparing postural strategy changes following adapted versus non-adapted responses in subjects with and without spinal stenosis. Manual Therapy. 2010;**15**(3):261-266

[7] Sung PS, Leininger PM. A kinematic and kinetic analysis of spinal region in subjects with and without recurrent low back pain during one leg standing. Clinical Biomechanics (Bristol, Avon). 2015;**30**(7):696-702

[8] Kuo YL, et al., Steadiness of spinal regions during single-leg standing in older adults with and without chronic low back pain. PLoS One. 2015;**10**(5):e0128318

[9] Abenhaim L, et al. The role of activity in the therapeutic management of back pain. Report of the International Paris Task Force on Back Pain. Spine (Phila Pa 1976). 2000;**25**(4 Suppl):1S-33S

[10] Bystrom MG, Rasmussen-Barr E, Grooten WJ. Motor control exercises reduces pain and disability in chronic and recurrent low back pain: A meta-analysis. Spine. 2013;**38**(6): E350-E358

[11] Kendall KD, et al. The effect of the addition of hip strengthening exercises to a lumbopelvic exercise programme for the treatment of non-specific low back pain: A randomized controlled trial. Journal of Science and Medicine in Sport. 2015;**18**(6):626-631

[12] Searle A, et al. Exercise interventions for the treatment of chronic low back pain: A systematic review and meta-analysis of randomised controlled trials. Clinical Rehabilitation. 2015;**29**(12):1155-1167

[13] Lee DC, Ham YW, Sung PS. Effect of visual input on normalized standing stability in subjects with recurrent low back pain. Gait Posture. 2012;**36**(3):580-585

[14] Sung PS, Yoon B, Lee DC. Lumbar spine stability for subjects with and without low back pain during one-leg standing test. Spine (Phila Pa 1976). 2010;**35**(16):E753-E760

[15] Tsao H, Hodges PW. Persistence of improvements in postural strategies following motor control training in people with recurrent low back pain. Journal of Electromyography and Kinesiology. 2008;**18**(4):559-567

[16] Scholtes SA, Gombatto SP, Van Dillen LR. Differences in lumbopelvic motion between people with and people without low back pain during two lower limb movement tests. Clinical Biomechanics (Bristol, Avon). 2009;**24**(1):7-12

[17] Hicks AL, Kent-Braun J, Ditor DS. Sex differences in human skeletal muscle fatigue. Exercise and Sport Sciences Reviews. 2001;**29**(3):109-112

[18] Hicks GE, et al. Absolute strength and loss of strength as predictors of mobility decline in older adults: The InCHIANTI study. The Journal of Gerontology A Biological Sciences and Medical Sciences. 2012;**67**(1):66-73

[19] Aberg AC, et al. Calculations of mechanisms for balance control during narrow and single-leg standing in fit older adults: A reliability study. Gait Posture. 2011;**34**(3):352-357

[20] Verhagen E, et al. The effect of a balance training programme on centre of pressure excursion in one-leg stance. Clinical Biomechanics (Bristol, Avon). 2005;**20**(10):1094-1100

[21] Hungerford BA, et al. Evaluation of the ability of physical therapists to palpate intrapelvic motion with the Stork test on the support side. Physical Therapy. 2007;**87**(7):879-887

[22] Shum GL, Crosbie J, Lee RY. Effect of low back pain on the kinematics and joint coordination of the lumbar spine and hip during sit-to-stand and stand-to-sit. Spine (Phila Pa 1976). 2005;**30**(17):1998-2004

[23] Shum GL, Crosbie J, Lee RY. Three-dimensional kinetics of the lumbar spine and hips in low back pain patients during sit-to-stand and stand-to-sit. Spine (Phila Pa 1976). 2007;**32**(7):E211-E219

[24] Howland J, et al. Fear of falling among the community-dwelling elderly. Journal of Aging and Health. 1993;**5**(2):229-243

[25] Vellas, B.J., et al., Fear of falling and restriction of mobility in elderly fallers. Age and Ageing, 1997;**26**(3):189-193

[26] Tinetti ME, Richman D, Powell L. Falls efficacy as a measure of fear of falling. Journal of Gerontology. 1990;**45**(6):P239–P243

[27] Fritz JM, George SZ. Identifying psychosocial variables in patients with acute work-related low back pain: The importance of fear-avoidance beliefs. Physical Therapy. 2002;**82**(10):973-983

[28] Ambrose AF, Cruz L, Paul G. Falls and fractures: A systematic approach to screening and prevention. Maturitas. 2015;**82**(1):85-93

[29] Austin N, et al. Fear of falling in older women: A longitudinal study of incidence, persistence, and predictors. Journal of American Geriatric Society. 2007;**55**(10):1598-1603

[30] Feipel V, et al. Development of kinematics tests for the evaluation of lumbar proprioception and equilibration. Clinical Biomechanics (Bristol, Avon). 2003;**18**(7):612-618

[31] Gill KP, Callaghan MJ. The measurement of lumbar proprioception in individuals with and without low back pain. Spine. 1998;**23**(3):371-377

[32] Koumantakis GA, Winstanley J, Oldham JA. Thoracolumbar proprioception in individuals with and without low back pain: Intratester reliability, clinical applicability, and validity. Journal of Orthopaedic & Sports Physical Therapy. 2002;**32**(7):327-335

[33] Ruhe A, Fejer R, Walker B. Center of pressure excursion as a measure of balance performance in patients with non-specific low back pain compared to healthy controls: A systematic review of the literature. European Spine Journal. 2011;**20**(3):358-368

[34] Intolo P, et al. The effect of age on lumbar range of motion: A systematic review. Manual Therapy. 2009;**14**(6):596-604

[35] Baldwin KM, Haddad F. Effects of different activity and inactivity paradigms on myosin heavy chain gene expression in striated muscle. Journal of Applied Physiology. 2001;**90**(1):345-357

[36] Tsao H, et al. Motor training of the lumbar paraspinal muscles induces immediate changes in motor coordination in patients with recurrent low back pain. Journal of Pain. 2010;**11**(11):1120-1128

[37] Rhee HS, Kim YH, Sung PS. A randomized controlled trial to determine the effect of spinal stabilization exercise intervention based on pain level and standing balance differences in patients with low back pain. Medical Science Monitor. 2012;**18**(3):CR174-189

[38] Cumming RG, et al. Prospective study of the impact of fear of falling on activities of daily living, SF-36 scores, and nursing home admission. The Journal of Gerontology A Biological Sciences and Medical Sciences. 2000;**55**(5):M299-305

[39] Salkeld G, et al. Quality of life related to fear of falling and hip fracture in older women: A time trade off study. British Medical Journal. 2000;**320**(7231):341-346

[40] Brumagne S, et al. Persons with recurrent low back pain exhibit a rigid postural control strategy. European Spine Journal. 2008;**17**(9):1177-1184

[41] Sung PS. Disability and back muscle fatigability changes following two therapeutic exercise interventions in participants with recurrent low back pain. Medical Science Monitor, 2013;**19**:40-48

[42] Brumagne S, Cordo P, Verschueren S. Proprioceptive weighting changes in persons with low back pain and elderly persons during upright standing. Neuroscience Letters, 2004;**366**(1):63-66

[43] Heidari P, et al. The role of ultrasound in diagnosis of the causes of low back pain: A review of the literature. Asian Journal of Sports Medicine, 2015;**6**(1):e23803

[44] Hides J, et al. An MRI investigation into the function of the transversus abdominis muscle during "drawing-in" of the abdominal wall. Spine (Phila Pa 1976). 2006;**31**(6):E175-E178

[45] Teyhen DS, et al. The use of ultrasound imaging of the abdominal drawing-in maneuver in subjects with low back pain. Journal of Orthopaedic & Sports Physical Therapy, 2005;**35**(6):346-355

[46] Hamaoui A, Do MC, Bouisset S. Postural sway increase in low back pain subjects is not related to reduced spine range of motion. Neuroscience Letters. 2004;**357**(2):135-138

[47] King DL, Zatsiorsky VM. Periods of extreme ankle displacement during one-legged standing. Gait Posture. 2002;**15**(2):172-179

[48] Jonsson E, Seiger A, Hirschfeld H. Postural steadiness and weight distribution during tandem stance in healthy young and elderly adults. Clinical Biomechanics (Bristol, Avon). 2005;**20**(2):202-208

[49] Elfving B, Dedering A, Nemeth G. Lumbar muscle fatigue and recovery in patients with long-term low-back trouble—Electromyography and health-related factors. Clinical Biomechanics (Bristol, Avon). 2003;**18**(7):619-630

[50] Johanson E, et al. The effect of acute back muscle fatigue on postural control strategy in people with and without recurrent low back pain. European Spine Journal. 2011;**20(12)**:2152-2159

[51] Tsao H, Danneels LA, Hodges PW. Smudging the motor brain in young adults with recurrent low back pain. Spine (Phila Pa 1976). 2011;**36**(21):1721-1727

[52] Tsao H, Galea MP, Hodges PW. Reorganization of the motor cortex is associated with postural control deficits in recurrent low back pain. Brain. 2008;**131**(Pt 8):2161-2171

[53] Shrout PE, Fleiss JL. Intraclass correlations: Uses in assessing rater reliability. Psychological Bulletin, 1979;**86**(2):420-428

[54] Izzo R, et al. Biomechanics of the spine. Part I: Spinal stability. European Journal of Radiology, 2013;**82**(1):118-126.

[55] Izzo R, et al. Biomechanics of the spine. Part II: Spinal instability. European Journal of Radiology, 2013;**82**(1):127-138

[56] Silfies SP, et al. Trunk muscle recruitment patterns in specific chronic low back pain populations. Clinical Biomechanics (Bristol, Avon). 2005;**20**(5):465-473

[57] Prieto TE, et al. Measures of postural steadiness: Differences between healthy young and elderly adults. IEEE Transactions on Biomedical Engineering, 1996;**43**(9):956-966

[58] Ham YW, et al. Kinematic analyses of trunk stability in one leg standing for individuals with recurrent low back pain. Journal of Electromyography and Kinesiology, 2010;**20(6)**:1134-1140

[59] Bogle Thorbahn LD, Newton RA. Use of the Berg Balance Test to predict falls in elderly persons. Physical Therapy, 1996;**76**(6):576-583; discussion 584-585

[60] Takahashi T, et al. Vertical ground reaction force shape is associated with gait parameters, timed up and go, and functional reach in elderly females. Journal of Rehabilitation Medicine, 2004;**36**(1):42-45

[61] Manaf H, Justine M, Omar M. Functional balance and motor impairment correlations with gait parameters during timed up and go test across three attentional loading conditions in stroke survivors. Stroke Research and Treatment. **2014**:439304

[62] Nagano K, Hori H, Muramatsu K. A comparison of at-home walking and 10-meter walking test parameters of individuals with post-stroke hemiparesis. Journal of Physical Therapy Science, 2015;**27**(2):357-359

[63] Springer BA, et al. Normative values for the unipedal stance test with eyes open and closed. Journal of Geriatric Physical Therapy. 2007;**30**(1):8-15

2

Role of the Neuroinflammation in the Degree of Spinal Cord Injury: New Therapeutic Strategies

Irene Paterniti, Emanuela Esposito and
Salvatore Cuzzocrea

Abstract

A case of spinal cord injury (SCI) is defined as the occurrence of an acute traumatic lesion of neural elements in the spinal canal (spinal cord and cauda equina), resulting in temporary or permanent sensory and/or motor deficit. Most studies on traumatic SCI show a bimodal age distribution, with a first peak in young adulthood and a second peak in older adults. Spinal cord trauma activates a cascade of events that exacerbates the damage such as activation of inflammatory process that determinates cytokine and chemokine production and that generates reduction in functional recovery resulting in necrosis or apoptosis of neurons. However, the precise mechanism of SCI-induced inflammatory response remains not fully understood at present. Current strategy to treat damage to the spinal cord is limited, only the treatment with methylprednisolone (MP), if administered in excessive dose during the acute phase of the damage, could ameliorate patients with severe SCI. However, associated to the beneficial effects, there are growing evidence that high-dose of MP is correlated to increased risk of infections, pneumonia and gastrointestinal bleeding. Therefore, there is a necessity to develop new therapies to treat SCI; one of these is to selectively reduce inflammation that possess unique role in the processes of injury and recovery.

Keywords: Immune response, oxidative stress, spinal cord injury, inflammation, neuroprotection

1. Inflammation response after spinal cord injury

Spinal cord injury (SCI) is damage caused to the spinal cord that compromise the major functions of the spinal cord and remains actually the most important cause of mortality in the society. In addition to its cost to the individual, physically as well as the health care system and society financially, SCI has profound psychosocial effects that are devastating for patients, families and friends. SCI usually begins with a sudden, traumatic blow to the spine that fractures or dislocates vertebrae; long-term mechanical compression of the spinal cord gradually causes various pathologic changes in neural tissue. The pathophysiology of SCI comprises both primary and secondary mechanisms of injury; the "primary injury" refers to the forces that impart the primary mechanical insult to the spinal cord, which in its mildest form causes a cord concussion with brief transient neurologic deficits and in its most severe form causes complete and permanent paralysis. The primary damage to tissue is followed by a second phase of tissue degeneration that might occur over weeks or even months and further generate progressive destruction of the tissue surrounding the necrotic core that expands from the injury "epicenter" and is known as secondary injury, that is a persistence of some crucial events of the acute phase such as edema and apoptotic cell death as well as generation of oxidative stress, activation of immune system response and inflammation process. In particular we focus our attention on some mechanisms that occur after spinal cord injury such as on the involvement of the inflammation process and immune system response.

Inflammation is a physiological process that removes damaged stimuli and initiates the healing process; however, if it persists and if it is over-activated, then the inflammation becomes devastating; inflammation is a key element in the pathophysiology of some disorders such as chronic pain, neurodegenerative pathology, trauma and spinal cord injury [1–5]. Principal pro-inflammatory markers that are both cellular components, such as neutrophils, macrophages and T cells, and non-cellular components, such as cytokines, prostaglandins and complement, have been found in spinal cord tissue that received a mechanical insult. Following spinal cord trauma, the site of injury is penetrated by neutrophils, that determinate release of cytokines that may progressive damage local tissue and recruit other inflammatory cells [6]; moreover, monocytes/macrophages are released and locally activated in microglia, that subsequently invade the injured tissue [7]. The pro-inflammatory cytokines that are produced at the site of injury, such as tumor necrosis factor (TNF-α), interleukins and interferons, mediate the inflammatory response and can generate further tissue damage [8,9]. Furthermore, cytokines can induce the expression of cyclo-oxygenase (COX) 2 and thus promote the breakdown of arachidonic acid into pro-inflammatory prostanoids (prostaglandins, prostacyclin and thromboxanes) that mediate vascular permeability/resistance and platelet aggregation/ adherance [10,11]. The involvement of the cyclo-oxygenases in the generation of these inflammatory mediators represents a potential target for intervention, because inhibitors of these enzymes are in widespread clinical use. Additionally, TNF-α contributes to the tissue injury induced by neutrophils by directly activating them [12,13] as well as by increasing the expression of such molecules as ICAM-1 and E-selectin, which cause the activated neutrophils to adhere to the surface of the endothelial cells; it has also been shown that the inhibition of neutrophil adhesion to the endothelial cell surface markedly reduces the severity of the SCI induced by compressive trauma [14]. These observations indicate that the interaction of activated neutrophils with the surface of the endothelial cells is another important mediator in the secondary tissue damage of the spinal cord.

1.1. Cytokine responses to inflammation

Cytokines are small and non-structural proteins with no amino acid sequence motif, their biological activities allow us in turn to group them into different classes: exit 18 cytokines called interleukin (IL), some of these promote inflammation and are named pro-inflammatory cytokines such as IL1β and IL1α, IL6, IL8 and TNF-α, whereas other cytokines suppress the activity of pro-inflammatory cytokines and are called anti-inflammatory cytokines such as IL-4, IL-10, TGFβ. The hypothesis that some cytokine functions primarily induce inflammation while others suppress inflammation is essential to cytokine biology and also to clinical medicine.

Cytokines are secreted by a variety of immune cells such as T-lymphocytes and macrophages, as well as b non-immune cells such as fibroblasts; the physiological effects mediated by cytokines comprise the stimulation or inhibition of cell growth, cytotoxicity/apoptosis, antiviral activity and inflammatory responses. The main function of cytokines is the regulation of T-cell differentiation from undifferentiated cells to T-helper 1 and 2, regulatory T cells, and T-helper 17 cells [15]. These regulatory proteins include ILs, interferons (IFNs) and TNFs. Many of these cytokines have already been shown to be produced by neurons or glia in central nervous system (CNS) disorders in which they are notably increased.

The cytokine class of inflammatory mediators is secreted by microglia and astrocytes and their production is increased in inflammatory states; moreover they act by modulating the intensity and duration of the immune response. Pro-inflammatory cytokines and chemokines up-regulate microbicidal activity of neutrophils, and they can be considered as additional immunomodulatory agents to treat serious or refractory infections in humans.

Through cytokines IL-1 the immune response is initiated, having a crucial role in the onset and expansion of a complex hormonal and cellular inflammatory cascade; the IL-1 family of cytokines includes IL-1α and IL-1β, which generate cell activation upon binding with specific membrane receptors and has been documented that IL-1 plays a role in neuronal degeneration. In astrocytes, IL-1 induces IL-6 production, stimulates iNOS activity [16], enhances neuronal acetylcholinesterase activity, microglial activation and additional IL-1 production, and astrocyte activation.

Another important pro-inflammatory cytokine is the IL-6, a multifunctional cytokine that plays an important role in host defence [17] and possesses main effects during the inflammatory response [18]. IL-6 is associated to the family of neuropoietin cytokine and it possesses direct and indirect neurotrophic effects on neurons [19]; moreover, IL-6 promotes astrogliosis [20], activates microglia [21], and stimulates the release of acute phase molecules.

1.2. Inflammatory mediator: crucial role of TNF-α

Through all the cytokines involved in the secondary damage, TNF-α plays a crucial role; in fact it releases shortly after injury, it can accumulate rapidly at the site of injury, and it is produced by a number of different cell populations, such as neutrophils, macrophages and microglia, astrocytes and T cells [22]. Several cell types are able to produce TNF-α, including macrophages after its activation, dendritic cells, monocytes, NK cells, CD4+ T cells, CD8+ T cells, microglia and astrocytes. Macrophages/monocytes are able to produce TNF-α in the acute phase of inflammation and this cytokines drives several range of signalling events within cells, leading to necrosis or apoptosis.

Several biological functions are ascribed to the TNF-α and for this reason the mechanism of action is somewhat complex; although it inhibits the growth of tumor cells and it has an enhancing effect on the proliferation of normal cells [23]. TNF-α takes part in septic shock, autoimmunity, and inflammatory disorders. The major role of TNF-α is explicated as mediator in resistance against infections; moreover, it was postulated that TNF plays a pathological role in a number of autoimmune pathology such as graft vs host rejection or rheumatoid arthritis. Moreover, TNF-α possesses potent pro-inflammatory effects that are associated to its capacity to generate endothelial cell adhesion molecules and subsequently support neutrophil adherence to vascular endothelium. Neutrophils are exquisite targets of TNF-α that is under certain conditions it strengthens their expression of adhesion molecules induces their degranulation and successive release of lysosomal enzymes, causing the production of highly reactive oxygen species. TNF-α induces the migration of neutrophils mediating the production of chemotactic factors, including IL-8; this testifies cytokine networking involvement in inflammatory cell recruitment and an active role in inflammation.

TNF-α works by binding and clustering high-affinity receptors that are present in a great numbers on most cell membranes [24], the ligand/receptor complex is easily internalised via clathrin-coated pits and ends up in secondary lysozymes where it is degraded. Interestingly, the binding of TNF-α to the 75 kDa TNFR-2 is not sufficient to reach cytotoxicity, but rather binding to the 55 kDa TNFR-1 is sufficient to reach TNF-α mediated cell killing. TNF-α exerts its effects by activating several secondary proteins that provoke a variety of responses within the cell such as activation of gene transcription and/or production of reactive oxygen or nitrogen radicals (e.g., NO). Activated proteins include Gprotein, transcription factors such as NF-κB and AP-1 and serine and cysteine proteases, known as caspases. Many members of the TNF receptor superfamily have intracellular "death domains" which represent protein interaction domains each consisting of 65–80 amino acids; these proteins participate in TNF-α mediated apoptosis process; many evidence demonstrated that TNF–TNFR interactions are implicated in the pathogenesis of CNS disorders such as EAE and MS. These interactions are able to monitor the disease outcome by modifying immune response and the interactions between CNS-resident cells and effector immune cells in the CNS.

However, recent studies showed a dual nature for TNF-α that it can be not only neurotoxic but also neuroprotective; a study conducted with transgenic mice for TNF-α receptors demonstrated that the mice lacking TNF-α showed more tissue loss and functional deficits compared to wild-type mice, implying that TNF-α mediated a neuroprotective effect [25]. The beneficial or deleterious effects of TNF-α dependent when it is being released and on cellular population that is acting on, the conflicting actions of TNF-α described above reflects a growing view of inflammation as a "dual-edged sword" having neurotoxic and neuroprotective properties [26].

Thus, comprehension of their profile, kinetics of expression and interactions between TNF-α ligands and their TNFRs on different CNS residents and infiltrating immune cells would aid to better design strategies to control neuroinflammation and CNS autoimmunity. Blockers of TNF-α have been acknowledged for human use in treating TNF-linked autoimmune and inflammatory disorders. Pathways downstream of receptor ligation supply critical points for interjection for planning new therapeutic strategies.

1.3. Microglia activation

Moreover, other important mediators of inflammation that respond rapidly to disturbances within the microenvironment by change in morphology are the microglia, the expression "activated microglia" is used to define cells that change their immunophenotype and their morphology after a specific stimuli; the principal role of microglia at the lesion site is a rapid phagocytosis of fragments and induction of apoptosis [27]. The different response of microglia *in vitro* suggests that these cells may elicit unique functional properties and consequently control the inflammatory response at the injury site. Microglial activation has been well-known in the spinal cord tissue that has received a trauma and has shown to occur from caudal to lumbar enlargement, based on that there are papers supporting the role of microglia in pain after injury and showing activation of microglia post-SCI.

Thus, we postulated that activated spinal microglia have a role in chronic pain after SCI.

Microglia activate the innate immune system and are key regulators of inflammatory processes in CNS pathologies such as trauma and neurodegenerative diseases participation in both acute and chronic phase of the inflammatory responses. Activated microglia secrete cytotoxic substances including various cytokines such as TNF-α, IL-1, reactive free radicals, and nitric oxide. However, the principal effects of microglia at the levels of the lesion core are probably rapid phagocytosis of debris rather than induction of apoptosis. Microglia when activated can cause neuronal and glial toxicity through the release of cytokines, free radicals, eicosanoids, activated neutrophils, and macrophages [28]. On the other hand, microglia activation leads to beneficial effects producing growth factors that are fundamental for neuronal and tissue restoration. Moreover, it has been demonstrated that transplantation of peripherally activated macrophages has beneficial effects on spinal cord regeneration.

1.4. Apoptosis

In the last decade the generation of apoptotic process after spinal cord trauma was also confirmed, apoptosis can be triggered by a variety of insults including cytokines, inflammatory injury, free radical damage, and excitotoxicity.

The apoptotic process after spinal cord trauma is activated in neurons, oligodendrocytes, microglia, and perhaps, astrocytes; apoptosis in microglia contributes to inflammatory secondary injury.

Two main pathways of apoptosis—extrinsic or receptor-dependent and intrinsic or receptor-independent—have been well characterized, and both appear to be active in SCI; the extrinsic or receptor-dependent pathway is mediated by Fas ligand and Fas receptor [29] and/or inducible nitric oxide synthase production by macrophages [30], while intrinsic or receptor-independent pathway is mediated via direct caspase-3 pro-enzyme activation [31] and/or mitochondrial damage, release of cytochrome c and activation of the inducer caspase-9, pathways of caspase-mediated apoptotic death [32].

Receptor-dependent apoptosis is evoked by extracellular signals, the most significant of which is TNF, so it is termed as "extrinsic" pathway; TNF is known to rapidly accumulate in the injured spinal cord, and activation of the Fas receptor of neurons, microglia, and oligodendrocytes induces a programmed sequence of caspase activation. Moreover, additional control of cell death/survival is provided by the balance between major pro-apoptotic proteins such as Bax, Bad, and Bid and anti-apoptotic proteins such as Bcl-XL and Bcl-2.

Apoptotic cells were reached in the grey matter after injury, starting from 1h with a proliferation during the other 8 h [33]. The number of apoptotic cells is increased at the site of injury and are related with axons degeneration [34].

Apoptotic process that is activated in the secondary injury in SCI has recently come under close study, and the precise contribution and potential therapeutic implications of apoptosis in SCI could be helpful to generate new therapeutic approach to treat the secondary events associated to spinal cord injury.

2. Inflammatory/immunologic response

The inflammatory and immunological response to injury within the CNS is different than that which is occurring in other tissues [35]. The inflammatory and immunologic responses to injury involve activation of innate immune cells that provide immediate defence against inflammatory stimuli and in turn help to recruit cells of the adaptive immune system (i.e., T- and B-lymphocytes). The activation of immune system is driven by interactions involving presentation of antigen and release of various inflammatory mediators [36]. Also, cells present at the injury site may sequester debris and carry CNS antigens to secondary lymphoid organs [37], where trigger lymphocyte activation. Recent studies done on mice showed that the number of activated T and B cells increases in the spleen and bone marrow within 24 hours of trauma [38].

2.1. Lymphocytes infiltration

T-lymphocytes are distributed in the intact spinal cord and gradually grow in number after trauma in parallel with the stimulation of microglia and influx of peripheral macrophages. Lymphocytes infiltrate the spinal cord tissue starting from 24 hours until 7 days after injury and return gradually back to normal levels in 4 to 5 weeks [14].

Under normal conditions, activated T cells can cross the Add Blood–brain barrier (BBB) and enter the CNS parenchyma. In contrast with other inflammatory cells enrolled after a trauma, the number of lymphocytes remains low [39]; however, T-lymphocytes play an important role in the CNS immune system, since on activation, T-lymphocytes may kill target cells and produce cytokines [40].

Once lymphocytes enter the lesion site, they persist indeterminately [38,41], whereas T and B cells increase at the lesion site at least 9 weeks post-injury [42,43], suggesting that cytokine/chemokine gradients exist chronically and regulate integrin expression on endothelia and cells [44,45]. These chemokine gradients and adhesion molecules represent molecular targets for manipulating the effects of intraspinal lymphocytes after SCI [46–48]; the progressive increase in lymphocyte numbers may also be justified by lymphocyte activation and proliferation within the injured centre of spinal cord.

Moreover, induction of immune response could be generated as impaired nerve transmission; increasing the production of pro-inflammatory cytokines in chronic phase of SCI could worsen the damage increasing the axonal injury and demyelination. Furthermore, there are evidences that autoreactive lymphocytes promote neuronal survival *in vivo* through activation not only of autoreactive T cell but also through activation of other non-CNS reactive T cells or B cells such as resident microglia and infiltrating macrophages.

Thus, because lymphocytes remain for long term at the site of the lesion; new strategy of treatment could orientate on these cells that possess a fundamental role in regulating degenerative and regenerative processes after injury.

3. Pharmacologic interventions for acute spinal cord injury

The temporal profile of the secondary injury cascade provides a window within which it is theoretically possible to reduce the pathophysiological processes; many of the current pharmacological and surgical strategies for the treatment of SCI are based on minimising secondary injury and preserving neurological function following trauma to the brain and spinal cord. Over the past couple of decades, a myriad of agents have been nominated as putative neuroprotective therapies, several of these have been tested in the pre-clinical and clinical studies.

The following section briefly highlights some of the most promising neuroprotective approaches that are being pursued.

3.1. Corticosteroids

In the last decade one of the most used approaches to treat patients with a severe SCI is the use of corticosteroids that possess a well-recognized anti-inflammatory properties reducing spinal cord edema. However, the exact mechanisms by which corticosteroids mediated neuroprotection are not yet completely understood but seems that they induce a reduction of inflammatory cytokines production, modulation of the inflammatory/immune cells, inhibition of lipid peroxidation and reduction of oxidative stress. In this regard, methylprednisolone (MP) appears to be particularly efficacious compared with other glucocorticoids. According to the National Acute Spinal Cord Injury Study 2 (NASCIS 2) protocol, MP is usually administered within 8 h after trauma in a high concentration of 30 mg/kg, followed by an infusion of 5.4 mg/kg/h for 23 hours [49,50]. MP is the only well-known pharmacological treatment of SCI injury patients; however, its administration has been shown to be controversial. Some toxic effects such as infection rates, pulmonary embolism, severe pneumonia and sepsis and even death secondary to respiratory complications appeared to be higher with steroid use.

The anti-inflammatory properties of MP are mediated by different mechanisms that are known as transrepression, this mechanism involves interference with pro-inflammatory transcription factor signalling (such as NF-κB) which is upstream of several inflammatory mediators including COX2, chemokines and cytokines.

Together with the minor functional improvement in humans and risk of adverse side effects, these studies highlighted the compelling need to develop better neuroprotective agents with more convincing efficacy.

3.2. Estrogen as a neuroprotective agent

At present, several effects have been associated to estrogen that acts with different mechanism of action [51]. Recently, the neuroprotective and anti-inflammatory effect of estrogen are of great interest; leukocyte adhesion and microglia activation are also sensitive to estrogen and show significantly decreased superoxide dismutase production and phagocytic activity when treated with estrogen *in vitro* [52].

Moreover, cell death is associated to decreases blood flow in spinal cord and estrogen are involved in increasing post-traumatic blood flow induced by ischemia [53] and TBI [54]. Thus, estrogen treatment has been related with increased expression of pro-apoptotic Bcl-2 in the spinal cord injured tissue, this anti-apoptotic increase in Bcl-2 may be mediated by Akt activation with downstream phosphorylation of cAMP response element binding protein (CREB) [55].

However, estrogen may also act on Add N-methyl-D-aspartate receptor (NMDA) receptors, indicating a potential to limit secondary cell death due to excitotoxicity [56].

3.3. Nuclear hormone receptors family: PPARs receptor

Other members of the nuclear hormone receptors family (NHRs) are now explored for their anti-inflammatory properties in experimental models, including SCI.

Peroxisome proliferator-activated receptors (PPARs) are part of the nuclear hormone receptor superfamily, upon ligand activation regulate gene expression and have been shown to be anti-inflammatory in different model of inflammatory pathology, including SCI. PPAR exists as three isoforms (α, β/δ and γ) that control many cellular functions including lipid metabolism, glucose absorption, cell growth and differentiation, and inflammation.

One mechanism involves direct interaction of PPAR with pro-inflammatory transcription factors, most importantly NFκB and AP-1, and the subsequent reduction of gene transcription. Pioglitazone and rosiglitazone are PPARγ agonists that are in common clinical use for type II diabetes. Beyond their metabolic effects, interest in PPAR γ ligand has grown due to their anti-inflammatory, neuroprotective, and even anti-neoplastic properties, suggesting its potential use after spinal cord trauma [57]. As such, PPAR agonists have already been clinically tested in other disorders with inflammatory pathology, such as Alzheimer's disease (AD), rheumatoid arthritis (RA), and ischemia reperfusion injury, but not in SCI yet. Moreover, in the last few years a great interest has been focused on other PPAR receptors agonist such as for PPARα and β/δ receptors. One of the first reports indicating that PPARα is involved in attenuating inflammation demonstrated that the eicosanoid LTB4 binds and activates PPARα [58]. Several studies on inflammatory cytokine produced in aged mice demonstrated an active interaction of PPARα with NFκB; in fact the oxidative stress in different tissue leads to active NFκB. Treatment with PPARα agonists were found to restore the alteration of oxidative mediators, to inhibit the activation of NFκB and to remove IL-6 and IL-12 produced [59,60].

These features were accompanied by enhanced functional motor recovery and reduced hyperalgesia.

Since PPAR agonists are currently used in medical treatment of diabetes, clinical studies for stroke and different CNS pathologies are to be expected. The knowledge about anti-inflammatory properties of PPAR ligands obtained from cell cultures and animal model of SCI demonstrate that PPARs signalling may be therapeutic targets after spinal cord injury.

4. Conclusion

Thus, recent researches are moving to develop new pharmacological approaches that may offer an effective neuroprotection after spinal cord injury. After spinal cord injury, inflammatory reactions account for a large proportion of the secondary damage to neurons and oligodendrocytes.

Promising research is being carried out to better understand the aspects of inflammation, lipid peroxidation and apoptotic cell death that may be the target of pharmacologic intervention.

Few agents have been studied demonstrating efficacy in animal models of spinal cord injury and may become appropriate for testing in the human setting in the near future.

Clearly, much effort has to be done to bring experimental strategies to clinical fruition, but they do represent promising potential interventions.

Thus, the current medical and surgical interventions for the acutely cord-injured patient attempt to minimize the inflammatory process that possess a crucial role in generating and maintaining secondary damage associated to injury and defend the neural cells that initially survived the mechanical injury.

Author details

Irene Paterniti, Emanuela Esposito* and Salvatore Cuzzocrea

*Address all correspondence to: eesposito@unime.it

Department of Chemical, Biological, Pharmaceutical and Environmental Sciences, University of Messina, Messina, Italy

References

[1] Giovannini MG, Scali C, Prosperi C, Bellucci A, Vannucchi MG, Rosi S, et al. Beta-amyloid-induced inflammation and cholinergic hypofunction in the rat brain in vivo: involvement of the p38MAPK pathway. Neurobiology of disease. 2002; 11(2): 257–74.

[2] Dauer W, Przedborski S. Parkinson's disease: mechanisms and models. Neuron. 2003; 39(6): 889–909.

[3] Tenorio G, Kulkarni A, Kerr BJ. Resident glial cell activation in response to perispinal inflammation leads to acute changes in nociceptive sensitivity: implications for the generation of neuropathic pain. Pain. 2013; 154(1): 71–81. doi:10.1016/j.pain. 2012.09.008.

[4] Najjar S, Pearlman DM, Alper K, Najjar A, Devinsky O. Neuroinflammation and psychiatric illness. Journal of neuroinflammation. 2013; 10: 43. doi: 10.1186/1742-2094-10-43.

[5] Iadecola C, Anrather J. The immunology of stroke: from mechanisms to translation. Nature medicine. 2011; 17(7): 796–808. doi:10.1038/nm.2399.

[6] Popovich PG, Wei P, Stokes BT. Cellular inflammatory response after spinal cord injury in Sprague–Dawley and Lewis rats. The journal of comparative neurology. 1997; 377(3): 443–64.

[7] Dusart I, Schwab ME. Secondary cell death and the inflammatory reaction after dorsal hemisection of the rat spinal cord. The European journal of neuroscience. 1994; 6(5): 712–24.

[8] Bartholdi D, Schwab ME. Expression of pro-inflammatory cytokine and chemokine mRNA upon experimental spinal cord injury in mouse: an in situ hybridization study. The European journal of neuroscience. 1997; 9(7): 1422–38.

[9] Klusman I, Schwab ME. Effects of pro-inflammatory cytokines in experimental spinal cord injury. Brain research. 1997; 762(1–2): 173–84.

[10] Tonai T, Taketani Y, Ueda N, Nishisho T, Ohmoto Y, Sakata Y, et al. Possible involvement of interleukin-1 in cyclooxygenase-2 induction after spinal cord injury in rats. Journal of neurochemistry. 1999; 72(1): 302–9.

[11] Dubois RN, Abramson SB, Crofford L, Gupta RA, Simon LS, Van De Putte LB, et al. Cyclooxygenase in biology and disease. FASEB journal : official publication of the Federation of American Societies for Experimental Biology. 1998; 12(12): 1063–73.

[12] Genovese T, Mazzon E, Di Paola R, Cannavo G, Muia C, Bramanti P, et al. Role of endogenous ligands for the peroxisome proliferators activated receptors alpha in the secondary damage in experimental spinal cord trauma. Experimental neurology. 2005; 194(1): 267–78. doi:10.1016/j.expneurol.2005.03.003.

[13] Paterniti I, Genovese T, Crisafulli C, Mazzon E, Di Paola R, Galuppo M, et al. Treatment with green tea extract attenuates secondary inflammatory response in an experimental model of spinal cord trauma. Naunyn-Schmiedeberg's archives of pharmacology. 2009; 380(2): 179–92. doi:10.1007/s00210-009-0414-z.

[14] Taoka Y, Okajima K. Role of leukocytes in spinal cord injury in rats. Journal of neurotrauma. 2000; 17(3): 219–29.

[15] Steinman L. A brief history of T(H)17, the first major revision in the T(H)1/T(H)2 hypothesis of T cell-mediated tissue damage. Nature medicine. 2007; 13(2): 139–45. doi: 10.1038/nm1551.

[16] Hausmann ON. Post-traumatic inflammation following spinal cord injury. Spinal cord. 2003; 41(7): 369–78. doi:10.1038/sj.sc.3101483.

[17] Okada S, Nakamura M, Mikami Y, Shimazaki T, Mihara M, Ohsugi Y, et al. Blockade of interleukin-6 receptor suppresses reactive astrogliosis and ameliorates functional recovery in experimental spinal cord injury. Journal of neuroscience research. 2004; 76(2): 265–76. doi:10.1002/jnr.20044.

[18] Roxburgh CS, McMillan DC. Therapeutics targeting innate immune/inflammatory responses through the interleukin-6/JAK/STAT signal transduction pathway in patients with cancer. Translational research: the journal of laboratory and clinical medicine. 2016; 167(1): 61–6. doi:10.1016/j.trsl.2015.08.013.

[19] Teng FY, Tang BL. Axonal regeneration in adult CNS neurons-signaling molecules and pathways. Journal of neurochemistry. 2006; 96(6): 1501–8. doi:10.1111/j. 1471-4159.2006.03663.x.

[20] Morales I, Farias G, Maccioni RB. Neuroimmunomodulation in the pathogenesis of Alzheimer's disease. Neuroimmunomodulation. 2010; 17(3): 202–4. doi: 10.1159/000258724.

[21] Inoue K. Microglial activation by purines and pyrimidines. Glia. 2002; 40(2): 156–63. doi:10.1002/glia.10150.

[22] Yan P, Li Q, Kim GM, Xu J, Hsu CY, Xu XM. Cellular localization of tumor necrosis factor-alpha following acute spinal cord injury in adult rats. Journal of neurotrauma. 2001; 18(5): 563–8. doi:10.1089/089771501300227369.

[23] Mandi Y, Endresz V, Krenacs L, Regely K, Degre M, Beladi I. Tumor necrosis factor production by human granulocytes. International archives of allergy and applied immunology. 1991; 96(2): 102–6.

[24] Loetscher H, Gentz R, Zulauf M, Lustig A, Tabuchi H, Schlaeger EJ, et al. Recombinant 55-kDa tumor necrosis factor (TNF) receptor. Stoichiometry of binding to TNF alpha and TNF beta and inhibition of TNF activity. The Journal of biological chemistry. 1991; 266(27): 18324–9.

[25] Kim GM, Xu J, Xu J, Song SK, Yan P, Ku G, et al. Tumor necrosis factor receptor deletion reduces nuclear factor-kappaB activation, cellular inhibitor of apoptosis protein 2 expression, and functional recovery after traumatic spinal cord injury. The journal of neuroscience : the official journal of the society for neuroscience. 2001; 21(17): 6617–25.

[26] Bethea JR. Spinal cord injury-induced inflammation: a dual-edged sword. Progress in brain research. 2000; 128: 33–42. doi:10.1016/S0079-6123(00)28005-9.

[27] Shuman SL, Bresnahan JC, Beattie MS. Apoptosis of microglia and oligodendrocytes after spinal cord contusion in rats. Journal of neuroscience research. 1997; 50(5): 798–808.

[28] Schwartz M. Autoimmune involvement in CNS trauma is beneficial if well controlled. Progress in brain research. 2000; 128: 259–63. doi:10.1016/S0079-6123(00)28023-0.

[29] Leskovar A, Moriarty LJ, Turek JJ, Schoenlein IA, Borgens RB. The macrophage in acute neural injury: changes in cell numbers over time and levels of cytokine production in mammalian central and peripheral nervous systems. The journal of experimental biology. 2000; 203(Pt 12): 1783–95.

[30] Satake K, Matsuyama Y, Kamiya M, Kawakami H, Iwata H, Adachi K, et al. Nitric oxide via macrophage iNOS induces apoptosis following traumatic spinal cord injury. Brain research molecular brain research. 2000; 85(1–2): 114–22.

[31] Citron BA, Arnold PM, Sebastian C, Qin F, Malladi S, Ameenuddin S, et al. Rapid upregulation of caspase-3 in rat spinal cord after injury: mRNA, protein, and cellular localization correlates with apoptotic cell death. Experimental neurology. 2000; 166(2): 213–26. doi:10.1006/exnr.2000.7523.

[32] Hartley CJ, Reddy AK, Madala S, Martin-McNulty B, Vergona R, Sullivan ME, et al. Hemodynamic changes in apolipoprotein E-knockout mice. American journal of physiology-heart and circulatory physiology. 2000; 279(5): H2326–34.

[33] Zurita M, Vaquero J, Zurita I. Presence and significance of CD-95 (Fas/APO1) expression after spinal cord injury. Journal of neurosurgery. 2001; 94(2 Suppl): 257–64.

[34] Casha S, Yu WR, Fehlings MG. Oligodendroglial apoptosis occurs along degenerating axons and is associated with FAS and p75 expression following spinal cord injury in the rat. Neuroscience. 2001; 103(1): 203–18.

[35] Schwartz M, Moalem G, Leibowitz-Amit R, Cohen IR. Innate and adaptive immune responses can be beneficial for CNS repair. Trends in neurosciences. 1999; 22(7): 295–9.

[36] Ling C, Sandor M, Fabry Z. In situ processing and distribution of intracerebrally injected OVA in the CNS. Journal of neuroimmunology. 2003; 141(1–2): 90–8.

[37] Karman J, Ling C, Sandor M, Fabry Z. Initiation of immune responses in brain is promoted by local dendritic cells. Journal of immunology. 2004; 173(4): 2353–61.

[38] Ankeny DP, Lucin KM, Sanders VM, McGaughy VM, Popovich PG. Spinal cord injury triggers systemic autoimmunity: evidence for chronic B lymphocyte activation and lupus-like autoantibody synthesis. Journal of neurochemistry. 2006; 99(4): 1073–87. doi: 10.1111/j.1471-4159.2006.04147.x.

[39] Schnell L, Fearn S, Klassen H, Schwab ME, Perry VH. Acute inflammatory responses to mechanical lesions in the CNS: differences between brain and spinal cord. The European journal of neuroscience. 1999; 11(10): 3648–58.

[40] Kierdorf K, Wang Y, Neumann H. Immune-mediated CNS damage. Results and problems in cell differentiation. 2010; 51: 173–96. doi:10.1007/400_2008_15.

[41] Sroga JM, Jones TB, Kigerl KA, McGaughy VM, Popovich PG. Rats and mice exhibit distinct inflammatory reactions after spinal cord injury. The journal of comparative neurology. 2003; 462(2): 223–40. doi:10.1002/cne.10736.

[42] Bilgen M, Dogan B, Narayana PA. In vivo assessment of blood-spinal cord barrier permeability: serial dynamic contrast enhanced MRI of spinal cord injury. Magnetic resonance imaging. 2002; 20(4): 337–41.

[43] Whetstone WD, Hsu JY, Eisenberg M, Werb Z, Noble-Haeusslein LJ. Blood-spinal cord barrier after spinal cord injury: relation to revascularization and wound healing. Journal of neuroscience research. 2003; 74(2): 227–39. doi:10.1002/jnr.10759.

[44] Lee YL, Shih K, Bao P, Ghirnikar RS, Eng LF. Cytokine chemokine expression in contused rat spinal cord. Neurochemistry international. 2000; 36(4–5): 417–25.

[45] Babcock AA, Kuziel WA, Rivest S, Owens T. Chemokine expression by glial cells directs leukocytes to sites of axonal injury in the CNS. The journal of neuroscience: the official journal of the society for neuroscience. 2003; 23(21): 7922–30.

[46] Bao F, Chen Y, Dekaban GA, Weaver LC. Early anti-inflammatory treatment reduces lipid peroxidation and protein nitration after spinal cord injury in rats. Journal of neurochemistry. 2004; 88(6): 1335–44.

[47] Eng LF, Lee YL. Response of chemokine antagonists to inflammation in injured spinal cord. Neurochemical research. 2003; 28(1): 95–100.

[48] Gonzalez R, Glaser J, Liu MT, Lane TE, Keirstead HS. Reducing inflammation decreases secondary degeneration and functional deficit after spinal cord injury. Experimental neurology. 2003; 184(1): 456–63.

[49] Bracken MB. Methylprednisolone in the management of acute spinal cord injuries. The medical journal of Australia. 1990; 153(6): 368.

[50] Bracken MB, Shepard MJ, Collins WF, Holford TR, Young W, Baskin DS, et al. A randomized, controlled trial of methylprednisolone or naloxone in the treatment of acute spinal cord injury. Results of the Second National Acute Spinal Cord Injury Study.

The New England journal of medicine. 1990; 322(20): 1405–11. doi:10.1056/NEJM199005173222001.

[51] Sribnick EA, Wingrave JM, Matzelle DD, Ray SK, Banik NL. Estrogen as a neuroprotective agent in the treatment of spinal cord injury. Annals of the New York Academy of Sciences. 2003; 993: 125–33; discussion 59–60.

[52] Bruce-Keller AJ, Keeling JL, Keller JN, Huang FF, Camondola S, Mattson MP. Antiinflammatory effects of estrogen on microglial activation. Endocrinology. 2000; 141(10): 3646–56. doi:10.1210/endo.141.10.7693.

[53] He Z, He YJ, Day AL, Simpkins JW. Proestrus levels of estradiol during transient global cerebral ischemia improves the histological outcome of the hippocampal CA1 region: perfusion-dependent and independent mechanisms. Journal of the neurological sciences. 2002; 193(2): 79–87.

[54] Roof RL, Hall ED. Estrogen-related gender difference in survival rate and cortical blood flow after impact-acceleration head injury in rats. Journal of neurotrauma. 2000; 17(12): 1155–69. doi:10.1089/neu.2000.17.1155.

[55] Honda K, Shimohama S, Sawada H, Kihara T, Nakamizo T, Shibasaki H, et al. Nongenomic antiapoptotic signal transduction by estrogen in cultured cortical neurons. Journal of neuroscience research. 2001; 64(5): 466–75.

[56] Nilsen J, Chen S, Brinton RD. Dual action of estrogen on glutamate-induced calcium signaling: mechanisms requiring interaction between estrogen receptors and src/mitogen activated protein kinase pathway. Brain research. 2002; 930(1–2): 216–34.

[57] Cuzzocrea S. Peroxisome proliferator-activated receptors gamma ligands and ischemia and reperfusion injury. Vascular pharmacology. 2004; 41(6): 187–95. doi:10.1016/j.vph.2004.10.004.

[58] Devchand PR, Keller H, Peters JM, Vazquez M, Gonzalez FJ, Wahli W. The PPAR alpha-leukotriene B4 pathway to inflammation control. Nature. 1996; 384(6604): 39–43. doi:10.1038/384039a0.

[59] Esposito E, Cuzzocrea S. Palmitoylethanolamide is a new possible pharmacological treatment for the inflammation associated with trauma. Mini reviews in medicinal chemistry. 2013; 13(2): 237–55.

[60] Esposito E, Cuzzocrea S. Targeting the peroxisome proliferator-activated receptors (PPARs) in spinal cord injury. Expert opinion on therapeutic targets. 2011; 15(8): 943–59. doi:10.1517/14728222.2011.581231.

3

CASP Methodology for Virtual Prototyping of Garments for People with Postural Disorders and Spinal Deformities

Andrej Cupar, Zoran Stjepanovič, Simona Jevšnik,
Rija Erveš and Andreja Rudolf

Abstract

"Nobody is Perfect" is a phrase we often hear and use for different purposes. It can relate to our physical appearances or behavioral properties. A great share of the world's population is faced with difficulties caused by postural disorders and spinal deformities. In our chapter we are not dealing with medical points of view. Instead, our intention is to highlight the problems and needs of affected people for suitable, well-fitted, and attractive garments. It is a fact that they need clothing items, not only for everyday use but also for special, festive occasions and sports. Finding suitable garments can be a nightmare for them. Normally, ready-made garments cannot be used if the postural disorders and spinal deformities are very expressive. Therefore, an individual approach is needed for planning, designing, and producing such garments. We propose virtual prototyping and CASP methodology for analyzing digitized geometry supported by computer-aided pattern designs for designing suitable, well-fitted garments for people with postural disorders and spinal deformities. "CASP" stands for Curvature, Acceleration, Symmetry, and Proportionality. It is used for methodology to analyze those four properties on surfaces in a virtual computer environment, as explained further on.

Keywords: CASP methodology, virtual prototyping, garments, postural disorders, spinal deformities

1. Introduction

Postural disorders and spinal deformities present major difficulties for affected people, not only from the medical point of view but also from the point of view of finding appropriate clothing. Without doubt, it can be stated that assuring garments with perfect fit and functionality taking into account the increased need for a modern design is not possible without an extensive use of modern computer-based technologies, above all three-dimensional (3D) body scanning, computer-aided design, and virtual prototyping. Moreover, additional methods for analyzing digitized geometry, such as CASP (Curvature, Acceleration, Symmetry, and Proportionality), are needed for assuring appropriate garment part designs and final fit of the garment. CASP methodology is a widely applicable approach in fields of use where a 3D virtual model is present. We have used it for virtual prototyping of garments for people with postural disorders and spinal deformities.

Nowadays, we can use virtual reality applications to produce digital prototypes of different garments and other textile forms, especially three-dimensional. The designers can alter their design creations with less time and cost. The aim of 3D virtual prototyping is to build a virtual model instead of developing a real product. Virtual garment prototyping is a technique which involves the application of computer-aided design systems used for the development of the garment pattern designs and the assessment of their fit to the 3D body model and virtual assessment of the appearance of the whole garment.

This chapter presents topics related to the multidisciplinary fields of computer graphics and analysis, 3D scanning, and 3D virtual modeling with the aim of supporting virtual prototyping of garments for people with postural disorders and spinal deformities. Mainly scoliosis and kyphosis are treated, because a significant share of the population is facing these problems, especially in the older population.

As a transformation tool between real world and virtual world, 3D scanning is used to capture and digitize real objects. 3D scans describe an object's shape. It makes sense to use precise 3D scanners for solid and rigid objects, where small details or deviations are important and can be measured, but for virtual prototyping, it is usually enough to have a rough shape of a person. Live persons are moving and changing shape literally with every breath and heart beat. Therefore, it is better to perform low-detail scans.

In this chapter, we present research relating to the applicability of CASP methodology to nonstandard body figures' garment pattern design with the aim of finding out whether CASP methodology is right for predicting the garment pattern design for persons with a curved spine, as well as for the construction of well-fitted garments.

After the theoretical background and study of the literature dealing with curves and shapes, CASP methodology is introduced and explained. Medical points of view regarding postural disorders and spinal deformities are detailed in order to highlight the need for adapted garment designs. Practical examples are discussed using CASP methodology, including three case studies dealing with curvature graphs, together with two examples related to the design and virtual prototyping of garments for people with postural disorders and spinal deformities. The chapter concludes with suggestions for further studies in this important and interesting research area.

2. Theoretical backgrounds

The human mind tries to order everything within the environment either in order to see specific patterns or just to try to understand something, as the Gestalt theory explains [1]. This "classification" is performed in every scientific field. The real world can be digitized very easily with 3D scanners and transformed into a virtual computer environment. Hence, it is important to treat 3D scans with proper tools for analysis or any further geometry extraction. To begin with, curves have already been explored widely and discussed; therefore, it is important to introduce a number of works from this field in the following paragraphs.

Curves with aesthetic impression are parts of logarithmic graphs [2–4], which have logarithmic horizontal axes with steps like 0.1/1/10/100/1000/10,000, and so on. The researchers in Ref. [2] observed graph curvature (K) in dependence of path (s)—K(s) in the logarithmic curvature histogram (LCH). They defined an aesthetic curve as a curve whose LCH is a straight line.

Researchers Kanaya et al. [3] used this method to determine objects' impressions by analyzing sections on objects' surfaces. They found that observed objects with Japanese origin have the so-called convergent impression and objects with European origin divergent impression. The word "convergent" comes from the graph in which the chart curve nears the horizontal line. Contrarily, "divergent" means a graph with a chart curve that goes away from the horizontal line. The authors provided a CAD system (computer-aided design system), which can feel the same impression on curved surfaces as those that human designers can. On the base of LCH, they proposed three types of surfaces by human impression: convergent, divergent, and neutral.

The authors Yoshida et al. in Ref. [4] have observed and analyzed spatial aesthetic curve segments drawn with completely mathematical functions. Curvature graphs and LCHs of those curves were plotted, analyzed, and classified.

Giannini, Monti, Podehl, and Piegl were leading researchers who participated in the project FIORES II [5–7]. They proposed several terms for styling properties and features in CAID (computer-aided industrial design. With observation of communication between stylists and engineers and technical meaning, they built a list of terms that describe styling properties; these are [5–7] as follows:

- Radius/blending
- Convex/concave
- Tension
- Straight/flat
- Hollow

- Lead-in
- Soft/sharp
- S-shaped
- Crown
- Hard/crude
- Acceleration

Not all researchers use all terms in their works, and they agree that the list is not complete or perfect. Some of the terms are similar, while some characteristics can be described with several terms [6].

2.1. CASP methodology

We tried to establish and improve the classification, but we developed a completely novel approach instead. Curvature graphs were not the main observation object any more. Rather, we observe the spatial surface, where distances from the created plane to the surface are valuated and collected in four values, which are characteristic for the observed surface. It is named CASP methodology [8]. The four properties that characterize surfaces are as follows:

- Curvature—C,
- Acceleration—A,
- Symmetry—S, and
- Proportionality—P.

Furthermore, combinations of quotients of those values have proven several charts and properties of observed parts of surfaces. CASP methodology is a widely applicable approach in fields of use where a 3D virtual model is present. CASP methodology was performed also on garments for people with postural disorders and spinal deformities.

First, we have to explain the meaning of the four properties.

Curvature goes from − to + sign. Zero determines a neutral curvature and represents a plane. Negative values determine a concave surface and positive values are for convex surfaces, as **Figure 1** shows. Values are calculated as the arithmetic average of normalized $n \times n$ distances, including a preposition sign. They are arranged in the $n \times n$ matrix. The $n \times n$ matrix follows natural directions, and is not the same as in mathematical writing. Mathematically, it has swapped rows over the middle row. The $n \times n$ matrix starts with entry (0,0) at the left bottom corner [8–11].

The starting point on the analyzed surface is also marked at the bottom left side. This enables us to locate the position of the same point in the 3D space and in the $n \times n$ matrix.

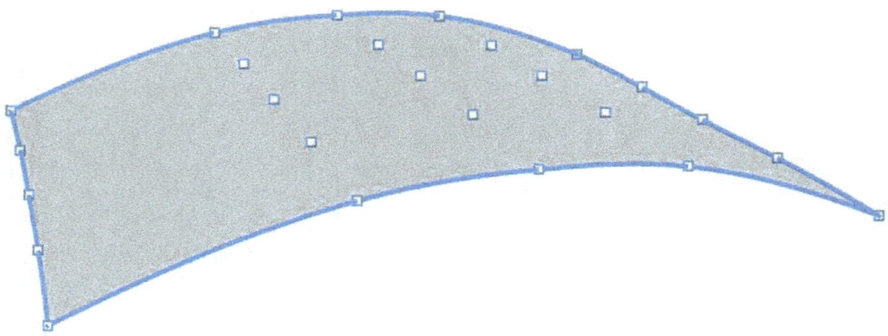

Figure 1. Curvature.

Acceleration is a property observed in a longitudinal direction and has higher values on curves where the curvature changes more. A typical accelerated surface is shown in **Figure 2**.

Symmetry compares the left and right sides of a surface. It takes just positive values. Zero means perfect symmetry of a surface. Values for *S* are observed over the middle column of the $n \times n$ matrix, as in **Figure 3**. Symmetry can be detected as the arithmetical average of differences between entities' pairs compared over the middle column in the $n \times n$ matrix.

Proportionality is the fourth property to indicate the size or width of the surface. It is calculated as a ratio between the length and width of the observed surface, as shown in **Figure 4**. As described in Ref. [12], it has to be projected on a triangular $n \times n$ plane.

The whole $n \times n$ procedure is based on the use of the graphical algorithm Grasshopper® (GH) [11], which is add-in integrated with the 3D modeling tool Rhinoceros (RH) [12]. Parametrical procedures are created by dragging components onto a canvas. Outputs of these components are then connected to the inputs of subsequent components, and so on. Grasshopper is used mainly to build generative algorithms and it acts like a programming tool. Many of Grasshopper's components create 3D geometry. Procedures may also process other types of algorithms, including numeric, textual, audiovisual or haptic applications. We used GH because of complex algorithms that can be connected and combined easily. Our procedure for analyzing digitized surface geometries exists in 10 steps [8–11].

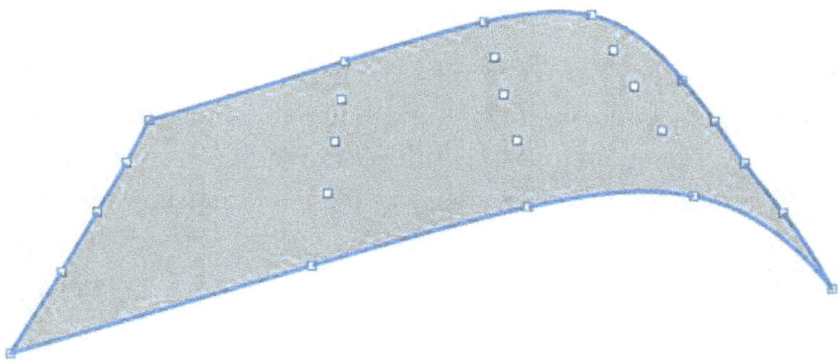

Figure 2. Accelerated surface.

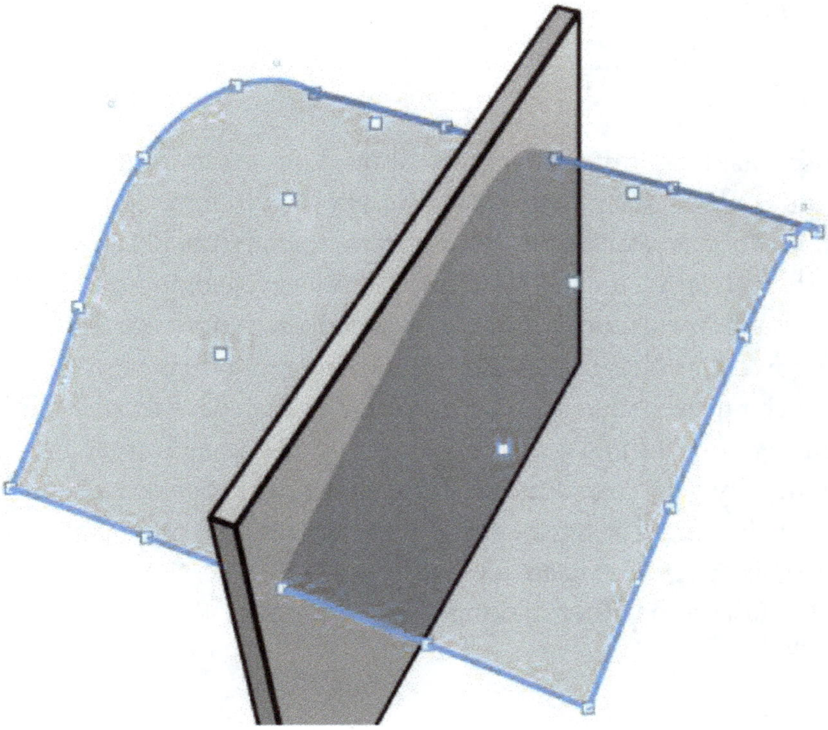

Figure 3. Symmetry.

2.2. Medical view of postural disorders and spinal deformity

2.2.1. Scoliosis

It is not easy to find appropriate, well-designed, and well-fitted garments for people with scoliosis. They are often faced with the problem of how to dress nicely and comfortably. Many different types of advice can be found in the source by Rudolf et al. [13] and, lately, these

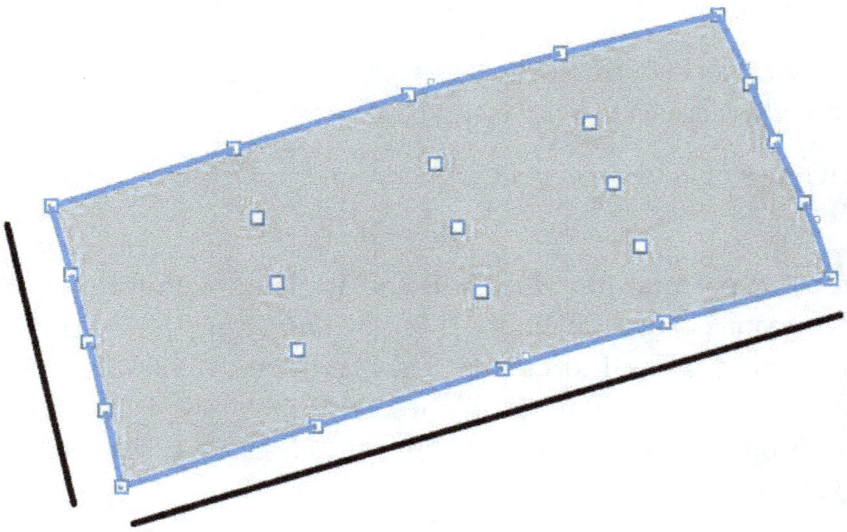

Figure 4. Proportionality.

can also be found on specialized webpages or blogs, as presented by Strauss [14] in "How to dress with scoliosis" or Munike Zanette Ávila [15] "Patternmaking for people with postural deviations."

Scoliosis can cause visible symptoms: uneven shoulders, uncentered, head, ribs at different heights, one shoulder blade that sticks out more than the other, uneven hips, one leg appearing shorter than the other, as well as the body leaning to one side. Because scoliosis causes this asymmetry in the body, imperfect and ill-fitting clothes can become a daily problem. The waist on pants or skirts may appear uneven, or shirts and dresses may not fit or hang on the body properly. Dressing in a way that makes the individual feel at their best and most secure with their scoliosis can become a challenge [15]. One of the easiest ways to mask scoliosis is to avoid tightly fitting clothing. Individuals with scoliosis tend to be small framed and long waisted, so their bones are generally very pronounced. Tight shirts can reveal the asymmetry more obviously. Not only can clothing like tight t-shirts and blouses emphasize the scoliotic deformity even more but also because there is an asymmetry on one side, the clothing might feel much tighter on one side than on the other making these types of clothing uncomfortable [14, 15].

2.2.2. *Kyphosis*

Kyphosis is the term used to describe an abnormal outwardly curved spine in the sagittal plane. The condition can contribute to a "hunchback" appearance, and may require exercise, braces, or spine surgery for treatment [16].

A certain degree of curvature is normal in the human spine. The gentle inward and outward curves of the neck, upper back, and lower back are necessary to maintain the body properly balanced and aligned over the pelvis. Kyphotic curved spines are the outward curves. Inward curved spines are called lordotic [16].

The term kyphosis is generally used to describe an excessive outward curve, or rounding, of the spine. Again, some kyphosis is normal—typically 20–50°; curves greater than 50° are considered abnormal. A spine with kyphosis can look normal, or it can develop a *"humpback"* appearance.

Mild kyphosis may cause few problems; however, severe kyphotic curvature can affect the lungs, nerves, and other tissues and organs, causing pain and other problems.

There are several types of kyphosis, and the condition can be found in children, adolescents, and adults.

Postural kyphosis, or postural round-back, is the most common form of kyphosis, and is often attributed to poor posture. Habitually, "slouching" can stretch spinal ligaments and contribute to abnormal vertebral formation. The condition usually appears during adolescence, and is more common in girls than in boys. Postural kyphosis is marked by a smooth, flexible curve that is not typically associated with pain, and usually does not lead to problems later in life [15, 16].

Scheuermann's kyphosis developed most commonly in teenage boys. It is characterized by a short, sharp curvature in the middle part of the upper spine, and may be associated with aching back pain. This type of kyphosis tends to be rigid on clinical examination. A mild degree of scoliosis is common in adolescents with Scheuermann's kyphosis.

Congenital kyphosis can be caused by a malformation of the spinal column during fetal development. Several vertebrae may be fused together or the bones may not form properly. This type of kyphosis may worsen as the child grows [16].

Self-image, or the way we feel about our bodies, can affect all aspects of our daily life. If we are wearing clothes that fit well and feel comfortable, this inevitably helps to boost our confidence. People with sustained spine deformity have problems with clothes that do not fit well in the back and front parts. They are tight across the back, too short in the back length (BL) and too long in the front length, open at the back of the neck and hemlines can become uneven, and so on [15].

3. Practical examples using CASP methodology

3.1. Curvature graphs

As we have already explained, the curvature graphs were not used directly, but were used just to show how they work. We will present some examples. Curvature graphs were used to determine non-symmetry on a real face scan as **Figure 5** shows. The highest peak on the curvature graph represents the nose, which is in the middle. The left and the right sides of the curvature graph will be symmetrically identical over this peak on a perfect symmetrical face, but it is not in this case. That way, we proof non-symmetry that is not obviously seen on a real face scan.

Figure 6 shows a series of increasing accelerated curves (a) with their curvature graphs (b) and a series of increasing decelerated curves (c) with their curvature graphs (d).

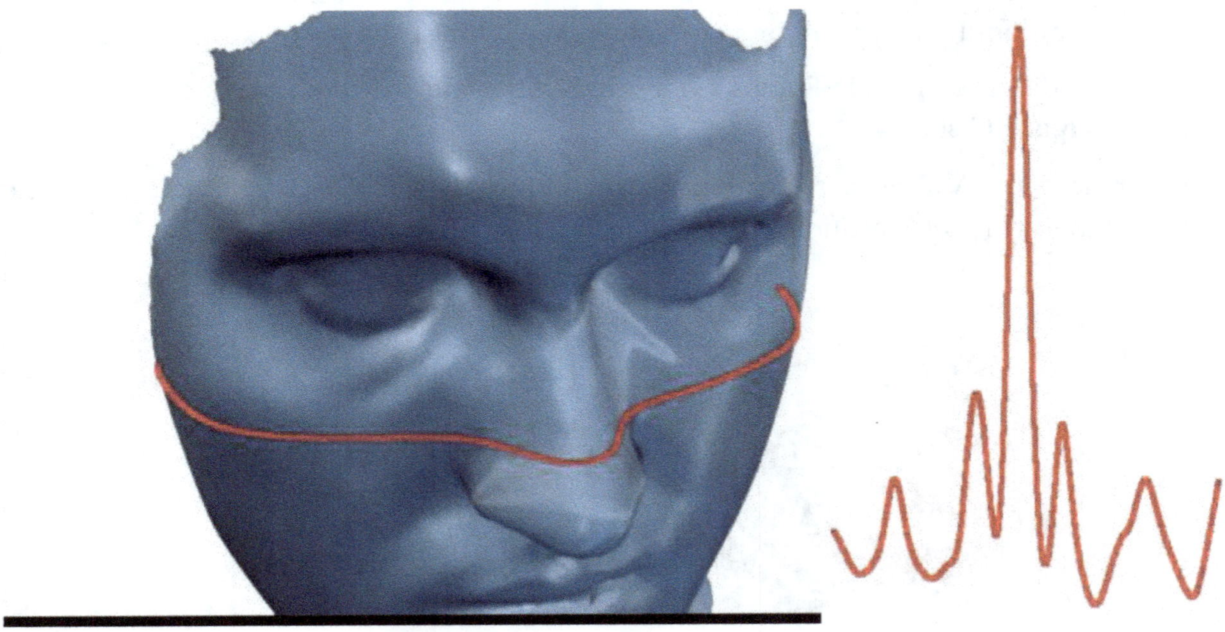

Figure 5. Symmetry on a cut-line of 3D-scanned human face. On the right side is the curvature graph [17].

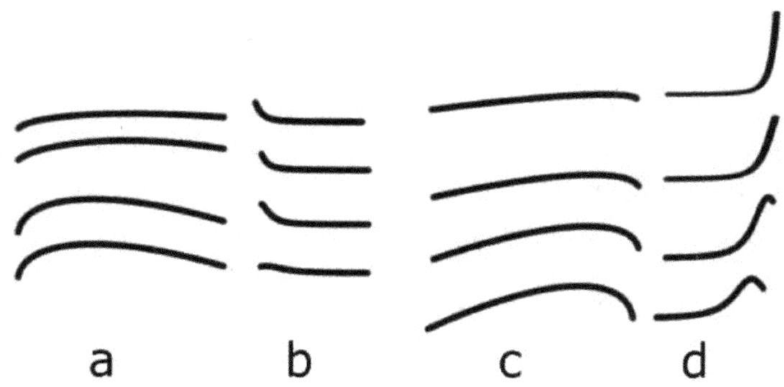

Figure 6. Increasing accelerated curves (a) and their curvature graphs (b). Increasing decelerated curves (c) and their curvature graphs (d) [18].

The last example of curvature graph use is the ergonomic fit of a thumb on the computer mouse as shown in **Figures 7** and **8**.

3.2. Virtual postural models

Virtual models were made using "Make Human" [19], an open-source program for human body creation. An open-source program "Blender" was used for posing [20], which means rotating or moving body parts virtually (in this case, the upper torso) to simulate not standard posture-scoliotic or kyphotic. 3D models that represent normal postures were used as reference and compared to models with postural deformity. The differences between them were determined with CASP values.

3.2.1. Scoliotic model

In our research on using the CASP methodology for virtual prototyping of garments for people with postural disorders and spinal deformities, we first created an artificial, symmetrical 3D female body without any deformity. Afterwards, this model was deformed in the left shoulder area. The deformity is typical for a girl or a woman with scoliosis, as shown in **Figure 9**.

Both body models presented in **Figure 9** were analyzed using the CASP method in the shoulder area as **Figure 10** shows.

The differences in CASP properties are primarily in the symmetry, which is expected, since we created the asymmetry artificially.

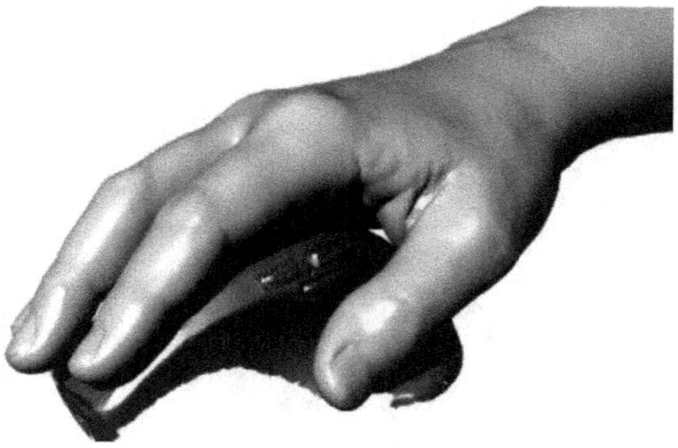

Figure 7. A user holds a computer mouse in the right hand [18].

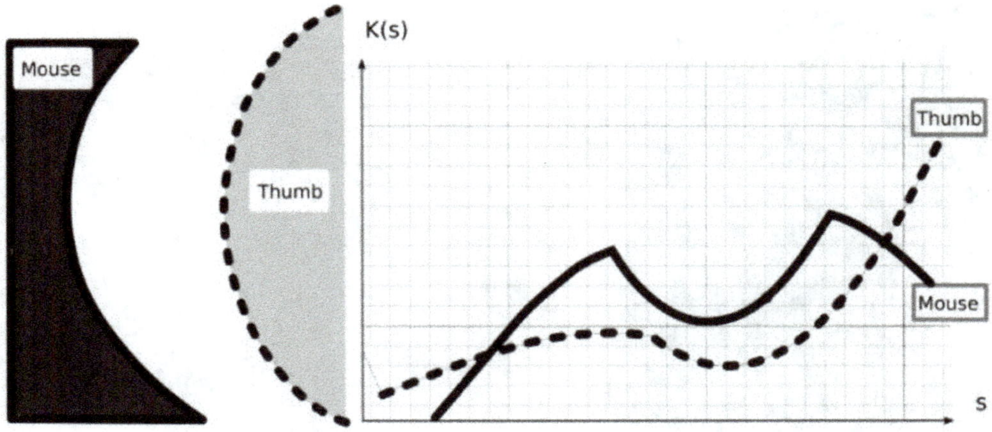

Figure 8. The shape of the thumb fits on the shape of the mouse and graph $K(s)$ on the right side [18].

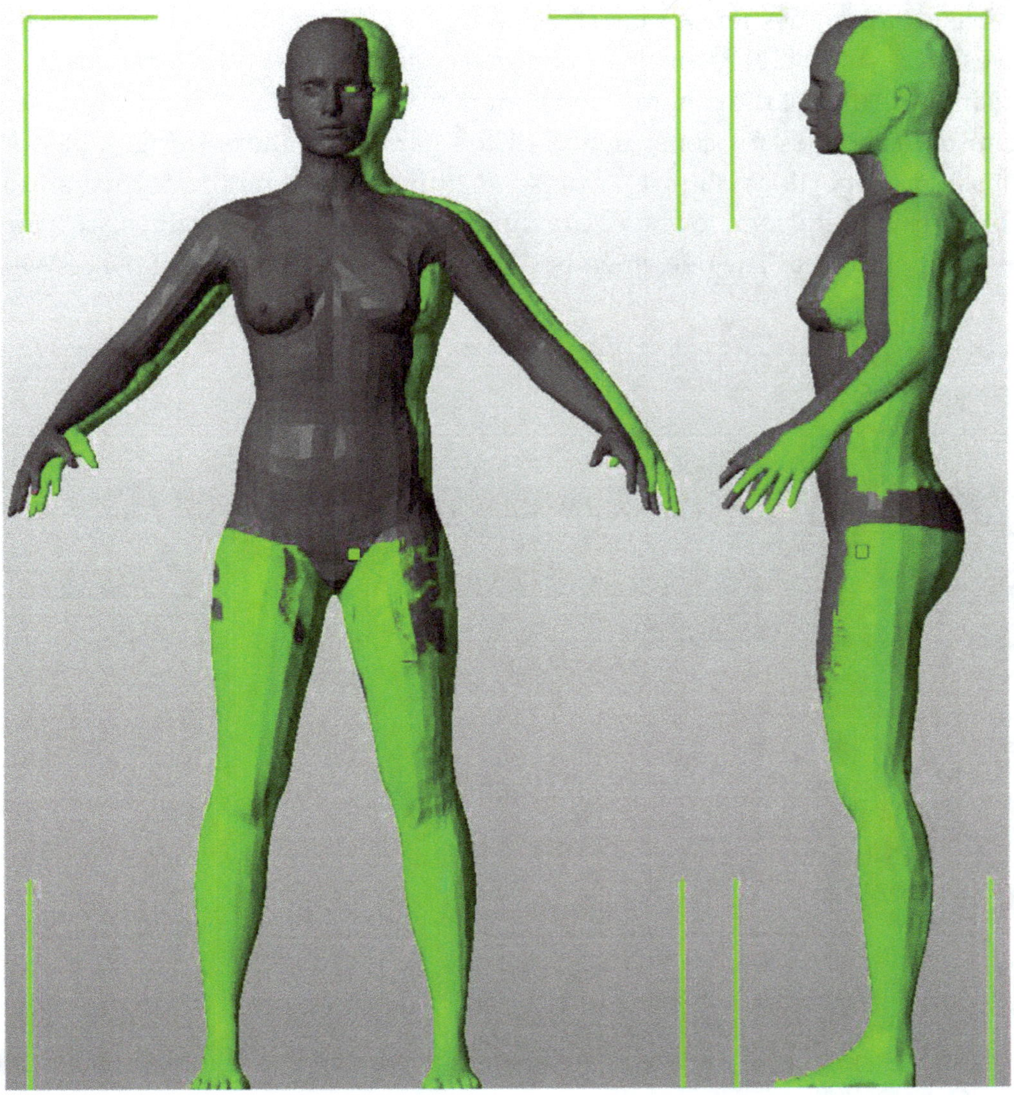

Figure 9. Normal (dark grey) and scoliotic synthetic female body (light grey) [21].

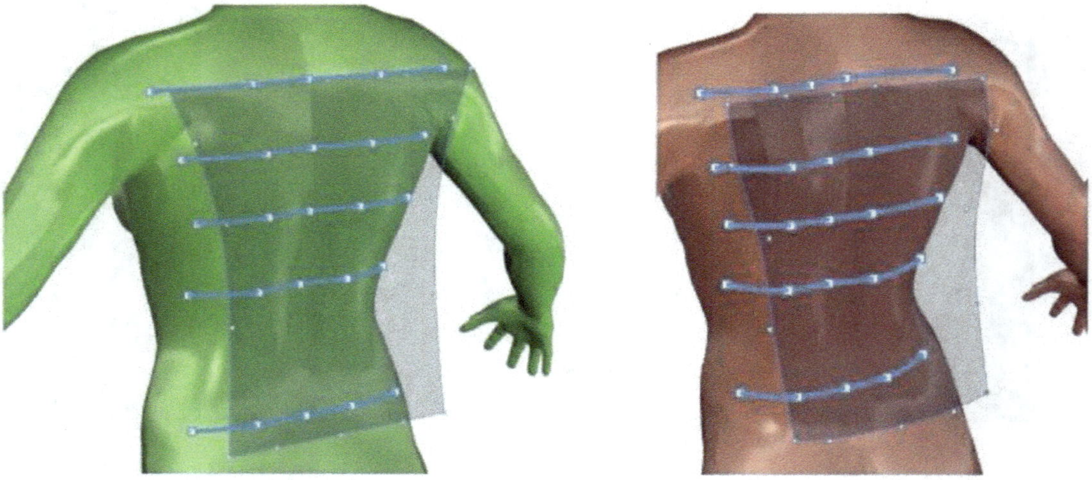

Figure 10. Cross-section parts on the back for a normal body (left) and a deformed body (right) [21].

The dress basic pattern design was constructed in the CAD computer program Optitex PDS (Pattern Design System) [22] according to normal (symmetric) synthetic female body dimensions by using the rules of the construction system by M. Müller and Sohn [23]. The construction system defines rules for construction of the garment pattern designs based on body dimensions and proportions. **Figure 11** presents fitting a dress on the normal and **Figure 12** on the scoliotic synthetic female body. The differences in the CASP values are also reflected in the dress's appearance. The deformed body is asymmetric. Because of the convex line, the

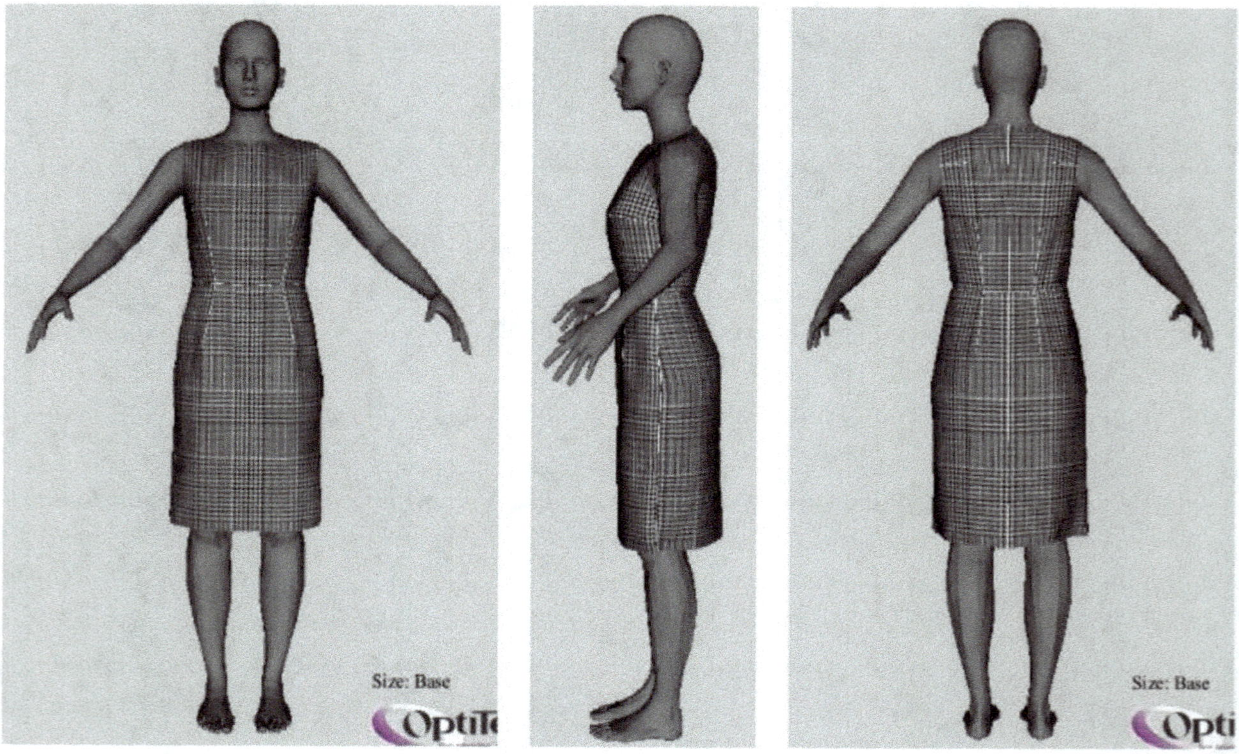

Figure 11. Basic dress pattern design on a normal synthetic body model [9].

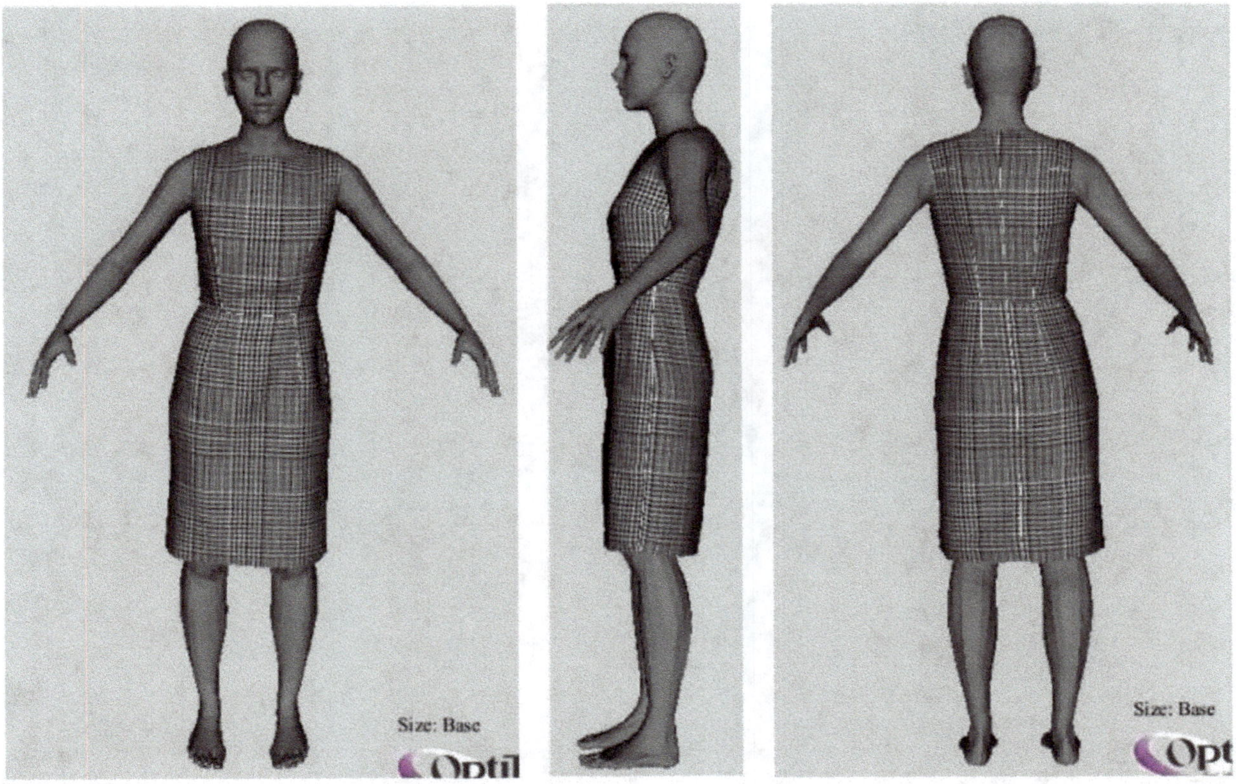

Figure 12. Basic dress pattern design on a synthetic scoliotic female body model [9].

straight seam in the middle of the back causes the appearance of the dress to increase the appearance of the asymmetry of the body. It is also observed in the movement of the parts and their asymmetry according to the body, and shortening of the dress on the right side of the body [9].

With reconstruction of the basic dress pattern design, we want to balance the appearance of the asymmetric body so that it looks as if the body is symmetrical. Contour corrections of the dress side seams, waist seams, and back middle seam in the blade area were performed, as well as contour corrections of the waist, breast, and blade darts, according to the fitting anomalies, as shown in **Figure 13**.

Adapted and not adapted basic dress pattern designs as virtual prototypes are presented in **Figure 14**. It is clearly visible that the reconstruction process of the basic dress pattern design improves the appearance and fit of the adapted dress to a deformed body. The seam in the middle of the back is aligned. Darts are symmetrical according to the center of the body. The seam line in the waist and dress edge are also aligned.

3.2.2. *Kyphotic model*

The body with a normal spine, and a kyphotic model with slightly curved, curved, and strongly curved spines, found in the case of kyphosis, were prepared in virtual space, as shown in **Figure 15**.

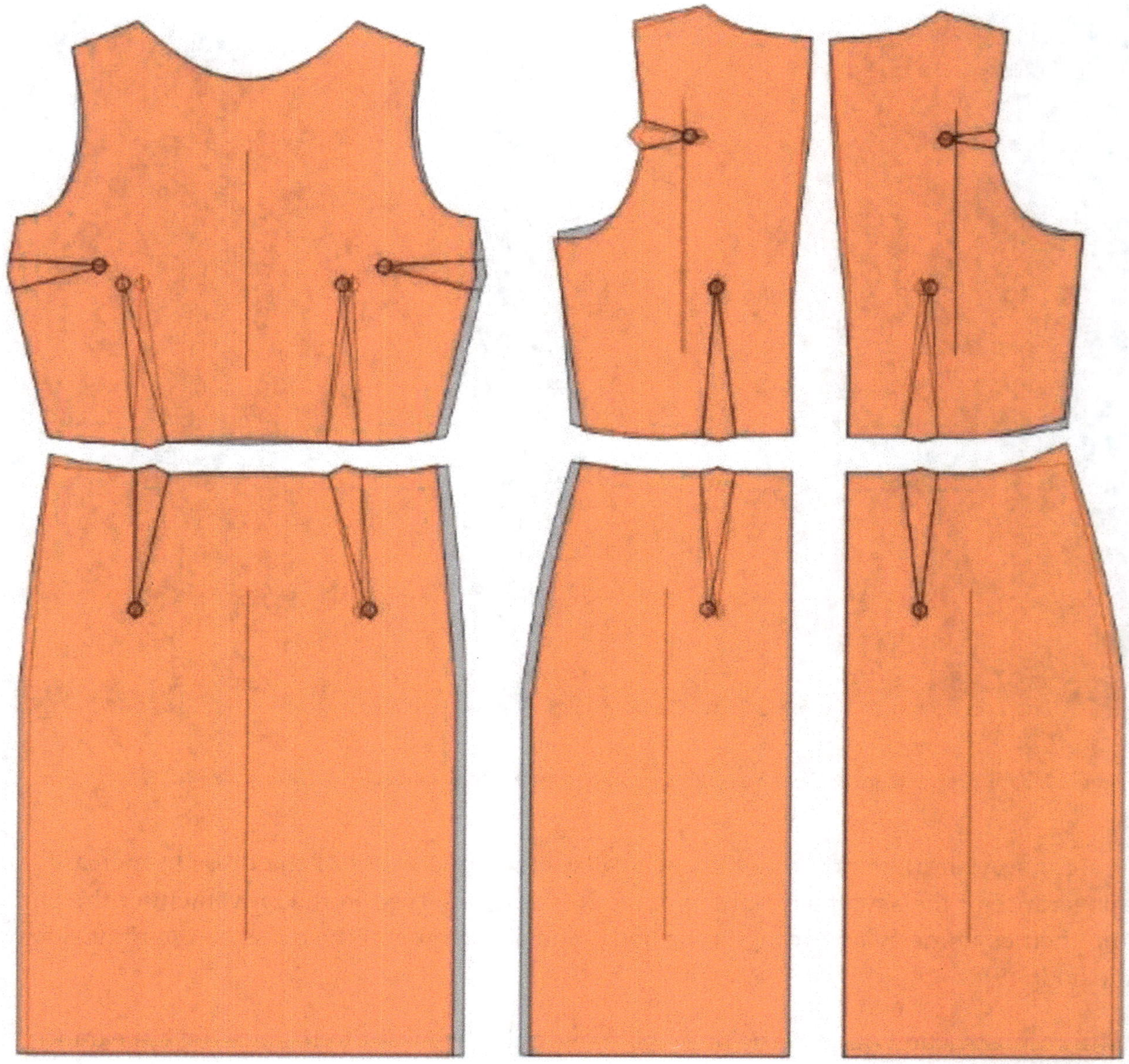

Figure 13. Comparison between basic dress pattern design (light grey) and adapted scoliotic dress pattern design (dark grey) [9].

All 3D body models were analyzed using the CASP methodology in the round-back area. The observation plane was projected on an imported body mesh model, as presented in **Figure 10**. Furthermore, calculations were executed by Grasshoppers' $n \times n$ procedure and values for CASP were obtained as a numerical result.

The virtual measurements of the back lengths were performed according to the Standard ISO 8559 [24] by using the Optitex PDS system [22]. The back length was measured precisely from the seventh cervical vertebra to the waist line. The waist girth in all 3D body models was 66.74 cm.

The results of the CASP analysis and measured back length are collected in **Table 1**.

In addition, differences were calculated between the normal spine and deformed spines for CASP parameters and back lengths, as well as quotients between the curvature differences

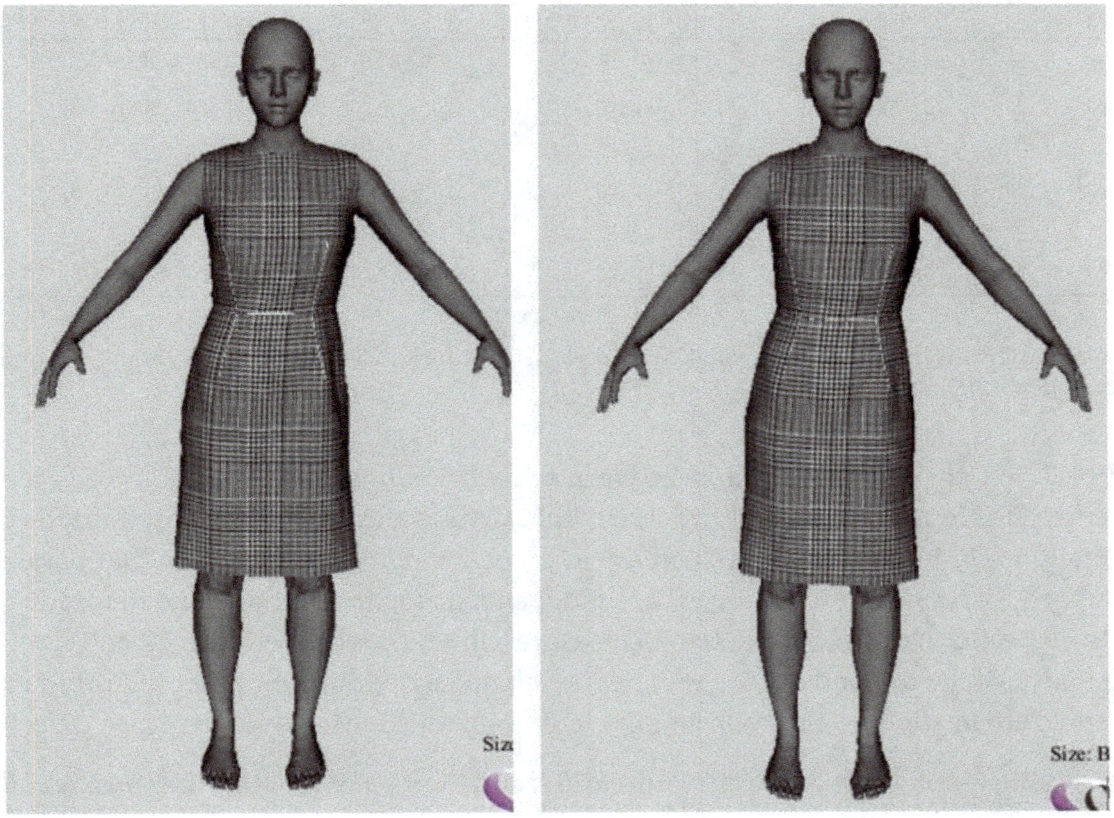

Figure 14. Not adapted and adapted (reconstructed) basic dress pattern design on a deformed body [9].

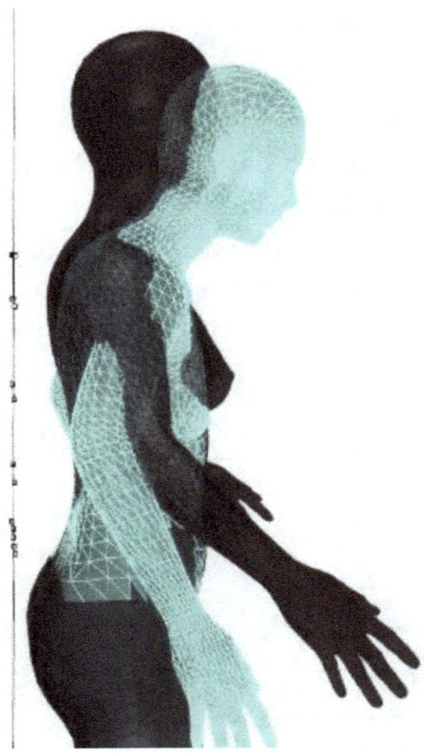

Figure 15. Normal (dark grey) and kyphotic (light grey) posture.

Spine	Normal	Slightly curved	Curved	Strongly curved
C	1.69	2.56	3.13	3.26
A	−3.73	−14.97	−55.79	−127.35
S	1.85	2.02	1/4	1.33
P	1.34	1.34	1.34	1.34
BL (cm)	33.19	34.95	36.14	36.31

Table 1. Values C (Curvature), A (Acceleration), S (Symmetry), P (Proportionality), and BL (back length) for normal and scoliotic models [25].

wand back lengths' differences, and between the acceleration differences and back lengths' differences, **Table 2**. The results show clearly that CASP values, especially Curvature—C and Acceleration—A, increase with an increase in the spine deformity. It seems that parameters Symmetry—S and Proportionality—P are independent regarding the spine deformity. This was also expected, because Symmetry—*S* measures differences between the left and right sides of the body. While the body was generated synthetically with a computer 3D program, the differences are negligible. The back length increases with an increase in the spine deformity.

A logarithmic graph chart of the **curvature difference** and **back length difference** was found when increasing the spine deformity. Logarithmic graphs have axes with logarithmic steps like 0.1/1/10/100/1000/10,000, and so on. The polynomial trend of the **acceleration difference** and the ratio DA/DBL was found with an increase in the spine deformity, **Figures 16** and **17**. Synthetically created body models were created with deformity of the upper spine with 5° steps. These equal steps caused chart trends of acceleration-dependent values presented in **Figure 15**.

The results show that the ratio DC/DBL is almost the same for all spine curvatures and equals 0.5, shown in **Table 2**. Therefore, it could be supposed that the back length difference is two times higher than the curvature difference. This means that it may be possible to include the CASP parameter for the curvature difference directly in the process of reconstruction of the garment pattern design to a specific body shape. The reconstruction of garment pattern

	Spine			
Parameter	**Normal**	**Slightly curved**	**Curved**	**Strongly curved**
DC	/	0.87	1.44	1.57
DA	/	11.24	52.06	123.62
DBL (cm)	/	1.76	2.95	3.12
DC/DBL (cm^{-1})	/	0.49	0.49	0.50
DA/DBL (cm^{-1})	/	6.39	17.65	39.62

Table 2. Values DC (curvature difference) and DA (acceleration difference). DBL (back length difference) and quotients DC/DBL and DA/DBL for scoliotic models [25].

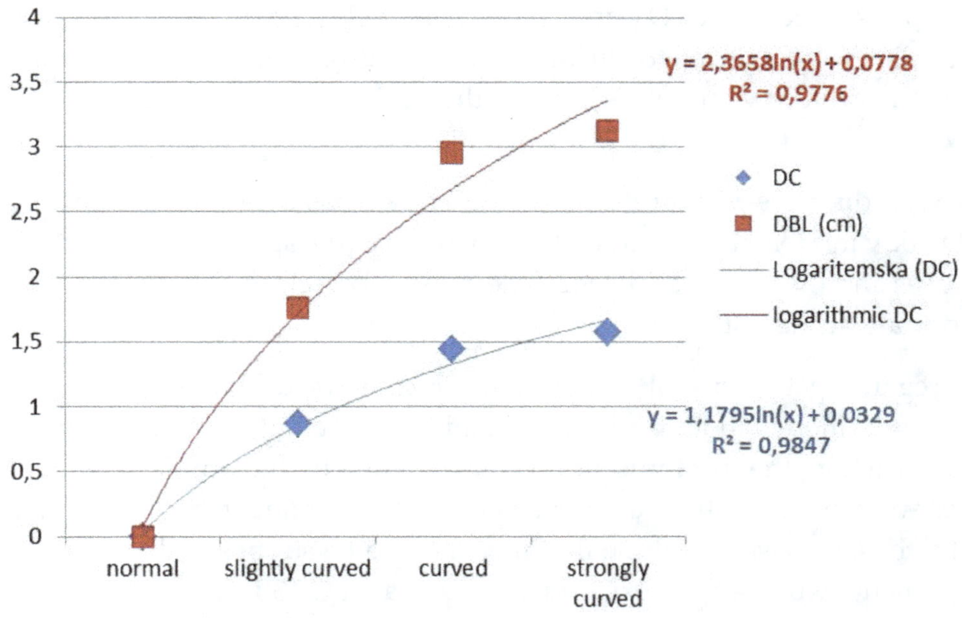

Figure 16. The curvature differences (DCs) and back length differences (DBLs) when increasing the spine deformity [25].

design is usually carried out by observation of the body shape and measuring of body dimensions, which is a lengthy process in terms of manufacturing and fitting clothing.

Based on the previous results, the constructed bodice basic pattern design was reconstructed according to the calculated value of the curvature difference for the slightly curved, curved, and strongly curved kyphosis spines. The virtual fittings of the bodice basic pattern design to a normal 3D body model and reconstructed bodice basic pattern

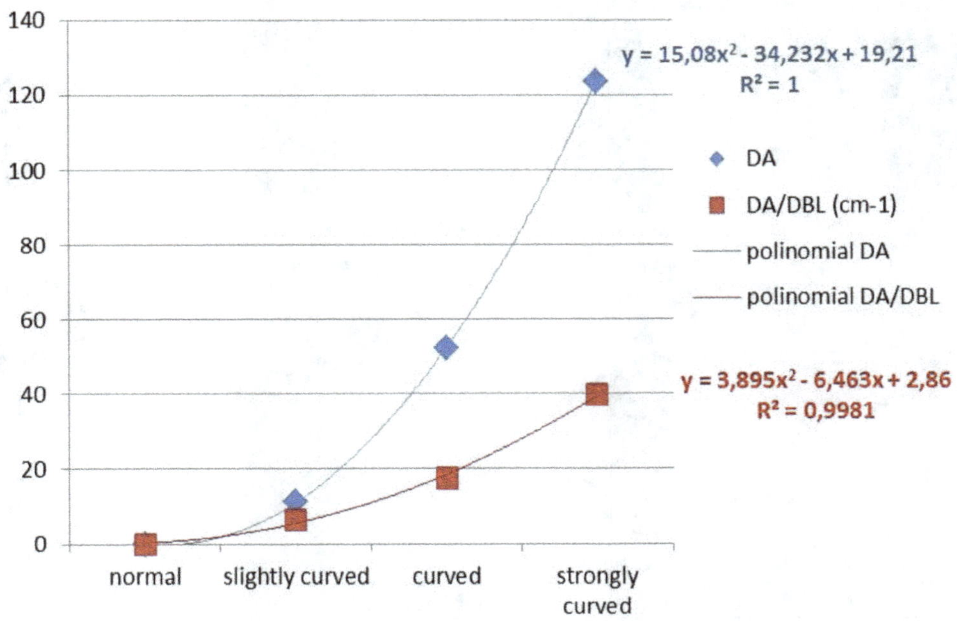

Figure 17. Acceleration difference (DA) and the ratio DA/DBL charts [25].

designs were performed to the 3D kyphosis body models, **Figure 18**. During reconstruction, the front middles were shortened for the double value of CD and the back middles were extended for the double value of DC, while the back darts were extended and raised for the CD.

The results regarding the virtual fitting of the bodice basic pattern design to normal and kyphosis 3D body models show that, with an increase in the spine curvature, the bodice front length increases and the bodice back length decreases. Therefore, the waistline is not straight, and inappropriate fitting appeared.

The results regarding the virtual fitting of the reconstructed bodice pattern designs to a kyphosis 3D body model show the straightened bottom edge of all the simulated bodices. During reconstruction, the front middles were shortened by the double value of CD and the back middles were extended by the double value of DC, while the back darts were extended and raised by the CD. Based on these findings, it could be supposed that, with a reconstruction of the garment by using the measured and calculated CASP values and the curvature differences for curved spines, respectively, improved garments fitting would be achieved and, at the same time, wearing comfort in terms of garment pattern design.

It can be concluded that the CASP methodology could be adequate for defining the appropriate garment pattern design for persons with a curved spine. Therefore, it is definitely

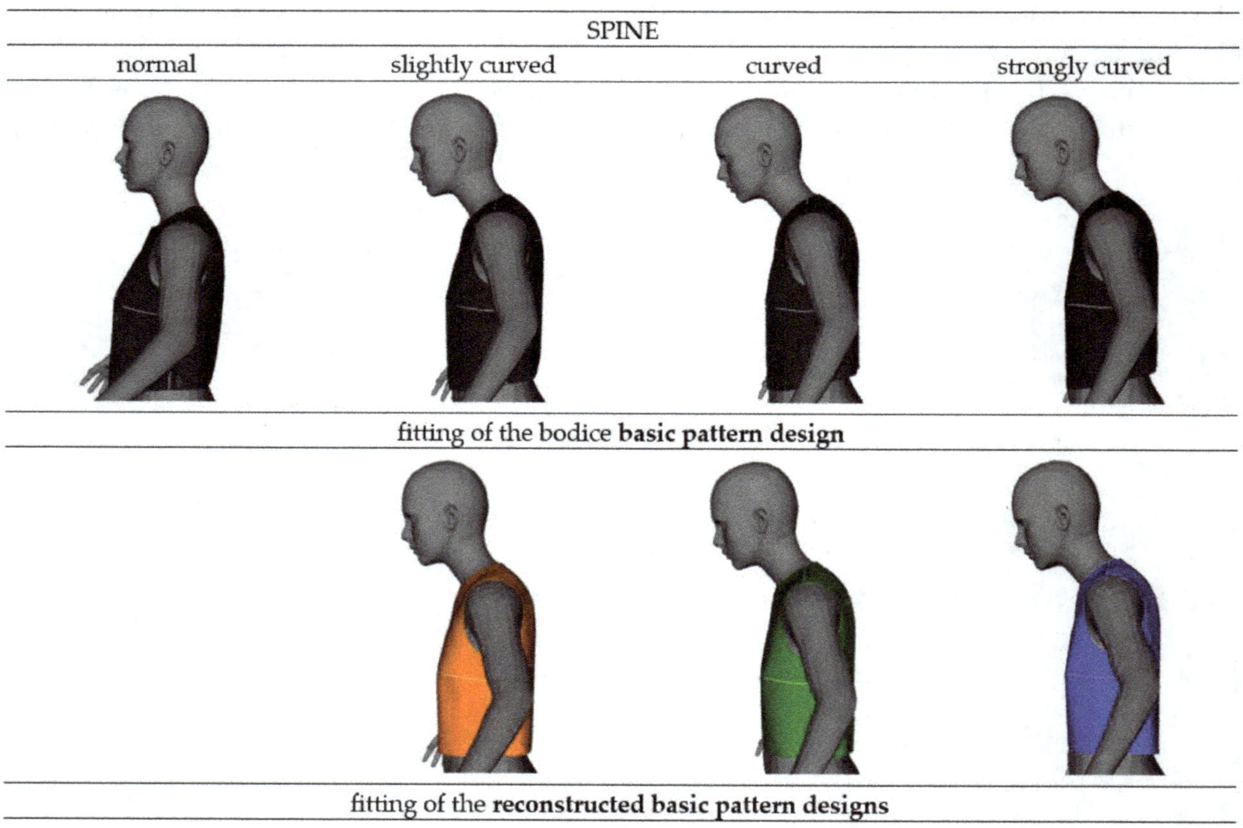

Figure 18. Fitting of the bodice basic pattern design (grey) and reconstructed bodice basic pattern designs [25].

necessary in the future to carry out additional research work on a larger number of diverse curvatures of the kyphosis spine with real persons, to confirm the findings of this research.

4. Results and discussion

The results of the CASP analysis and measured back length are collected in **Table 1**. It is evident that CASP values, especially Curvature—C and Acceleration—A, accrue with an increase in the spine deformity. It seems that parameters Symmetry—S and Proportionality—P are independent of spine deformity, which was expected, because Symmetry—S measures differences between the left and right sides of the body. While the body was generated synthetically with a 3D computer program, the differences are negligible. The proportionality—P depends on the observation frame, where the quotient is calculated between the length and width. In this case, the frame was the same for all models [25].

With an increase in the spine deformity, the back height increased, **Table 1**. The back length was measured with a computer program on a virtual model and was 33.19 cm for the normal spine, for the slightly curved spine 33.51 cm, and it increased for the strongly curved spine up to 36.31 cm. With an increase in the spine deformity, the bodice length on the back is too short and on the front too long. Therefore, the bodice in the front moves back to the neck, and thus compensates for the lack of the bodice length on the back. The result is an increase in the bodice tension in the area of neck and armholes when the deformity of the spine increases.

Virtual 3D models and virtual prototyping present an important approach to individual design and manufacturing. However, an individual treatment requires both sufficient time and suitably qualified people; therefore, not everybody can afford it. The future purpose is to enable virtual prototyping, including the design, construction, and visualization of adapted garments for people with postural disorders and spinal deformities to become more automated with 3D scanning, CASP methodology, and an established protocol.

The size of an object does not matter while CASP methodology performs normalization. For a scoliotic case, not all four parameters are observed, but just *C* and *A* while they show the curvature and acceleration of the back shape.

The ideal human body is symmetrical. The producers of ready-made garments cannot consider the deformity of a body caused by scoliosis, because they are specific and differ from case to case. Therefore, the only solution to improve the appearance and fit of the garment seems to be to adapt the garment pattern design to individual people.

5. Conclusions

In this chapter, advanced approaches such as virtual prototyping and multipurpose methodology CASP were used for designing dress patterns for people with postural disorders and spinal deformities such as scoliosis and kyphosis. Individuals can be analyzed with this methodology and the values obtained can be considered while the garment patterns are constructed. Dress fit is shown on virtual synthetic models. First, we took completely symmetrical designs for a normal body and prepared a dress that fitted well. Second, a digital scoliotic model was created and a third kyphotic model was designed with several increasing steps of spine deflection. The same dress used for a normal body did not fit well; therefore, an adapted dress pattern was developed. A satisfying correlation between the spine curvature and CASP values was obtained; therefore, it can be concluded that the CASP methodology could be adequate for defining the appropriate garment pattern designs for persons with a curved spine. In the future, we plan to carry out additional research work on a larger number of diverse body shapes of real people with postural disorders and spinal deformities to confirm the findings of this research.

Author details

Andrej Cupar[1]*, Zoran Stjepanovič[2], Simona Jevšnik[3], Rija Erveš[4] and Andreja Rudolf[2]

*Address all correspondence to: andrej.cupar@um.si

1 Faculty of Mechanical Engineering, Institute of Structures and Design, University of Maribor, Maribor, Slovenia

2 Faculty of Mechanical Engineering, Institute of Engineering Materials and Design, University of Maribor, Maribor, Slovenia

3 Inlas, Slovenske Konjice, Slovenia

4 Faculty of Civil Engineering, University of Maribor, Maribor, Slovenia

References

[1] Koffka K. Principles of Gestalt Psychology. Mimesis International, Milano, Italy; 2014

[2] Harada T, Yoshimoto F, Moriyama M. An aesthetic curve in the field of industrial design. In: Proceedings of the IEEE Symposium on Visual Languages, IEEE Computer Society Press, New York; 1999

[3] Kanaya I, Nakano Y, Sato K. Classification of aesthetic curves and surfaces for industrial designs, Design Discourse, Vol. II, no. 4; 2007;**4**:1-8

[4] Yoshida N, Fukuda R, Saito T. Log-aesthetic space curve segments. In: 2009 SIAM/ACM Jt. Conference on Geometric and Physical Modeling, SPM '09, San Francisco, California; 2009. p. 35-46

[5] Giannini F, Monti M, Podehl G. Styling properties and features in computer aided industrial design. Computer-Aided Design and Applications. 2004;**1**(1-4):321-330

[6] Giannini F, Monti M, Podehl G. Aesthetic-driven tools for industrial design. Journal of Engineering Design. Jun 2006;**17**(3):193-215

[7] Podehl G. Terms and measures for styling properties. In: International Design Conference—Design, Proceedings of the 7th International Design Conference Dubrovnik, Croatia, Zagreb; 2002. pp. 879-886

[8] Cupar A. Development of Classification Methodology of Perceptional Surfaces in Product Design. University of Maribor, PhD thesis; 2015

[9] Stjepanovič Z, Cupar A, Jevšnik S, Kocjan-Stjepanovič T, Rudolf A. Applying CASP method for construction of adapted garments for people with scoliosis. In: 7th TEXTEH International Conference Proceedings; Bucharest, Romania; October 22-23, 2015. pp. 276-285

[10] Cupar A, Stjepanovič Z, Kaljun J, Pogačar V. Methodology framework for surface shape evaluation. In: New Developments in Mechanical Engineering, editor: Mastorakis N.E. Proceedings of the International Conference on Mechanical Engineering (ME 2015) Vienna, Austria; 2015. pp. 58-65

[11] Scott D. Grasshopper [Online]. Available from: http://www.grasshopper3d.com/. Accessed: April 25, 2017

[12] McNeel R, et al. Rhino5 [Online]. Available from: http://www.rhino3d.com/. Accessed: April 25, 2017

[13] Rudolf A, Stjepanovič Z, Cupar A. Designing of functional garments for people with physical disabilities and postural disorders by using 3D scanning, CASP and computer simulation techniques. Forthcoming

[14] Strauss A. How to Dress with Scoliosis [Online]. Available from: http://www.hudsonvalleyscoliosis.com/clothing-for-scoliosis/. [Accessed: December 18, 2016]

[15] Ávila MZ. Patternmaking for People with Postural Deviations [Online]. Available from: http://www.well-women.com/Clothing.html. [Accessed: July 1, 2015]

[16] Spinedoc. [Online]. Available from: http://myspinedoc.com/conditions-diagnosis/conditions/kyphosis. [Accessed: December 18, 2016]

[17] Cupar A, Pogačar V, Stjepanovič Z. Methodology for surfaces analysis and classification. University of Journal of Mechanical Engineering. 2014;**2**:64-70

[18] Cupar A, Pogačar V, Stjepanovič Z. Methodology for analysing digitised geometry. In: Katalinic B, Tekic Z, editors. Vienna: Daaam International Scientific Book; 2013. pp. 903-920

[19] Make Human [Online]. Available from: http://www.makehuman.org/. [Accessed: December 2, 2016]

[20] Blender [Online]. Available from: http://wiki.blender.org/index.php/Doc:2.6/Manual/Modeling/Meshes/Editing/Sculpt_Mode. Accessed: April 25, 2017

[21] Stjepanovič Z, Cupar A, Jevšnik S, Kocjan Stjepanovič T, Rudolf A. Construction of adapted garments for people with scoliosis using virtual prototyping and CASP method. Industria Textila. 2016;**67**(2):141-148

[22] Optitex [Online]. Available from: http://www.optitex.com/. [Accessed: December 7, 2015]

[23] System M. Müller & Sohn: Schnittkonstruktionen für Kleider und Blusen, Deutsche Bekleidungs-Akademie München. München: Rundschau Verlag; 1992

[24] I. O. for Standardization. ISO 8559:1989: Garment construction and anthropometric survey: Body dimensions = Confection des vetements et releves anthopometriques: Mesures du corps humain. Geneva: International Organization for Standardization; 1989

[25] Rudolf A, Stjepanovič Z, Jevšnik S, Cupar A. Research on the Applicability of CASP Methodology for Nonstandard Body Shapes' Garment Pattern Design. In: Autex; 2016. pp. 1-7

4

Limits of Normality and Symmetry in Standing Back Shape and Posture: 3D Mapping and Analysis of Young Adults

Josette Bettany-Saltikov,
Gokulakannan Kandasamy, Dariusz Czaprowski and
Lukasz Stolinski

Abstract

Abnormalities of posture are a common cause of pain and disability. Objective measurement systems for postural evaluation are not widely accessible in the UK especially on the National Health Service. Within physiotherapy practice one of the most common methods of assessing posture and/or back shape is by visual observation which is prone to error and lacks objectivity. The study has sought to produce normative values for back shape and posture indices in young asymptomatic adults. A convenience sample of 100 Teesside University (TU) students were recruited. This study used a 3-D Digitizer. Data was analyzed using SPSS. The acromion and the inferior scapular angle in the dorsal frontal plane differed between the right and left shoulders of the back in females. The distance between the inferior angle of the scapula and the apical thoracic vertebrae also differed. No other statistically significant differences were found in distances between key landmarks. Overall young adults are very symmetrical. Frontal plane angles showed that overall healthy young adults have relatively straight spines. The left inferior angle of the scapula in females was found to be rotated anteriorly in comparison to the right shoulder. Results will provide a normative database for clinicians who routinely assess back posture.

Keywords: posture, assessment, gender differences, normative values, digitizer

1. Introduction

Abnormalities of back shape and posture are a common cause of pain and disability with the range of effect from discomfort to incapacitating disability being related to both the **severity** as well as to the **persistence** of the faults [1]. While the terms "back shape" and "back posture" are sometimes used interchangeably it is important to be clear of what precisely is meant by each term. The focus of the term "posture" is on **muscular and skeletal balance** as seen from the definition provided by the American academy of orthopedic surgeons. The society define "good" posture as "that state of muscular and skeletal balance which protects the supporting structures of the body against injury or progressive deformity irrespective of the attitude [sitting, lying erect] in which these structures are working or resting." Under such conditions the muscles will function most efficiently and the optimum positions are afforded for the thoracic and abdominal organs [2]."

The focus of the term "back shape" on the other hand is on the **back surface** and generally refers to the surface topography of the back. "Topography [from Greek topo-, "place," and graphia, "writing"] is the study of the back's surface shape and includes the measurement of parameters that may or may not be similar to those measured for back posture." For instance, thoracic kyphosis and lumbar lordosis are usually measured when assessing both back shape and back posture.

The measurement of the surface equivalent of the spinal curvature [Cobb angle] in the frontal plane, however is usually measured solely during the assessment of spinal deformities within orthopedic clinics or private practices. A further key difference is that different professional health practitioners traditionally use different terminologies. Spinal deformity clinics within orthopedic medical practice generally refer to back shape whereas within physiotherapy practice the term 'posture' is usually the term of choice.

The assessment of back shape and posture is common practice in a number of disciplines within rehabilitation [1]. Within physiotherapy practice one of the most common methods of assessing posture and/or back shape is by visual observation of standing posture as viewed from the back and sides and is a routine part of all back assessments for patients with low back pain and/or spinal dysfunctions. Kipling et al. [3] in a survey on Common methods of assessing posture in Physiotherapy practice, found that up to 82% of physiotherapists reported using observation alone to evaluate patients posture.

A more recent survey was developed very recently in 2016 by Johnson et al. [4] who created the "The Postural Assessment Survey." The authors surveyed a group of manual therapists (chiropractors, physical therapists, osteopaths and sports therapists) to ascertain whether or not they actually used postural assessment within their practice, and if so what type of assessment they used. 432 therapists answered the question about which method of postural assessment they used. The large majority of therapists (98.15% n = 424) said that they used visual postural assessment.

Back shape/postural assessment is also part of the clinical examination for patients with spinal deformities in musculoskeletal clinics. Within Physiotherapy and Orthopedic clinical settings, the parameters evaluated may differ. Physiotherapists primarily evaluate asymmetries in standing back posture at four key areas; the shoulder level, scapular level, pelvic level and the posterior superior iliac spines (PSIS) levels [5]. In the orthopedic setting however the assessment of back shape and posture is predominantly focused on the assessment of the skeletal measurement of spinal curvature on x-ray together with the measurement of the maximum trunk inclination values in forward bending [5].

Normative values of back shape and posture values may assist in classifying back shape types and provide normal ranges of different back surface parameters for the purpose of research or clinical decision making.

Two key studies in this area are those by Bettany-Saltikov [6] and Duff and Draper [7]. Bettany-Saltikov conducted a study evaluating normal back shape in young adults using the Integrated spinal imaging system (ISIS1). This is an optical computer system that is able to measure the 3D surface topography of the back. We were able to produce a representative scan for the interpretation of the back shape for all participants included in the study. This study found a mean *thoracic kyphosis* of 24.9 mm (median 24 mm, deciles: 6.8–47.2 mm). The thoracic kyphosis values found in this group of young adults are very similar to the children in Duff and Draper's study [7] who reported a median value for thoracic kyphosis of 27.8 mm (17–40 mm).

Carr et al. [8] reported these values in degrees and therefore values were not directly comparable. In this study the mean *lumbar lordosis* was 14.9 mm (median 14 mm). The lumbar lordosis values were found to be greater in Saltikov's study [6] that evaluated young adults compared to the Duff and Draper study (median 9 mm) that evaluated children. This suggests the possibility that lumbar lordosis may increase during growth from young adolescence to young adulthood. Carr et al. [8] however reported no significant differences in lumbar lordosis angles between children and adults. It is possible that these changes may be due to variables such age, race and other population differences.

Duff and Draper [7] conducted a survey of back shape in children using the Integrated spinal imaging system (ISIS1). with a sample of 105 boys and 101 girls, with an age range of 12.28–13.69 years. It was noted by the authors that these parameters were specific to the age group of the subject's used. Duff and Draper [7] also commented on the need for a standardized value for what should be considered a "normal" degree of back shape and spinal curvature that may be used as a reference against which back posture and shape parameters can be measured in young teenagers.

Within both fields therefore uncertainly still remains as to what constitutes "normality" within the context of standing back shape and/or posture. More pertinently the question remains "what are the limits of normality in standing back shape and posture?" In other words, how do physiotherapists and other clinicians know when a patient's posture is abnormal, if the ranges of normality are not known? Knowledge of what actually constitutes normality would significantly benefit clinicians in this field as it would enable them to decide when postural retraining exercises or other treatment modalities are warranted.

A further problem with regards to the quantification of back shape is that no boundaries of "normality" have been established that are ***universally accepted***. Sahrmann [9] comments on the need for establishing normative values with standard deviations for spinal curvature that would benefit the analysis of extreme variations of spinal alignment and better inform the clinician as to the nature of the condition as a whole. However, in the literature while numerous spinal deformities have been defined, sparse information is available on the quantification of normal back parameters in standing. Kawchuk and McArthur comment that the primary limitation in the study and treatment of scoliosis is the lack of an accurate, reliable, convenient and completely safe form of scoliosis quantification [10]. Indeed, normative data of standing back shape and posture for comparison and reference in young adults is not currently available.

2. Objectives

1. To identify the limits of normality and symmetry/asymmetry of back shape and posture in a group of healthy young male and female subjects (i.e., to establish normative reference values).
2. To evaluate the symmetry/asymmetry between key anatomical landmarks and distances between the left and right sides of the back in normal young female and male subjects.
3. To compare back shape and posture in normal young males and females.

3. Materials and methods

3.1. Subjects

A convenience sample of 100 TU students were recruited for this study (n = 59 females and 41 males). Their ages ranged from 18 to 40 years old. Subjects were excluded if they had any lower limb or back injury that prevented the subject standing for the duration of data collection, any vestibular problems that prevented the subject maintaining normal balance for the duration of data collection or a known allergy to self-adhesive stickers when in contact with the skin. Ethical approval was granted by Teesside University School of Health and Social Care ethics committee.

3.2. Instrumentation

The Middlesbrough Integrated Digital Assessment System (MIDAS) (**Figure 1**) is a tool for acquiring a static 3-D computer recording of a physical object. A counterbalanced mechanical arm has optical sensors in each joint for X, Y, Z coordinate awareness with a mean accuracy of 0.23 mm. A footplate was created with marks to standardize foot position and a chart was placed on the wall in front of the subject with markers to focus on [11–13].

Through assessment with an anatomical mannequin this system demonstrated very high intra-rater reliability (ICC > 0.999, p < 0.0001) [12], with a sample of 50 human subjects (r = 0.92–0.99, p < 0.001). Further intra and inter rater reliability were also found excellent when evaluated by McAlpine et al. [14]. Additionally previous work has found improvements

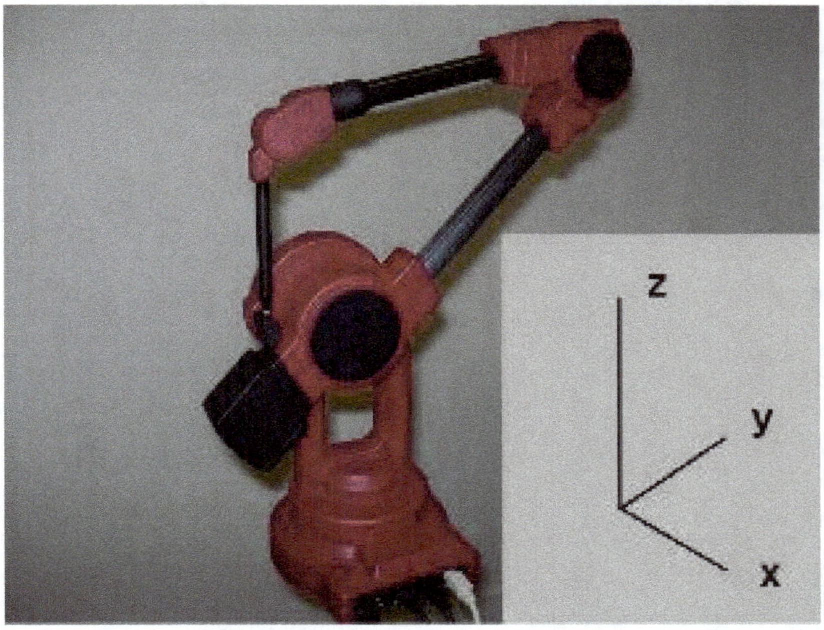

Figure 1. The microscribe digitizer in resting position.

in repeat measurements with foot and vision standardization [10]. The MIDAS was placed on an adjustable tripod for positioning and connected via a serial port to a laptop PC for data storage. A set of scales and a stadiometer were used to obtain weight and height measurements of subjects.

3.3. Procedure

Subjects read the subject information sheet and after consenting to participate were attired so that their back was visible for landmark identification. Subjects stood and fixed their vision to a point on a wall chart, in agreement with other studies of postural assessment tools [14]. The landmarks used were identical to those used in previous MIDAS studies [11, 15]. Landmarks were identified as shown in **Table 1**. Selection of anatomical landmarks.

The landmarks above were carefully chosen from current clinical methods, back shape studies as well as studies related to spinal deformities [16]. The intention was to produce a map of the back for cervical, thoracic and lumbar regions that enabled the two sides of the back to be identified and produced a "normal" back shape profile in three dimensions. To date it is still unclear what "normal" back shape is although attempts have been made in school children [8]. The spinal vertebrae chosen were those at the ends of the apices of each curve, i.e., VP TA and T12 in the cervical thoracic and lumbar regions. For landmarks on either side of the back, bony points were chosen that were as far from the spine as possible to enable a total picture of back shape to be produced. It needs to be remembered that this is a work in progress and changes could be made in future in response to the results obtained.

Data collection involved the tester touching the MIDAS stylus tip to each of the marked points in a standardized order dictated by the software and pressing the foot pedal of the MIDAS to store the position on the computer. Data was analyzed using the Statistical Package for Social Sciences (SPSS) version 23.

Label	Anatomical point
AL	Left acromion processes
AR	Right acromion process
SL	Left inferior angle of scapulae
SR	Right inferior angle of scapulae
ICL	Left iliac crest
ICR	Right iliac crest
PSL	Left posterior superior iliac spine
PSR	Right posterior superior iliac spine
C2	2nd cervical vertebra
CA	Anterior cervical vertebra
VP	Vertebra prominens
TA	Anterior thoracic vertebra
T12	12th thoracic vertebra
LA	Anterior lumbar vertebra
SA	Sacral point

Table 1. Key to standing back anatomical landmarks measured.

4. Results

4.1. Frontal plane values

4.1.1. Mean distances between key anatomical landmarks in male and female subjects

In the frontal plane, the mean distances between key anatomical landmarks can be seen in **Table 2**. The only statistically significant differences found between the two sides of the back in females were the distances between the acromion and the inferior scapular angle; with the right side distance (AR-SR) being significantly smaller than the left side distance AL-SL as seen in **Figure 2**. The other statistically significant difference found was between the inferior angle of the scapula and the apical thoracic vertebrae. For this parameter the right side distance (TA-SR) was significantly greater than the left sided value (TA-SL). No other significant differences in the distances between key anatomical landmarks between the left and right sides of the back were found. Further no significant differences were found for all key anatomical landmark distances in male subjects between the two sides of the back. The mean female and male distances and standard deviations on the left and right sides of the back can be seen in **Tables 2** and **3**. The back landmarks positions and representation of key anatomical landmarks on a mannequin are presented in **Figures 3** and **4**. Normative values of analysed parameters can be seen in **Tables 4** and **5**.

Frontal plane back shape distances between key anatomical landmarks for female subjects	Female left side (mm and SD)	Male left side (mm and SD)	Female right side (mm and)SD	Male right side (mm and SD)	Mean diff between left and right side distances mm		P value	
					F	M	F	M
Distance between vertebra prominans and the acromion (VP-AL; VP-AR)	174.6 ± 16.6	195.2 ± 26.2	171.9 ± 14.2	198.2 ± 29.1	2.7	3.12	NS	NS
Distance between the acromion and the inferior scapula	175.9 ± 12.1	191.1 ± 14.4	171.3 ± 16.7	190.1 ± 14.8	4.6	0.97	0.003	NS
Distance between the inferior scapular angle and iliac crest	221.3 ± 18.9	234.8 ± 28	220.7 ± 21.8	238.9 ± 33.1	0.5	−4.14	NS	NS
Distance between the iliac crest and the PSIS	63.8 ± 17.9	73.4 ± 58.3	63.5 ± 17.8	63.7 ± 19.7	.33	9.61	NS	NS
Distance between the PSIS the sacral point	55.1 ± 11.9	59.7 ± 12.08	53.8 ± 12.8	60.4 ± 21.4	1.24	−0.65	NS	NS
Distance between the inf. angle of the scapula and the apical thoracic vertebrae	88.4 ± 12.2	116.7 ± 54.2	92.3 ± 13.5	115.9 ± 30.8	3.96	.75	0.046	NS
Distance between the iliac crest and the lumber apical vertebra	65.8 ± 19.8	76.8 ± 47.3	65.4±16.9	71.1 ± 25.5	0.46	5.72	NS	NS

Table 2. The distance between the acromion and the inferior scapula on the left side is statistically longer than the right side and the distance between the inf. angle of the scapula and the apical thoracic vertebrae on the right side is significantly longer on the right side than on the left side.

4.1.2. Differences in female and male height values between the left and right sides of the back for key anatomical landmarks in the frontal plane

The set of values below **Table 3** refers to the differences in height levels between specific key anatomical landmarks on the two sides of the back. The only significant differences found were at the level of the shoulders; The left shoulder acromion was significantly higher than the right (AL > AR). Otherwise no other staticatically significant differecnes were found at the levels of the inferior scapular angle, the iliac crests and the PSIS. In males there were no stat sign difference at any level, however at the PSIS level the left PSIS showed a trend toward being higher than the right PSIS

4.2. Dorsal frontal plane spinal angles

The mean frontal plane angles values showed that overall healthy young adults have relatively straight spines. The mean thoracic curvature value was +2.38° and the mean lumber curve was +1.65°.

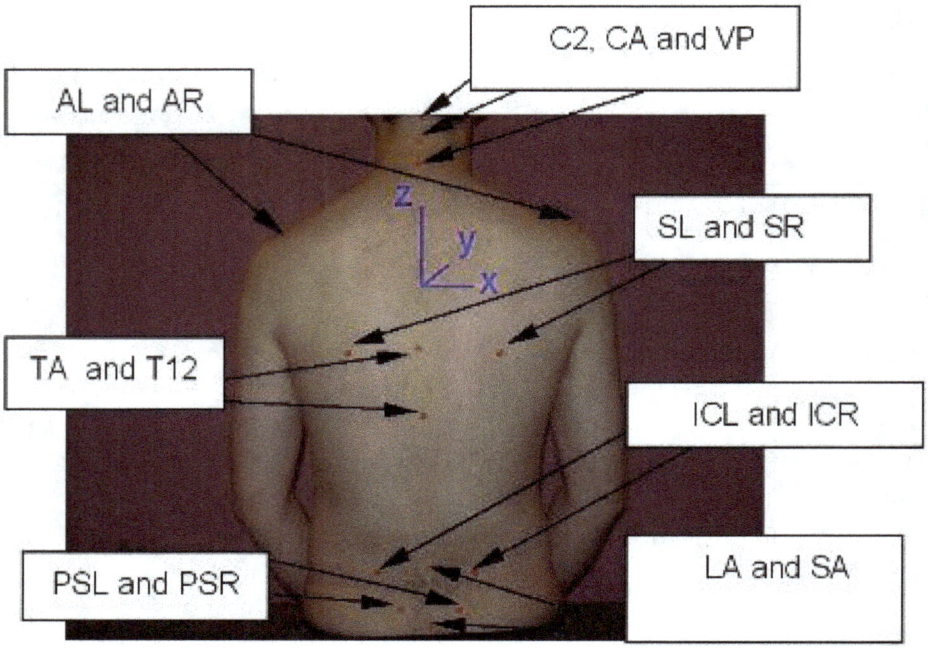

Figure 2. Back landmarks identified with self-adhesive marker.

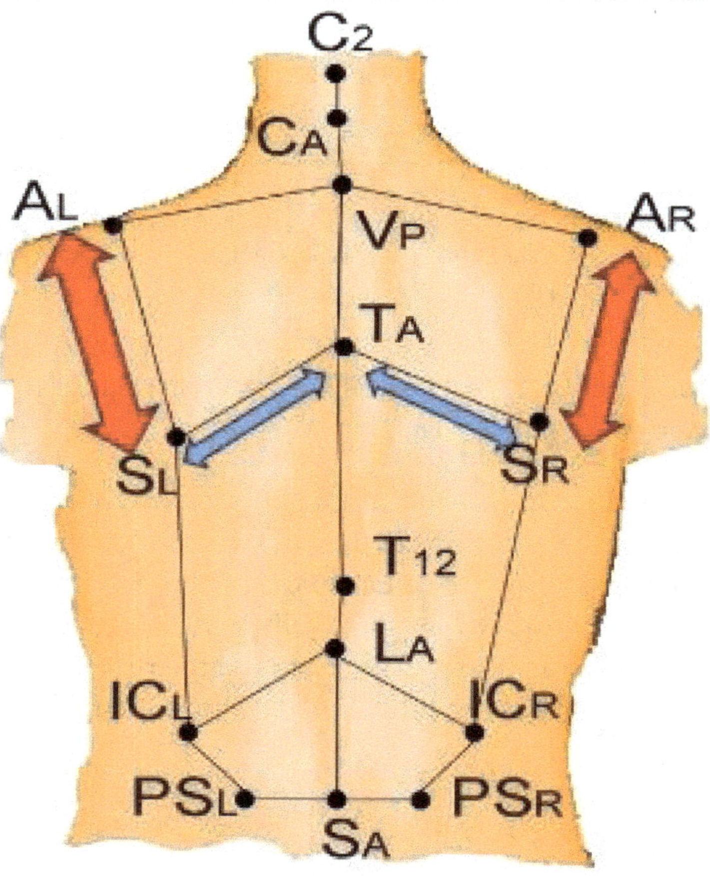

Figure 3. Representation of key anatomical landmarks on a mannequin, with a description below.

1. AL is higher than AR in the frontal plane
2. Distance AL-SL greater on left side than on right side
3. Right side distance (TA-SR) was significantly greater than the left sided value (TA-SL) for females
4. No significant differences were found for all key anatomical landmark distances in male subjects between the two sides of the back

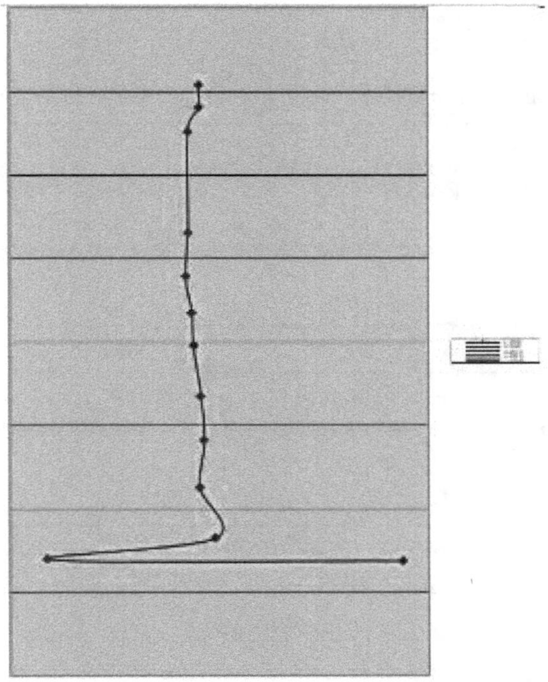

Figure 4. Frontal plane lateral asymmetry value for one female subject [surface equivalent to Cobb angle].

Differences in height levels between the two sides of the back in males and females Left side minus right side	Females			Males		
	Height difference and SD in mm	95% CI of the difference	P value	Height difference and SD in mm	95% CI of the difference	P value
Shoulder level (acromium) ALz-ARz	4.48 ± 10.98	1.63–7.35	.003	−1.34 ± 13.07	−5.71 to 3.01	NS
Inf. angle of scapula SLz-SRz	0.12 ± 7.6	−1.86 to 2.11	NS	−2.43 ± 9.06	−5.44 to 0.59	NS
Iliac crests ICLz-ICRz	−0.22 ± 7.2	−2.24 to 1.78	NS	−5.7 ± 9.11	−3.61 to 2.47	NS
PSIS PSLz-PSRz	0.53 ± 4.10	−5.3 to 1.6	NS	1.38 ± 4.91	−0.25 to 3.02	NS (0.09)

Table 3. Differences in height levels between the two sides of the back in males and females.

Mean spinal distances between spinal anatomical landmarks in the frontal plane	Mean values and SD in mm	
	For female subjects	For male subjects
Distance between C2 and the apical cervical vertebra CA	27.9 ± 8.1	44.2 ± 73.5
Distance between the apical cervical vertebra and the vertebra prominens	49.5 ± 29.7	66.6 ± 41.8
Distance between the vertebra prominens and the thoracic apical vertebra	371.0 ± 51.2	388.6 ± 67.6
Distance between the thoracic apical vertebra and the 12th Thoracic vertebra	227.9 ± 32.6	241.1 ± 40.6
Distance between the 12th Thoracic vertebra and the lumber apical vertebra	90.5 ± 29.6	88.9 ± 40.7
Distance between the lumbar apical vertebra and the sacral point	89.5 ± 25.8	96.3 ± 27.5

Table 4. Normative values for the mean spinal distances between spinal anatomical landmarks in the frontal plane for female and male subjects.

Differences in depth levels between the two sides of the back in males and females Left side minus right side	Females			Males		
	Height difference and SD in mm	95% CI mm of the difference in mm	P value	Height difference and SD in mm	95% CI of the difference in mm	P value
Shoulder level (acromium) ALy-ARy	5.85 ± 40.05	−4.58 to 16.29	NS	11.55 ± 34.9	−0.10 to 23.19	P = 0.05
Inf. angle of scapula SLy-SRy	5.82 ± 23.24	−0.23 to 11.88	P = 0.05	6.22 ± 18.64	0.01 to 12.44	P = 0.05
Iliac crests ICLy-ICRy	2.08 ± 13.81	−1.52 to 5.69	NS	−0.298 ± 34.2	−14.41 to 8.45	NS
PSIS PSLy-PSRy	2.45 ± 13.84	−1.15 to 6.06	NS	3.29 ± 12.54	−0.89 to 7.47	NS

Table 5. Female and male normative values and mean differences between the left and right side of the back in the horizontal plan.

4.3. Horizontal plane values (rotation)

The left inferior angle of the scapula in females was rotated forward in comparison to the right shoulder. No other statistically significant differences at the acromium, iliac crests or PSIS were found (see **Table 5**).

4.4. Sagittal plane values for female and male subjects

The mean thoracic kyphosis angle was 29.37 + 3.94° and the mean lumbar lordosis angle was -37.7.

5. Discussion

The purpose of this study was to produce normative data for asymptomatic standing back shape and posture in young adults, against which significant postural deformity could be defined. Although numerous commercial optical and computer systems are available [17–20] data on normal adolescent and adult back shape have so far been scarce [12, 13]. This will affect the clinical certainty with which we can establish an observed spinal curve as abnormal and therefore be able to initiate appropriate treatment.

Overall young adults in the current study were very symmetrical. The mean distances between the left and right sides of the back and the average values were calculated. Overall only the distance between the scapula and the acromion process was significantly smaller on the right side than the left side of the back. It is possible that this is related to the fact that most subjects were right handed and asymmetry can be related to the upper limb dominance influence. In a typical posture pattern the right shoulder is lower than left in right-handed people [1, 21]. Additionally, as the body is not perfectly symmetrical, some deviations may have no clinical implications [5].

"Normal" standing posture is generally described as one with a straight back and no trunk asymmetries [22]. Comparison between studies using quantitative results is difficult because of the wide diversity of tools used within other studies. A further challenge is that different quantitative variables have been measured in different studies through different approaches; for example, the different back shape instruments that have been used in previous studies, such as non-tactile optoelectronic systems like the formetric and ISIS2 systems where a light beam is shone onto the back [23–25]. The microscribe digitizer used in this study is a tool for acquiring a static 3-D computer recording of a physical object based on optical sensors in each joint of the instrument and is capable of measuring all three X, Y, Z coordinates. The methods for measuring angles or distance used by these different systems has meant that comparison of "normal" values between different systems is very difficult as the individual parameters are calculated in different ways.

With regards to the methodological aspects of this study, the sample size of 100 individuals comprised a homogenous population of young adults. The results have provided a template or framework of the range and limits of normative values for specific back variables of young adults in a standing posture. We acknowledge that a hundred subjects is not usually considered to be a large sample size and agree that a larger sample size of a few hundred subjects would have increased the external validity of this study (the degree to which the results can be transferred to the general population of young adults).

The other statistically significant difference was the distance between the inferior angle of the scapula and the apical thoracic vertebrae. For this parameter the right side distance was significantly greater than the left sided value. No other significant differences in the distances between key anatomical landmarks between the left and right sides of the back were found in females. For male subjects however no statistically significant differences were found between the left and right sides of the back for all the key anatomical landmark distances. To the best of our knowledge no similar studies using the Microscribe have been conducted that have measured similar variables so it was not possible to compare the results of this study with previous studies.

In the frontal plane the key difference in height levels between specific key anatomical landmarks on the two sides of the back was at the level of the shoulders; the left shoulder acromion was found to be significantly higher than the right. Further, no statistically significant differences were found at the levels of the inferior scapular angle, the iliac crests and the PSIS. In males there were no statistically significant differences between the two sides of the back. However, at the PSIS level, the left PSIS showed a trend toward being higher than the right PSIS.

With regards to the measurement of the frontal plane spinal angles, the mean frontal plane angles values showed that overall healthy young females have relatively straight spines. As stated previously, in this current study the mean thoracic curvature value was +2.38° and the mean lumbar curve was +1.65°. This supports the textbook "Ideal" of adults having a relatively straight spine [1]. These results however differ to the results we obtained previously using the surface topography equipment ISIS to measure a similar cohort of young adult students [6]. In this study, the mean thoracic curvature value found was 16.1° + 6.9° and the mean lumbar curvature value was 13.4° + 6.9°. It is the authors belief that the differences in values obtained from the ISIS2 scanner and the microscribe digitizer are due to the fact that the ISIS2 scanner has previously been shown to overestimate the magnitude of small curves [26].

In our study and in this population of young asymptomatic adults we found a mean thoracic kyphosis of 29.37° and lumbar lordosis of −37.7° in the sagittal plane. These values support the values provided by the Scoliosis Research Society who suggest that the normal range of thoracic kyphosis is between 20 and 40° on X-ray measurement [18, 26]. Our results also support the study by Betz [27] who found that the normal range for lumbar lordosis on X-ray ranged between −20 and −60°. Propst-Proctor and Bleck and Stagnara et al. evaluated the sagittal profile of a group of normal subjects aged 20–29 years old [28, 29]. The mean values of thoracic kyphosis ranged from 30 to 50° and the mean values of lumbar lordosis was calculated to be 55° which was greater than the lumbar lordosis in our group of subjects.

Bernhardt and Bridwell [30] conducted a segmental analysis of sagittal plane alignment of the normal thoracic and lumbar spines as well the thoracolumbar junction on X-rays. Within this study a wide range of healthy subjects (n = 102) aged between 5 and 29 years old were included. The authors reported a mean value of thoracic kyphosis at 40°, and mean of lumbar lordosis at −44°. While the thoracic Kyphosis in our study support the results obtained in the Bernhardt study, the lumbar lordosis reported in the Bernhardt study is much higher than the mean lumbar lordosis in our study. This may possibly be attributed to the fact that Bernhardt study included a wide range of ages comprised of children, adolescents and adults.

6. Limitations

The Microscribe is a manual measurement tool and although is very easy to use in a research setting it is not really ideal to use in a clinical setting at the current time. More research as well as instrument development is needed before this Microscribe can be used within a clinical setting. It should be particularly well suited to use in small clinical units owing to its simplicity of operation, size and cost. In today's climate of evidence based medicine there is an increasing emphasis on objective assessment to monitor treatment effectiveness. Our results stress the need for clinicians to objectively assess back shape and posture in three dimensions, as our study shows that changes in one dimension are associated with changes in other dimensions.

Future studies should focus on measuring normal back shape and posture throughout the life cycle as well as evaluating the effectiveness of different management strategies on back shape and posture. This is necessary to provide a positive shift toward a more objective and evidence based profession. More work is necessary to determine an appropriate set of clinically relevant measures to be implemented for use in clinical practice.

7. Conclusions

Ranges for normality of back shape and posture suggest that overall young asymptomatic males and females are very symmetrical, with the exception of shoulder values in young females. The normative ranges provided should help clinicians decide when postural retraining exercises or conservative treatment is warranted.

The results will also provide a normative database for clinicians (physiotherapists, chiropractors, spinal surgeons) who routinely assess back posture. Additionally, this method of assessment will provide an evidenced based objective alternative to other crude methods of assessment or just "eyeballing" back posture during clinical evaluation. Accurate recording of intervention or efficacy of treatment, if scientifically based on reliable measures can be used to credibly validate treatment effectiveness.

Author details

Josette Bettany-Saltikov[1*], Gokulakannan Kandasamy[2], Dariusz Czaprowski[3,4] and Lukasz Stolinski[5]

*Address all correspondence to: j.b.saltikov@tees.ac.uk

1 School of Health and Social Care, Teesside University, Victoria Road, Middlesbrough, UK

2 School of Social Sciences Business and Law, Teesside University, Middleborough, UK

3 Department of Physiotherapy, Józef Rusiecki University College, Olsztyn, Poland

4 Center of Body Posture, Olsztyn, Poland

5 Spine Disorders and Pediatric Orthopedic Department, University of Medical Sciences, Poznan, Poland

References

[1] Kendall FP, McCreary EK, Provance PG, Rodgers MM, Romani WA. Muscles; Testing and Function with Posture and Pain. Seoul. Hanmi Medical Publishing Co.; 2006

[2] Core Standards of Physiotherapy Practice, London. The Chartered Society of Physiotherapy. 2000;**10**:1c

[3] Kipling Kay, Bettany-Saltikov J. Survey of Postural Assessment by Physiotherapists. Teesside University, Middlesbrough. 2001

[4] Johnson Jane, Bettany-Saltikov, Josette Newell, David Van-Schaik, Paul; Cordry J. The Postural Assessment Survey, Teesside University, Middlesbrough. 2017

[5] Magee DJ. Orthopedic Physical Assessment. Elsevier Health Sciences, Missouri. 2014

[6] Saltikov JA, Van Schaik P, Bell JA, Warren JG, Wojcik AS, Papastefanou SL. 3D back shape in normal young adults. Studies in Health Technology and Informatics. 2002;**88**:81-85

[7] Duff ES, Draper R. Survey of normal adolescent back shape as measured by ISIS. Stokes, Pekelsky IF, Moreland, M S Surf Topogr Spinal Deform IV. Stuttgart, New York: Gustav-Fisher; 1987. pp. 163-169

[8] Carr AJ, Jefferson RJ, Turner-Smith AR, Beavis A. An analysis of normal back shape measured by ISIS scanning. Spine (Phila, Pa 1976). 1991;**16**(6):656-659

[9] Sahrmann SA. Does postural assessment contribute to patient care? Journal of Orthopaedic & Sports Physical Therapy, Inc. JOSPT 2002;**32**(8):376-379

[10] Kawchuk G, McArthur R. Scoliosis quantification: An overview. The Journal of the Canadian Chiropractic Association. 1997;**41**(3):137

[11] Warren JG, Bettany-Saltikov JA, van Schaik P, Papastefanou SL. Evidence-based postural assessment for use in therapy and rehabilitation. International Journal of Therapy and Rehabilitation. 2005;**12**(12):527-532

[12] Warren JG, Bettany-Saltikov JA, Van Schaik P, Papastefanou SL. 3-D measurement of posture and back shape using a low cost, portable system—A reliability study. Studies in Health Technology and Informatics. 2002; Jan 1:100-104

[13] Immersion Corporation (online) Microscribe digitizer [Internet]. 2005. [cited 24 Nov 2008]. Available from: http://www.immersion.com/digitizer/docs/MSG2_0704_V1.pdf

[14] McAlpine RT, Bettany-Saltikov JA, Warren JG. Computerized back postural assessment in physiotherapy practice: Intra-rater and inter-rater reliability of the MIDAS system. Journal of Back and Musculoskeletal Rehabilitation[Internet]. Jan 2009 [cited 23 Feb 2012];**22**(3):173-178. Available from: http://www.ncbi.nlm.nih.gov/pubmed/20023347

[15] McEvoy MP, Grimmer K. Reliability of upright posture measurements in primary school children. BMC Musculoskeletal Disorders. 2005;**6**(1):35

[16] Fortin C, Feldman DE, Cheriet F, Gravel D, Gauthier F, Labelle H. Reliability of a quantitative clinical posture assessment tool among persons with idiopathic scoliosis. Physiotherapy [Internet]. Mar 2012 [cited 16 Mar 2012];**98**(1):64-75. Available from: http://www.ncbi.nlm.nih.gov/pubmed/22265387

[17] Van Schaik P, Bettany-Saltikov Ja, Warren JG. Clinical acceptance of a low-cost portable system for postural assessment. Behaviour & Information Technology [Internet]. Jan 2002 [cited 23 Feb 2012];**21**(1):47-57. Available from: http://www.tandfonline.com/doi/abs/10.1080/01449290110107236

[18] Cobb D. Controllability, observability, and duality in singular systems. IEEE Transactions on Automatic Control. 1984;**29**(12):1076-1082

[19] Scutt ND, Dangerfield PH, Dorgan JC. The relationship between surface and radiological deformity in adolescent idiopathic scoliosis: Effect of change in body position. European Spine Journal. 1996;**5**(2):85-90

[20] Posture Score Sheet Orthopedic Assessment and Treatment of the Geriatric Patient. Reedco, Mosby, St Louis. 1974

[21] Milanesi JM, Borin G, Corrêa ECR, da Silva AMT, Bortoluzzi DC, Souza JA. Impact of the mouth breathing occurred during childhood in the adult age: Biophotogrammetric postural analysis. International Journal of Pediatric Otorhinolaryngology. 2011;**75**(8): 999-1004

[22] Fidler C, Turner-Smith AR, Gant CA. Repeatability of ISIS analysis in normal subjects. Annual Report of Oxford Orthopaedic Engineering Centre. 1984;**11**:45-48

[23] Schroder J. Posture analysis: Variations and reliability of biomechnical parameters in bepedal standing by means of Formetric-system. In: 14th Annual Congress of the European College of Sports Science, Oslo. 2009

[24] Lason G, Peeters L, Vandenberghe K, Byttebier G, Comhaire F. Reassessing the accuracy and reproducibility of diers formetric measurements in healthy volunteers. International Journal of Osteopathic Medicine. 2015;**18**(4):247-254

[25] Berryman F, Pynsent P, Fairbank J, Disney S. A new system for measuring three-dimensional back shape in scoliosis. European Spine Journal [Internet]. May 2008 [cited 20 jul 2011];**17**(5):663-672. Available from: http://www.pubmedcentral.nih.gov/articlerender.fcgi?artid=2367415&tool=pmcentrez&rendertype=abstract

[26] Bettany-Saltikov, Josette, Forbes H, Edgar, Michael, Harrison D. The ISIS experience at the Royal national orthopaedic hospital. In: Alberti, Drerup, Hierholzer, editor. Surface Topography and Spinal Deformity. VI. 1992: pp. 70-75

[27] Betz RR. Kyphosis of the thoracic and thoracolumbar spine in the pediatric patient: Normal sagittal parameters and scope of the problem. Instructional Course Lectures. 2003;**53**:479-484

[28] Propst-Proctor SL, Bleck EE. Radiographic determination of lordosis and kyphosis in normal and scoliotic children. Journal of Pediatric Orthopaedics. 1983;**3**(3):344-346

[29] Stagnara P, De Mauroy JC, Dran G, Gonon GP, Costanzo G, Dimnet J, Pasquet A. Reciprocal angulation of vertebral bodies in a sagittal plane: Approach to references for the evaluation of kyphosis and lordosis. Spine (Phila Pa 1976). 1982;**7**(4):335-342

[30] Bernhardt M, Bridwell KH. Segmental analysis of the sagittal plane alignment of the normal thoracic and lumbar spines and thoracolumbar junction. Spine (Phila Pa 1976). 1989;**14**(7):717-721

5

Postural Restoration: A Tri-Planar Asymmetrical Framework for Understanding, Assessing, and Treating Scoliosis and Other Spinal Dysfunctions

Susan Henning, Lisa C. Mangino and Jean Massé

Abstract

Current medical practice does not recognize the influence of innate, physiological, human asymmetry on scoliosis and other postural disorders. Interventions meant to correct these conditions are commonly based on symmetrical models of appearance and do not take into account asymmetric organ weight distribution, asymmetries of respiratory mechanics, and dominant movement patterns that are reinforced in daily functional activities. A model of innate, human asymmetry derived from the theoretical framework of the Postural Restoration Institute® (PRI) explicitly describes the physiological, biomechanical, and respiratory components of human asymmetry. This model is important because it gives an accurate baseline for understanding predisposing factors for the development of postural disorders, which, without intervention, will likely progress to structural dysfunction. Clinical tests to evaluate tri-planar musculoskeletal relationships and function, developed by PRI, are based on this asymmetric model. These tests are valuable for assessing patient's status in the context of human asymmetry and in guiding appropriate exercise prescription and progression. Balancing musculoskeletal asymmetry is the aim of PRI treatment. Restoration of relative balance decreases pain, restores improved alignment, and strengthens appropriate muscle function. It can also halt the progression of dysfunction and improve respiration, quality of life, and appearance. PRI's extensive body of targeted exercise progressions are highly effective due to their basis in the tri-planar asymmetric human model.

Keywords: human physiological asymmetry, spinal disorders, scoliosis, neutral posture, right-side dominance, muscle chain activity, biomechanical model of scoliosis, sagittal plane dysfunction, hyper lumbar lordosis, scoliosis specific exercises, postural restoration, etiology of scoliosis, kyphosis, respiratory mechanics, postural disorders

1. Introduction

Recognition of inherent physiological asymmetry has not yet been applied to the understanding, assessment, or treatment of scoliosis or other spinal and postural disorders. Even without an accurate baseline model of human form and function, interventions to correct dysfunction can be successful; however, while a local dysfunction may be rectified, the underlying biomechanical imbalance will persist as will the musculoskeletal strategies developed to compensate for the imbalance.

The Postural Restoration Institute® (PRI) methodology is a theoretical framework, which describes a model of universal human anatomical and physiological asymmetry. This unique model provides a new baseline for understanding common postures, movement patterns, and respiratory mechanics, which generate from our asymmetrical bias. It also explains the factors that support human right-side dominance. While human asymmetry can be understood as a positive factor that facilitates movement, overuse or misuse of the dominant muscle pattern will promote progressive imbalance within the body and will likely result in dysfunction. The treatment goal for dysfunction resulting from musculoskeletal imbalance needs to be restoration of the baseline in which there is relative balance between the dominant and nondominant muscle patterns [1–4].

Scoliosis is an example of a tri-planar, biomechanical dysfunction. In its most common form (90% of the cases), right thoracic convexity and left lumbar convexity [5–7], it exemplifies the extreme progression of normal human asymmetry according to the PRI model, which will be described in this chapter. Other postural disorders such as kyphosis and lordosis, exhibiting primary sagittal plane dysfunction, also belong to the spectrum of disorders developing from unbalanced human asymmetry. These conditions result in musculoskeletal stress, subsequent structural damage, loss of efficiency in movement and in respiratory function, as well as in a diminished quality of life.

This chapter introduces the fundamental concepts of PRI's theoretical framework and its baseline model. It will then describe how PRI's clinical tests can more accurately evaluate a patient's status by taking into account the inherent human asymmetry. These tests guide exercise prescription and treatment progression. Some examples of exercises used in the treatment of scoliosis have been selected to demonstrate activity progression from supported target muscle isolation, to complex, unsupported, multiple muscle integration, all with a major emphasis on respiration. Three case studies are presented here to illustrate this process. Many similarities exist between PRI rehabilitation concepts and exercises and the well-known Schroth methodology [8, 9].

2. Fundamental PRI concepts

The following fundamental concepts provide a new perspective on effective restorative techniques for treating scoliosis, other spinal dysfunctions, and postural disorders. The concepts explain the PRI baseline model of innate human asymmetry. Each is discussed in detail in this chapter: (1) human asymmetry arises from our innate anatomy and physiology and exerts significant influence on human posture and movement. (2) Ideal or neutral posture results from relative musculoskeletal balance of our asymmetrically organized body. (3) Anatomical and physiological asymmetries evident in the respiratory system are powerful contributors to our biomechanical function. (4) Right-side dominance is the functional result of physiological asymmetry. (5) The movement of the respiratory diaphragm and the pelvic diaphragm (pelvic floor muscles) is synchronized during breathing. The pelvis is a primary structure that facilitates gait. The synergistic activity of these two diaphragms links respiration and gait. (6) Gait requires integrated muscle activity, different on two sides of the body, in order to stay erect on one leg as the other advances the body through space. In the context of human asymmetry, right-side stance phase and left-side swing phase will be most competent. (7) Biomechanical dysfunction begins in the sagittal plane.

2.1. Innate physiological human asymmetry

Studies of many aspects of human asymmetry abound in the literature [10–15]. Much of this fascinating material is beyond the scope of this chapter. However, asymmetries of the internal organization of the body, organ weight distribution, muscle mass, and muscle attachments are all factors that contribute significantly to human asymmetrical posture and movement patterns. For example, the heart and its vessels share the left upper quadrant with two lobes of the lung. The right upper quadrant is less full, housing three lung lobes. The weight of the heart is offset by the large, heavy liver, which sits—lower than the heart—in the right lower quadrant [14]. This weight distribution and placement difference facilitates a gravitational shift of the body onto the right lower extremity, thereby promoting right stance. The left lower quadrant is less weighty because of the small spleen and usually empty stomach [1–4] (see **Figure 1**).

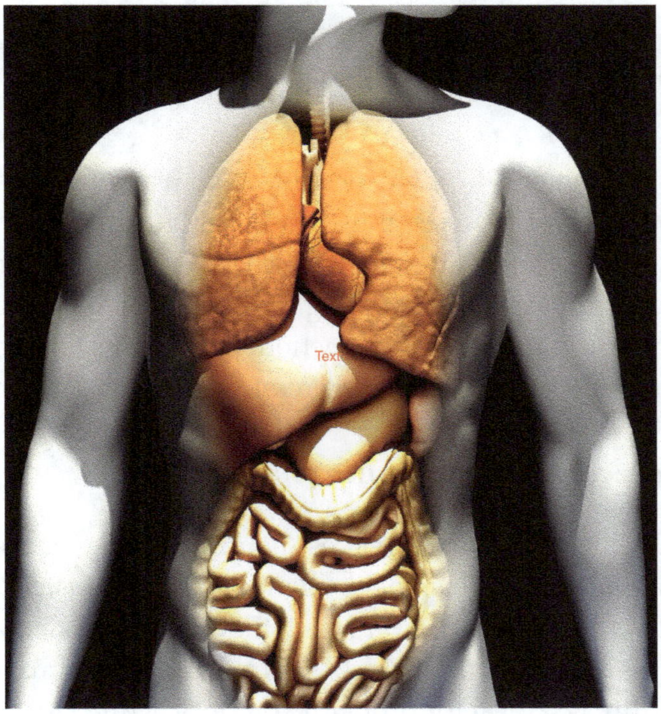

Figure 1. Asymmetrical organ distribution. Scottff72 copyright 123RF.com

The upper and lower quadrants are separated by the respiratory diaphragm, a unique muscle that spans the internal dimension of the body. The diaphragm is comprised of a stronger, larger, and better-supported right leaflet, and a smaller, less efficient, left leaflet. The diaphragm's respiratory mechanics exert a powerful asymmetrical influence on the torso. The crura of the right leaflet, which inserts onto three lumbar vertebrae L1–3, is also stronger and thicker than the left crura, which inserts on only two lumbar vertebrae L1, 2 [16] (see **Figure 2**). This distribution exerts a right rotational influence on the lumbar spine, orienting it to the right. Articulation of the lumbar spine with the sacrum orients the sacrum to the right. Strong ligaments bonding the sacrum to the pelvis effect right rotation of the pelvis as well. This right rotational orientation of the lower spine and pelvis is enhanced by the gravitational shift of the body over the right leg due to the weight of the liver on the right side of the body [1–4].

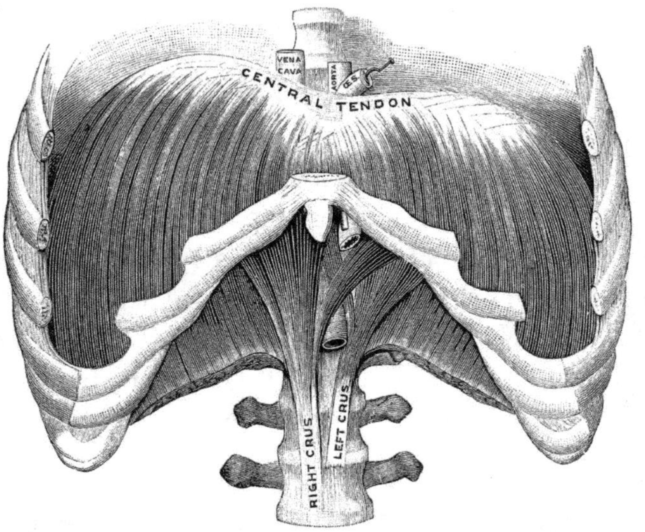

Figure 2. Diaphragm with crura. Florida Center for Instructional Technology copyright 2004–2017.

Asymmetry facilitates movement. In a balanced system, asymmetry is a positive, vitalizing force. In the human body, loss of balanced musculoskeletal function precipitates and reinforces overuse of dominant postures and patterns because of the underlying structural bias toward right stance, influenced by organ placement, weight distribution, and muscle attachment. Habit and repetition perpetuate and reinforce dysfunction. Innate physiological human asymmetry may well be a factor in the onset and development of scoliosis and other postural disorders.

2.2. Neutral posture reflects relative musculoskeletal balance

Webster's New World Medical Dictionary defines "neutral posture" as the stance that is attained when the "joints are not bent and the spine is aligned and not twisted" [17]. Neutral posture gives rise to the concept of "ideal posture" in which the alignment of body segments involves a minimal amount of stress and strain and which is conducive to maximal efficiency in use of the body [18, 19]. Ideal posture is critical for proper respiratory action [20]. When the body is in its ideal or neutral alignment, diaphragmatic respiratory mechanics are optimized [16].

Due to physiological asymmetry, a neutral posture does not imply strict symmetry; rather, it describes a position of relative structural balance and a readiness for movement in any direction. Loss of relative musculoskeletal balance reflects persistence of a structural bias resulting from habitual, repetitive muscle activity. For example, hyper lumbar lordosis is a frequently seen, sagittal plane, postural disorder. Positional alignment of the ribcage and pelvis has become imbalanced. The lumbar paraspinals have shortened and tightened, and the abdominal muscles have become overlengthened and weak [19, 21]. Neither of these muscle groups exists in their neutral or rest position. The neutral position of a muscle is equivalent to physiological rest [19]. With hyper lumbar lordosis, all future movements will initiate from this unbalanced basis of the skeleton (ribcage and pelvis) now supported and reinforced by adaptive muscle imbalance. Movement into any direction will require compensation by other muscles or will not be accomplished. Compensatory muscle activity is less efficient, energy demands increase, and stress accumulates on poorly aligned joints. Restoration of musculoskeletal balance would address these multiple issues [1–4].

Respiration is a key component of posture [22–27]. Our ability to breathe efficiently affects all aspects of our daily function and our endurance for activity. Through its anatomic attachments, the position and functional efficiency of the respiratory diaphragm is highly dependent on musculoskeletal posture as well as on tonic muscular activity [23]. The average person takes 21,000 breaths per day [28] with the respiratory diaphragm as a key muscle of respiration [22, 25]. Thus, the respiratory pattern is powerful in its contributions to posture. Efficient respiratory mechanics are dependent on neutral body position and muscle function [16].

When the diaphragm is compromised, it not only causes inefficient breathing patterns but also becomes a key contributor to the persistence and progression of postural disorders, including hyper lumbar lordosis, [29] kyphosis, forward head posture [20], and changes in ribcage symmetry [9, 16] as seen in scoliosis.

2.3. Asymmetries of respiration

The influence of the respiratory system is significant and often underlies or is complicit with scoliosis and other postural disorders. Understanding the mechanisms of breathing and how the loss of diaphragmatic competency can precipitate biomechanical dysfunction is not sufficiently appreciated in most current rehabilitation practices. Since the ability to exchange air is crucial to life, the respiratory system is a core motivator for muscle activity to insure adequate oxygenation. Within the respiratory system, the diaphragm is considered the primary muscle of respiration; however, there are numerous accessory muscles of respiration to assist when supplemental ventilation is needed. For instance, running places higher oxygen demands on the body to support a higher level of physical exertion. The accessory muscles of respiration are designed to accommodate such needs. Loss of diaphragmatic effectiveness due to postural or biomechanical dysfunction will result in pathological, compensatory accessory muscle recruitment [30].

The respiratory diaphragm is centrally located in our asymmetrically organized trunk. It is highly asymmetrical in form, in muscle attachment, and in function. Most importantly, it is uniquely positioned to directly influence every aspect of the postural, skeletal, and muscular core, and it influences the position and function of all other body systems [31]. The respiratory diaphragm is comprised of two muscles: a right and left hemidiaphragm [32], each with its own central tendon and each innervated by a right and left phrenic nerve, respectively [16].

Together, these two muscles span the internal dimension of the body just below the lungs. They insert on the xiphoid process, on the inner surfaces of ribs 7–12, and on the anterior aspect of the spine. The right leaflet is larger in diameter, it has a thicker and larger central tendon, its dome is higher, and it is better supported than the left by the liver beneath it and by strong right eccentric abdominal activity [31]. The right crura anchors to L1–3 on the right, the left crura to L1, 2 on the left [16]. The diaphragm leaflets also insert into the fascia overlying quadratus lumborum and to the psoas muscles via the arcuate ligaments, creating a strong functional linkage between these muscles. The superior strength, position, and function of the right hemidiaphragm supports and is supported by the physiological right orientation via right stance [1–4] (see **Figure 3A**).

The respiratory "Zone of Apposition" (ZOA) is the region of interface between the hemidiaphragm and the inner surface of ribs 7–12 [16, 33]. Apposition refers to multiple layers of muscles with differing fiber orientation lying adjacent to one another. The ZOA facilitates inhalation by generating tension between the muscle layers, which promotes external rotation of the ribs, complementing the action of the external intercostals. As the central tendons contract and descend, the hemidiaphragms displace caudally while the ribcage expands and externally rotates. The ZOA diminishes in volume with this activity. Simultaneously, the abdominal viscera are displaced caudally enabling lung expansion [16, 33] (see **Figure 3B**). Exhalation reverses this process. Shortening of the internal intercostals and of the lateral abdominal musculature reduces ribcage dimension. The hemidiaphragms relax and recoil upward returning to their domed configurations. Then, in a position of potential energy, the hemidiaphragms are ready to piston down again, thereby creating a vacuum, which will draw air into the lungs. Additionally, the diminished volume of the pleural cavity aids in expelling depleted air from the lungs [16, 33] (see **Figure 3B**).

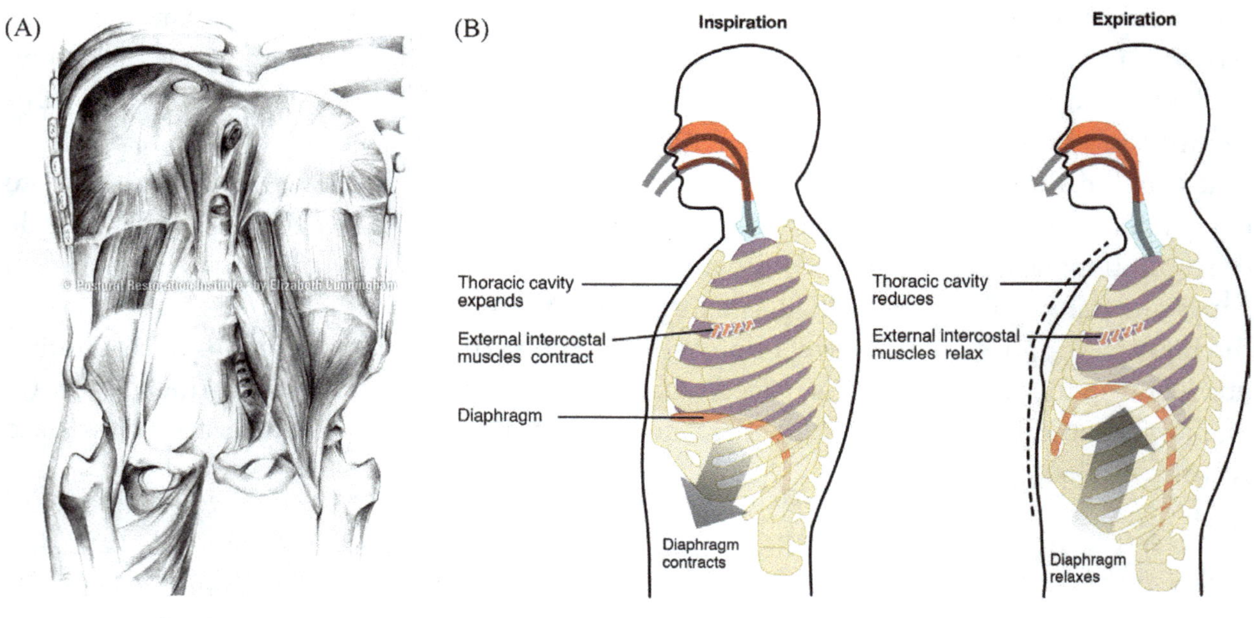

Figure 3. (A) Functional relationship of diaphragm, psoas, quadratus lumborum, and right stance illustration created by Elizabeth Noble for the PRI copyright. Used with permission from the PRI. Copyright 2017, www.posturalrestoration.com. (B) Respiratory mechanics of inspiration and expiration. www.wikimedia.org

Application of these respiratory mechanics to the biomechanical model of innate human asymmetry gives a more realistic understanding of our functional baseline. The three layers of lateral abdominals: transverse abdominis, internal, and external obliques, taken together, insert cephalically on the costal cartilage of ribs 5–12 and caudally on the ipsilateral iliac crest. These lateral abdominal muscles link the ribcage and pelvis, and they are critical components of posture and respiration [25, 26]. As described previously, shifting of weight to the right leg and orientation of the lumbar spine and pelvis to the right result in anterior rotation of the left hemipelvis. When the left hemipelvis is chronically anteriorly rotated, these lateral abdominal fibers will be adaptively overlengthened and weak. (In some cases, the right hemipelvis will also rotate anteriorly to avoid the strain of this asymmetry, resulting in bilateral compensatory and pathologic anterior pelvic rotation). The weakened, lateral abdominal muscles cannot maintain balance between the anterior ribcage and the pelvis. Without the anchoring action of the lateral abdominals, the anterior ribcage migrates further into elevation and external rotation mimicking thoracic position on inhalation [1–4].

This positioning has consequences for respiratory mechanics. When the left ribcage is in a chronic state of inhalation (expanded ribcage), the diaphragm is obligatorily in its descended state of inhalation as well. This chronic positioning limits diaphragmatic ascension on exhalation, thereby reducing the left ZOA. Consequently, the diaphragm loses its effectiveness for inspiration. Additionally, as the left anterior ribcage elevates, the diaphragm's domed configuration decreases and its fibers take on a more flattened, diagonal orientation, elevated anteriorly, resulting in further loss of the left ZOA. In this altered state, when the diaphragm contracts, it pulls the lumbar spine forward and reinforces anterior ribcage elevation. Having lost efficiency as a respiratory muscle, the diaphragm now functions more as a postural extensor muscle promoting progressive lumbar lordosis [29] (see **Figure 4**). Left anterior ribcage flares are commonly seen clinically and are exaggerated in patients with scoliosis. These flares indicate hyperinflation of the left lung due to insufficiency of the left lateral abdominals.

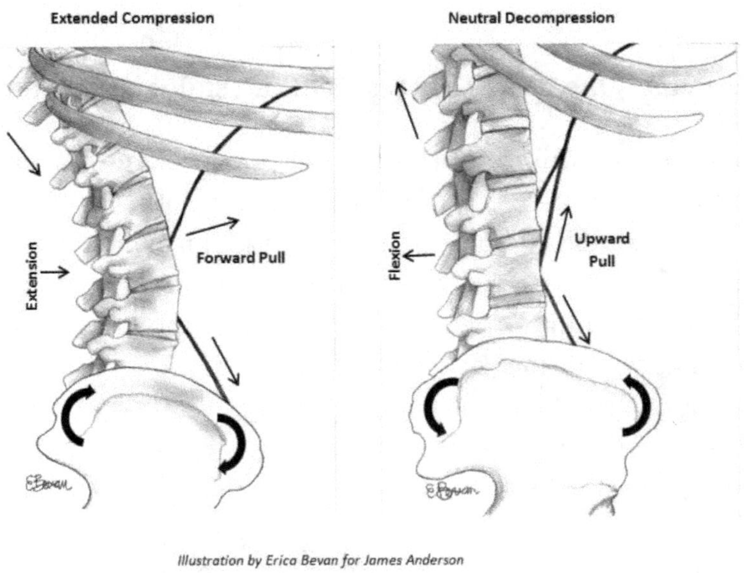

Figure 4. Positional consequences for respiratory mechanics. Illustration by Erica Bevin for James Anderson and the PRI. Copyright 2017 PRI®.

The right hemipelvis configuration is opposite relative to the left; it is posteriorly rotated. The right lateral abdominals are better positioned to exhale, but are more restrictive to inhale. Compensatory strategies to maximize breathing capacity in order to meet respiratory need will then rely on the accessory muscles of respiration, including the psoas, paraspinals, muscles of the upper back, chest, and anterior neck. With these compensatory changes in breathing mechanics, left anterior ribcage flares and right anterior ribcage restriction may progress along this diagonal trajectory, resulting in the common scoliosis pattern of right posterior ribcage prominence and left posterior ribcage concavity [1–4] (see **Figure 5A** and **B**).

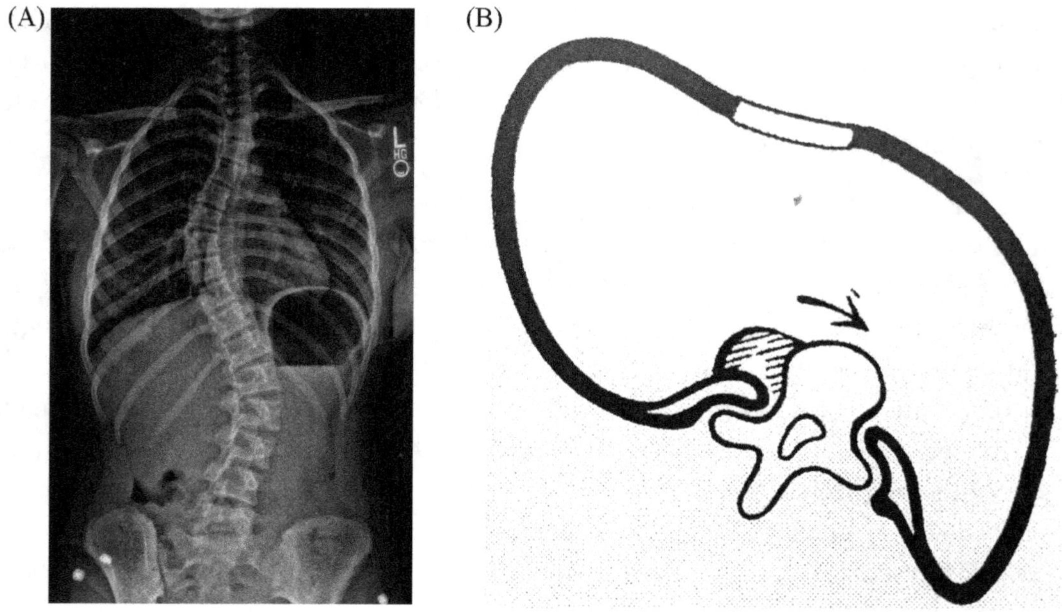

Figure 5. (A) EOS of common scoliosis pattern used with permission. (B) Common costal deformity in scoliosis used with permission from The Martindale Press, Three Dimensional Treatment for Scoliosis, 2007 by Lehnert-Schroth, C.

2.4. Right-side dominance, the functional result of physiological asymmetry

Humans almost universally exhibit right-dominant postural and movement patterns resulting from physiological asymmetry. Preferential standing on the right leg and increased breathing efficiency of the right hemidiaphragm are major contributors to this fundamental bias. Additionally, 90% of the population is right-handed, a defining characteristic of humans [11, 15]. Use of the right upper extremity for manipulative and reach activity dates far back in human history and has been correlated with early human brain asymmetrical development [11]. Right arm swing accompanies right stance phase of gait and coordinates with left leg swing-through. Right arm swing, consistent with right reach activity, promotes left trunk rotation to balance lumbar spine and pelvis right orientation, present in right unilateral stance. However, it is important to emphasize that handedness does not define side dominance [34]. Left-right asymmetry is a fundamental, ancient characteristic of animal development present in the earliest large multicellular organisms according to fossil records [14, 34]. Strong right-hand preference for manipulative and expressive tasks is thought to correspond to the emergence of language. These developments occurred with cerebral cortical lateralization at a much later date [11, 13, 35] and differ from inherent left-right organism asymmetry [34].

2.5. Synchronicity of respiration and gait

During breathing, the thoracic diaphragm and the pelvic diaphragm (pelvic floor muscles) function synergistically, linking gait and respiration [4, 36]. Internal obliques and transverse abdominis muscles are key participants in this process. Acting as a force couple, these lateral abdominals assist the hamstring's postural activity to maintain a neutral pelvis position as they simultaneously assist ribcage position and motion [25, 26, 31, 37]. Concurrently, lateral abdominal and hamstring lengths are determined by pelvic position due to their respective pelvic insertions.

When the thoracic diaphragm descends for inhalation, the abdominal muscles and the muscles of the pelvic floor *eccentrically* lengthen to allow for visceral displacement caudally [16]. As the abdominal muscles elongate, the ribcage expands and externally rotates, and the pelvic crest migrates forward into anterior rotation, abduction, and external rotation, while the ischial tuberosities approximate, allowing the pelvic floor to descend. The femur remains oriented anteriorly to keep the feet in a forward trajectory. Relative to the acetabulum, the femur is in an externally rotated *unlocked* position, described as "Acetabular Femoral External Rotation" (AFER), which facilitates the swing phase of gait [1–4] (see **Figure 6**).

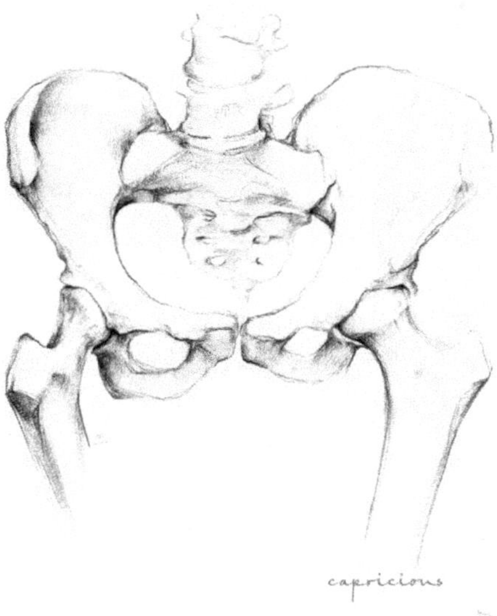

Figure 6. Frontal view of left AFER and right AFIR illustration created by Elizabeth Noble for the PRI copyright. Used with permission from the PRI®. Copyright 2017, www.posturalrestoration.com

Active exhalation relies on *concentric* activation of the internal obliques and transverse abdominis muscles to assist ribcage contraction, internal rotation, and thoracic diaphragmatic ascension. As the lateral abdominals shorten, they assist posterior rotation, adduction, and internal rotation of the pelvis. This pelvic position assists ascension of the pelvic floor as the ischial tuberosities move laterally as pelvic crests move medially [4, 25, 26]. The two diaphragms coordinate their pistoning activity, moving as a unit cephalically on exhalation and caudally on inhalation. While the pelvis rotates posteriorly with adduction and internal rotation, the stance leg maintains its forward orientation. The now internally rotated configuration of femur to acetabulum, described as "Acetabular Femoral Internal Rotation" (AFIR), *stabilizes* the hip joint (see **Figure 6**). Muscles of the hip—hamstrings, adductors, and gluteals—synchronize with lateral abdominals to stabilize the pelvis [1–4].

These functional relationships occur during gait. Gait is a highly complex movement task, which requires multisystem coordination and integration. Visual-vestibular, somatosensory, respiratory, and cardiovascular systems all give input and guidance [38]. Biomechanically, the challenge is to stay upright as the body advances through space balanced over one limb. When one side is in stance phase of gait, the contralateral side is in swing phase. The opposite arm and leg swing forward together (see **Figure 7**). This reciprocal extremity activity balances the torso around a vertical axis and assures nonstressful upright balance. In stance phase, the pelvis and lumbar spine are rotated toward the stance leg. The trunk is rotated opposite to the stance leg at or above the upper aspect of the diaphragm and is side bent ipsilaterally due to ipsilateral forward arm swing and ribcage kinematics [39]. This configuration mechanically supports shortening of the stance leg side abdominals, further assisting ribcage contraction and diaphragmatic ascension. Efficient gait requires the right and left sides of the body to be relatively equally competent in both stance and swing phases of gait. Gait is the best measure of balanced, biomechanical asymmetry [2].

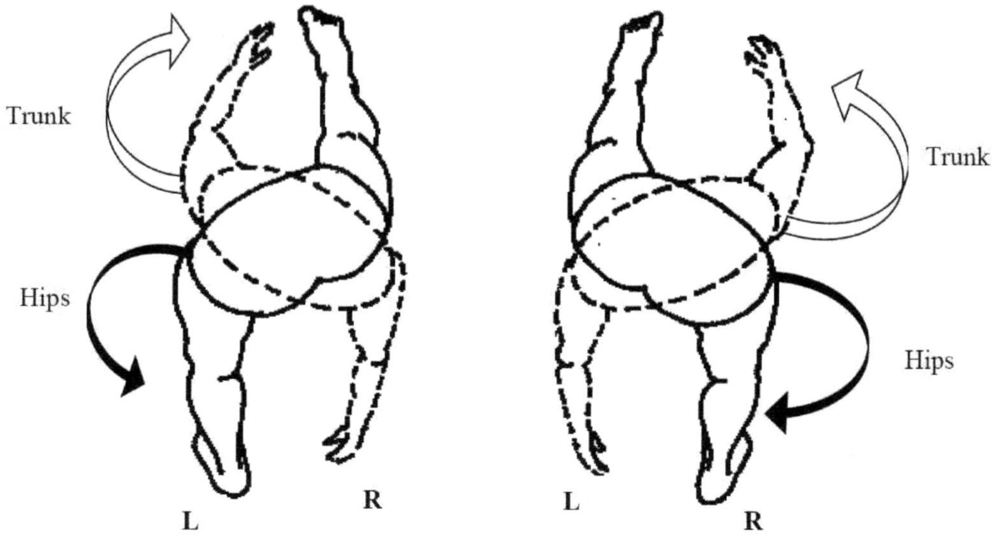

Figure 7. Alternating reciprocal gait viewed from above used with permission from the Postural Restoration Institute®. Copyright 2017, www.posturalrestoration.com

However, anatomical and physiological asymmetry biases the body toward greater competency in right stance. When musculoskeletal function is not relatively balanced, the left side does not achieve full stance phase of gait or full exhalation phase of respiration, and the right side will likely not achieve effective swing phase of gait or efficient inhalation phase of respiration. The daily repetitive nature of these basic activities of life reinforces and strengthens unbalanced asymmetrical function. Without intervention, the unequal stresses placed on musculoskeletal elements will likely progress to structural changes.

2.6. Muscle chain activity of the right-side dominant pattern

The development of muscle compensation follows a predictable pattern based on the model of human right-side dominance. Interventions to restore balance to a dysfunctional system will be maximally effective if the underlying baseline is understood and accounted for in the intervention. To this end, PRI describes muscle patterns based on a right-side dominant model. These patterns identify polyarticular muscle chains within the body, defined as a series of muscles, which overlap one another having fibers in the same direction and spanning multiple joints and thereby working synergistically together [2].

The anterior interior chain (AIC) governs the pelvis, lumbar spine, and lower extremities (see **Figure 8A**). It is so named because it is comprised of muscles located anterior to the spine and situated within the abdominal cavity. Muscles of the AIC are active during swing phase of gait (see **Figure 8B**). Swing phase of gait corresponds to the left nondominant muscle bias. The left-side pattern is, therefore, exemplified by the body's configuration during swing phase of gait.

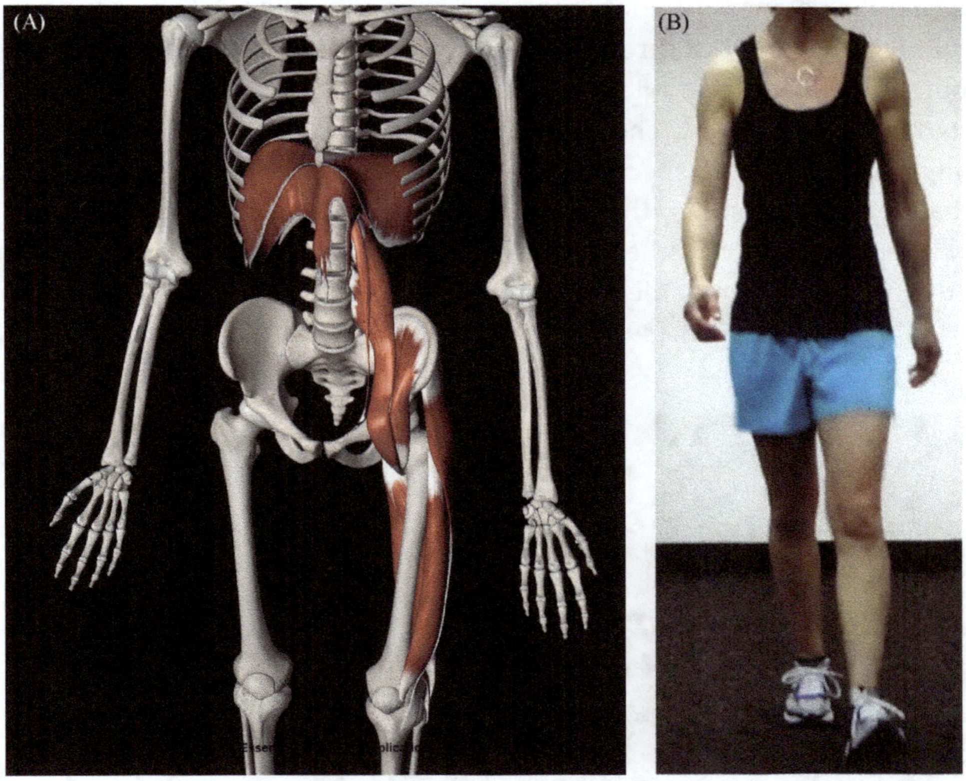

Figure 8. (A) Muscles of the left anterior interior chain. Copyright—3D4 medical modified with permission by the Postural Restoration Institute®. (B) Left anterior, interior chain in left swing phase of gait.

The biomechanical elements are already familiar from earlier description: the lumbar spine, sacrum, and pelvis orient to the right. The left hemipelvis rotates anteriorly, abducts and externally rotates, facilitating muscles that promote left swing through. These AIC muscles include the left diaphragm, the left psoas major, the left iliacus, the left tensor fasciae latae, the left biceps femoris, and the left vastus lateralis. Simultaneously, the left anterior ribcage elevates and externally rotates as the left diaphragm flattens into an inhalation position. The left lumbar spine is pulled forward and downward by the psoas and forward and upward by the diaphragm, resulting in increased lumbar lordosis [3] (see **Figure 4**).

This is the normal swing through configuration. However, when body neutrality is lost, the left AIC pattern remains tonically active. Persistence of the left swing through pattern interferes with full recruitment of its opposite, the muscles of left stance [31]. Consequently, left stance performance is weakened and less stable. Left AIC patterning thereby reinforces right-side dominance that is neurologically encoded as the new normal posture. Biomechanical strategies to compensate for this maladaptive left stance phase often involve overuse of the right lower extremity and/or malpositioning and stress of the left lower extremity joints. The right AIC muscle chain is not constrained by underlying positional insufficiency, and it supports right stance well. However, the efficiency of right swing through may be limited due to left-side instability during left stance as well as due to persistent overactivity of the right adductors and lateral abdominals.

The upper trunk muscle chain described by PRI is named the "Brachial Chain" (BC) (see **Figure 9A**). The BC balances rotational forces generated by the AIC by counterrotating the spine and ribcage to a forward direction. A right BC pattern complements the left AIC pattern by promoting left thoracic rotation (see **Figure 9B**). Counterrotation takes place in the approximate region of T7–9 [1]. The respiratory diaphragm inserts on the inner surfaces of ribs T7–12 and to the anterior aspect of vertebrae L1–3 on the right and L1,2 on the left. In its normal, exhalatory rest position, the dome of the diaphragm is at about T8. Therefore, the trunk could be considered to be the portion of the torso above the diaphragm. This counterrotation of the trunk is accompanied by ipsilateral side bend due to ipsilateral forward arm swing and to ribcage kinematics [39].

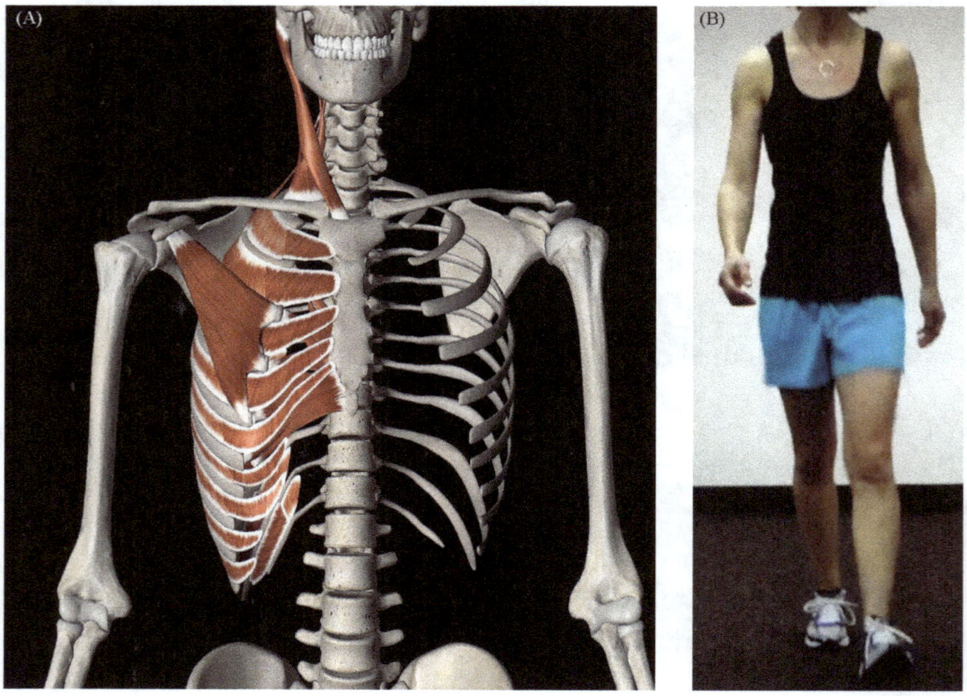

Figure 9. (A) Muscle of the right brachial chain. Copyright—3D4 medical modified with permission by the Postural Restoration Institute®. (B) Right brachial chain in left swing phase of gait.

Right arm reach is facilitated by this configuration. As the mid and upper trunk turn leftward, opposite to the right rotation of the lumbar spine and pelvis, ribcage kinematics re-form the shape of the ribcage and its muscular attachments. Left trunk rotation results in right ribcage approximation and internal rotation, and left ribcage expansion and external rotation [39]. This configuration encourages airflow from inhalation to the already-expanded left ribcage and lung while decreasing airflow to the right internally rotated approximated side. Muscles of the BC supporting right ribcage internal rotation include the right triangularis sterni, right sternocleidomastoid, right scalenes, right pectoralis minor and right intercostals, and also muscles of the right pharynx and anterior neck.

The "left AIC, right BC" pattern can be understood as the normal configuration of one half of the gait cycle, i.e., right stance. A *right* AIC, *left* BC pattern would reflect the other half of the gait cycle, i.e., left stance (see **Figure 10**). Human physiological asymmetry and right-side dominance predispose the body for greater right competency. Although left-side function will never be as efficient as the right, left stance can achieve near-equal stability with musculoskeletal balance or body neutrality.

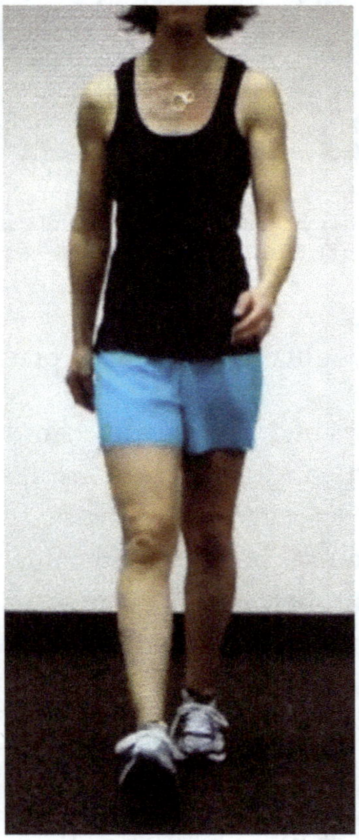

Figure 10. Right swing phase of gait illustrating the right anterior interior chain and left brachial chain.

This Left AIC, right BC pattern explains the biomechanics predisposing the development of a right thoracic, left lumbar spinal curvature, which describes 90% of curves [5–7] (see **Figure 11A**). The left AIC, right BC pattern underlies all human posture and movement (see **Figure 11B**). While different circumstances may result in different pathological compensations, generating a variety of stresses and/or structural changes, this innate human asymmetrical bias will be present [1–4].

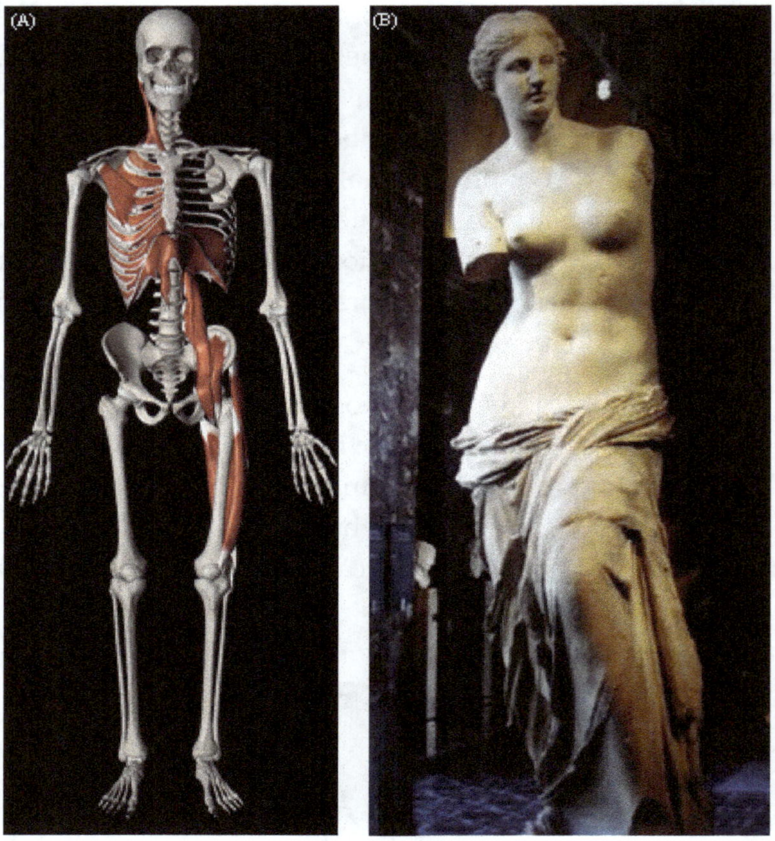

Figure 11. (A) Muscles of the left anterior interior chain and right brachial chain. Copyright—3D4 medical modified with permission by the Postural Restoration Institute®. (B) A classic example of a Left AIC, right BC pattern.

2.7. Biomechanical dysfunction begins in the sagittal plane

The sagittal alignment of the pelvis and ribcage affects muscle length and strength throughout the body. With any activity, the positional relationships of the structures and of the muscles that attach to them change. However, when the body is at rest, the ribcage and pelvis should be in a relative sagittal neutral position with muscle groups at their resting length. In an alternating reciprocal activity such as gait, there should be a moment of relative sagittal plane neutrality as weight shifts from one side to the other.

When this relative state of neutrality is no longer possible due to overactive right-dominant patterning, the left AIC, right BC pattern takes precedence. The left hemipelvis chronically positioned in swing phase of gait is anteriorly rotated. The spine balances this forward momentum with backward tilting as tonic, shortened paraspinal muscles take on the responsibility of keeping the spine erect. The left psoas and iliacus muscles adaptively shorten as the left transverse abdominis and internal oblique muscles are stretched between their insertions on the anterior lower ribs and the now more distal iliac crest. The left anterior ribcage flares, further weakening the overstretched left lateral abdominal muscles. With diminished opposition to left diaphragm recoil, because of lengthened abdominals and a loss of ZOA, the fibers of the left diaphragm orient more vertically, and the diaphragm assumes a greater role as a back extensor muscle than as a respiratory muscle. Its directional pull on the spine is forward and upward, while the psoas pulls the spine forward and downwards. The action of these two muscle groups encourages an exaggerated lumbar lordosis, reinforced by the lumbar paraspinals [16] (see **Figure 4**).

Exaggerated lordosis in the sagittal plane precedes a cascade of compensatory muscle and respiratory activity, as the brain encodes alternative strategies for continuing upright function. Further sagittal plane dysfunction follows, for example, the development of thoracic kyphosis to rebalance weight distribution over the pelvis. Another common strategy is the development of thoracic lordosis with reversal of the cervical spine to assist inhalation as cervical respiratory accessory muscle use increases to support the inefficient diaphragm position. According to the Hueter-Volkmann Law, epiphyseal bony growth is inhibited by compression and facilitated by tractioning [40]. In a young spine, exaggerated lordosis compressing the posterior vertebral segments would facilitate the development of relative anterior spinal overgrowth (RASO). This sagittal plane flattening of the thoracic kyphosis is an acknowledged precursor of scoliosis [41, 42].

Human physiological asymmetry expressed as right-side dominance via the left AIC, right BC pattern, demonstrates biomechanical challenges to maintaining neutrality of the pelvis and ribcage in the sagittal plane. Other factors contributing to loss of neutrality may include prolonged static positioning, especially sitting, hypermobility especially when participating in extreme sports or dance, and impaired somatosensory input. In the absence of pathology, right stance is a common default stance position. Respiration and gait will reinforce imbalance once neutrality is lost.

3. PRI tests to evaluate tri-planar musculoskeletal relationship and function

Taking into account the universal predisposition for human left AIC, right BC patterning, PRI tests accurately assess structural relationships such as sagittal plane position of the hemipelvis and ribcage and rotational orientation of the lumbar, thoracic, and cervical spines. Other palpatory tests reveal the patients' ability or inability to expand both apical lungs fields and both posterior mediastinal spaces. Initial testing exposes underlying patterning based on the left AIC, right BC model. Therefore, patients who exhibit typical findings for these patterns are not in a neutral state. It has to be understood that results from any further testing of range of motion, or strength, including core strength, would be based on their compensatory strategies. Deviation from predictable configuration implicates pathological compensation.

Neutral posture is defined by an alignment of body segments involving minimal amount of stress and strain and which is conducive to maximal efficiency in use of the body. It also optimizes diaphragmatic respiration. The neutral position of a muscle is equivalent to physiological rest [19]. This equates with musculoskeletal relative balance in a body, which is physiologically and functionally asymmetric. It is, therefore, imperative to first restore this neutrality. Once accomplished, further testing will give accurate information about weaknesses or restrictions in joints limiting appropriate frontal plane and transverse plane balance and function. Only with the restoration of musculoskeletal neutrality can appropriate, compensatory-free strengthening be initiated.

Over 25 PRI tests are available for initial assessment and to guide exercise progression as the patient progresses toward functional strength, respiratory competence, and upright alternating reciprocal activity. During treatment, the PRI tests are often applied before and after therapeutic exercise to determine its effectiveness, to reveal weakness or improvements in strength, and to further guide appropriate exercise progression. Three basic tests are described below.

3.1. The adduction drop test (ADT)

This is an example of a positional test for hemipelvic position in the sagittal plane. This side-lying test position facilitates a neutral hemipelvic position by flexing the hips and knees, thereby taking potential overstretch off the hamstring muscles. If the hemipelvis is in its neutral range, the ipsilateral femoral head will align with the acetabular groove allowing the femur to achieve full passive adduction as it is lowered by the clinician. If the hemipelvis is anteriorly rotated despite the test position of bent hips and knees, the femoral neck will impinge on the acetabular rim. The femur will not achieve full passive adduction (see **Figure 12**).

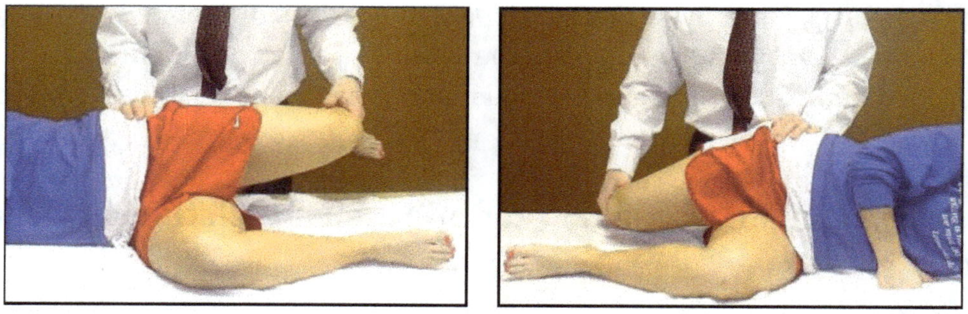

**Positive* *Negative*

Figure 12. Adduction drop test used with permission from the Postural Restoration Institute®. Copyright 2017, www.posturalrestoration.com

3.2. The humeral glenoid internal rotation test (HGIR)

This positional test assesses ribcage alignment. The posterior ribcage, as the foundation for the scapulae, determines scapular position and glenoid orientation, and therefore, humeral-glenoid mechanics. In the supine, bent knees test position, the humeral head is abducted to 90°, the elbow is flexed to 90°, and the forearm is pronated. Neutral alignment of the hemiribcage will allow full passive humeral internal rotation within the glenoid fossa. If the ribs of the anterior ribcage are internally rotated and the intercostals adaptively shortened, the apical chest wall will exhibit restriction and limited expansion with inhalation. The scapula is pulled forward by pectoralis minor and positioned in a state of upward rotation, abduction, internal rotation, and protraction. Consequently, the humeral head is now in external rotation relative to the glenoid fossa. Passive internal rotation of the humerus will result in impingement on the glenoid fossa and the range of motion will be limited (see **Figure 13**).

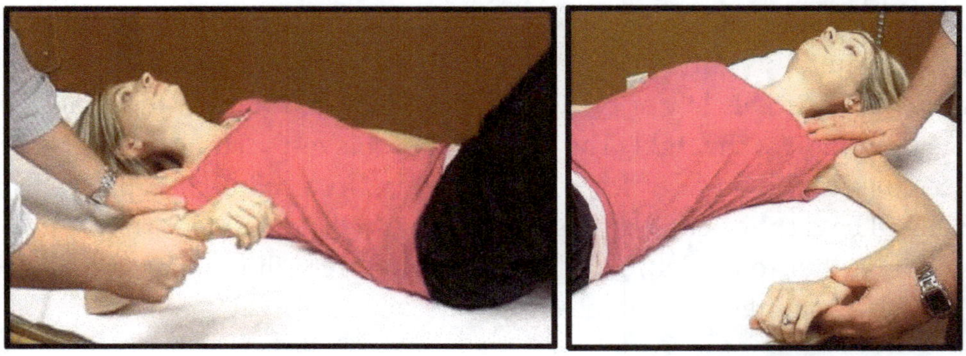

Positive Test *Negative Test*

Figure 13. Humeral glenoid internal rotation test used with permission from the Postural Restoration Institute®. Copyright 2017, www.posturalrestoration.com

3.3. Trunk rotation test (TRT)

This test assesses the integrity of the right iliolumbar ligament and the stability of the lumbopelvic junction. In patients with scoliosis, it is used to classify curve patterns. A "nonpathological" curve indicates this ligament is intact and the pelvis moves with the lumbar spine. A "pathological-compensatory" curve refers to an overstretching of the ligament, allowing the pelvis to move opposite to the lumbar spine and indicating laxity of this lumbopelvic stabilizing ligament. The nonpathological curvature is similar to the Schroth Barcelona[1] 3 curve or non 3-non 4; the pathological-compensatory curve is similar to the 4 curve or thoracolumbar curve. A positive TRT corresponds to countertilts identified by X-ray.

The test position is supine with knees bent and with ankles together. As the bent legs are passively rotated to one side, the clinician monitors the contralateral lower ribcage feeling for a movement of the ribcage away from the supporting surface. The beginning of ribcage movement indicates that the pelvis has reached its end of range and the spine is beginning to assist the rotation. Because the ribs articulate with the spine, the initiation of spinal rotation can be palpated. The range of motion is recorded and compared with motion to the other side (see **Figure 14**).

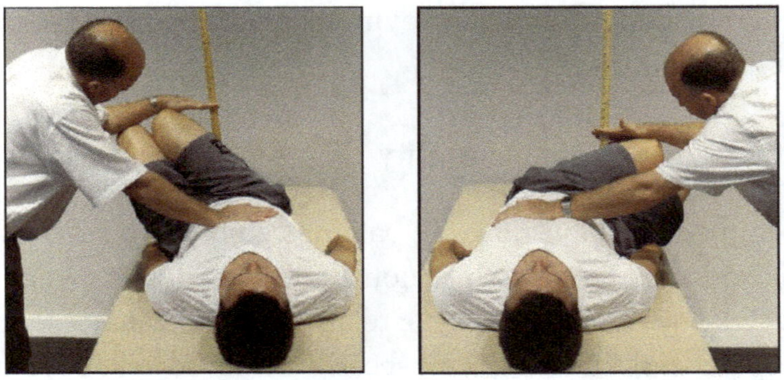

Right Trunk Rotation (limited) *Left Trunk Rotation*

Figure 14. Trunk rotation test used with permission from the Postural Restoration Institute®. Copyright 2017, www.posturalrestoration.com

[1]C2 certified.

Findings from this test must be correlated with the ADT for accurate assessment. If the ADT demonstrates a bilaterally neutral pelvic position, the rotational range to right and left should be equal. If the ADT reveals left or bilateral anterior pelvic rotation, the legs should have a greater range of motion to the right. The rationale for this test assumes a right-side dominant pattern unless the ADT demonstrates neutral balance. In a right-side dominant person, the lumbar spine will be right-oriented; therefore, the legs will appear to turn further to the right. If the legs move farther to the left, it indicates that the right iliolumbar ligament is compromised and does not maintain lumbopelvic stability.

These few examples give an idea of how the findings from PRI clinical tests correlate with one another to give an understanding of the patient's position and biomechanical function. These physiological details are otherwise hard to assess and factor into treatment protocols.

4. Exercise progressions for restoration of musculoskeletal balance

Exercises, termed "nonmanual techniques" in PRI, are powerful tools for proprioception and physiological transformation for patients with scoliosis of all ages. Based on the model of right-side dominance due to human asymmetry, and taking into consideration the patient's unique configuration and function revealed by the evaluation tests, exercises are carefully chosen to most appropriately meet the tri-planar needs of that patient. Some of the greatest similarities between the methodology of Schroth Barcelona and PRI are in the application of exercises. Both place emphasis on exercise position, breath, and stabilization in the corrected tri-planar position [8, 9].

Exercise progression begins in fully supported positions to isolate and recruit underused or misused muscles. Supported positions are also favored for the introduction of multimuscle integration. When the patient demonstrates competence in activating correct muscle chain activity while supported, challenge is intensified by progression to more upright activities. Repetition of challenging positions, held through multiple breathing cycles, promotes proprioceptive familiarity with new alignment and stabilization in new muscle patterns. Increased self-awareness and more precise muscle and breath control enable the patient to self-correct in activities of daily living. Achieving true alternating, reciprocal movement, as required in gait, is a final challenge.

4.1. Repositioning for sagittal plane neutrality

The PRI protocols begin with establishing the patient's ability to achieve sagittal plane neutral position of the pelvis and the ribcage. As previously described, this means that in a position of rest, their musculoskeletal system is in a state of relative muscle balance following a "repositioning" activity. Sagittal plane repositioning is most easily achieved in supported positions. Gravity is thereby eliminated and underused muscles can be positionally isolated and challenged.

Recruitment of the hamstring muscles is the most common starting point for repositioning exercises. The hamstring muscles insert proximally on the ischial tuberosity and distally on the medial tibial condyle and on the head of the fibula and the lateral tibial condyle. When the pelvis tilts anteriorly, the ischial tuberosity moves proximally and away from the tibia, resulting in overlengthening and weakening of the hamstring complex. Consequently, this powerful muscle group is unable to perform its postural function of stabilizing the pelvis, especially during stance phase of gait. Assessing ADT or another relevant test, prior to and following the activity, demonstrates whether that activity was helpful in restoring correct hamstring length and neutral pelvic alignment. If so, it is useful to ask the patient to stand and describe their body sensation to assure a definitive, proprioceptive experience of difference. Some patients, especially people with hypermobility, have difficulty noticing subtle differences. Others notice new sensations: "I feel lighter, taller, more weight on my heels."

The skill of sensing, i.e., the ability to focus attention on subtle sensations, is a potent tool for reshaping one's alignment from within. These sensations include awareness of the ground, of the body's orientation in space, internal structural relationship, and subtle changes in muscle tone. Most empowering is the ability to achieve expansion of targeted thoracic regions on inhalation.

4.2. Balancing the frontal plane

As the patient becomes stronger and more proficient at maintaining sagittal plane ribcage and pelvic alignment via hamstring and lateral abdominal integration, work begins on balancing muscles of the frontal plane. The pelvis and hips are key components. For example, in the stance phase of gait, the femur should be internally rotated relative to the acetabulum to insure stability. The right leg is typically better positioned to achieve stable stance. The pelvis is typically oriented right, positioning the right femur in stance and the left femur in swing phase of gait. Muscle chain activity supporting left stance is weak. Exercise progressions to recruit, strengthen, and integrate the left nondominant muscle chain are initiated. Target muscles to promote frontal plane balance include, but are not limited to the left adductor, the left anterior gluteus medius, the right gluteus maximus, and right serratus anterior.

Frontal plane exercise progressions often begin with sidelying to assist isolation, strengthening, and neural encoding of underused muscles. More upright positions challenge the patient's ability to maintain sagittal control with the addition of appropriate abduction and adduction movements. Exercise complexity and challenge increases as isolated muscles are integrated together in activities that require frontal plane muscle chain activity. Isolated left nondominant muscles are gradually integrated together in increasingly complex and challenging exercises in the frontal plane.

Muscle inhibition is another powerful technique utilized by PRI to rebalance patterned systems. Recruitment of an antagonist to an overactive muscle will neurologically inhibit that muscle's firing. Overactive and overused muscles are inhibited by the exercise position as well as by the action of the exercise.

4.3. Restoring the transverse plane (via the left zone of apposition)

As we see in right-side dominant posture and in almost every patient with scoliosis, irrespective of curve pattern, the left anterior ribcage is prominent and flared. The anterior left lateral abdominals are lengthened and weak, and the right abdominals are often restricted anteriorly. The left diaphragm is maintained in a position of inhalation. Activities to restore and to achieve greater left diaphragm respiratory effectiveness require a neutral pelvis and relative frontal plane balance. Mobilizing muscles to promote left anterior ribcage internal rotation targets left internal obliques and transverse abdominis. Right and left lower trapezius, left serratus anterior, and right subscapularis are important muscle chain agonists.

Retraining of alternate, reciprocal, upright gait is the ultimate goal. Balanced asymmetry in gait requires sagittal core strength to maintain neutrality of the pelvis and ribcage, with frontal plane competence to achieve *left* AFIR in stance phase and *right* AFER in swing phase, and the ability of the left diaphragm to fully exhale and the right to fully inhale. This exemplifies normalized function of the nondominant *right* AIC (see **Figure 10**). Although not all patients can achieve full-balanced asymmetry, especially in the presence of structural change, balancing triplanar muscle activity will enhance functionality, improve respiration, and in most cases, halt curve progression.

4.4. Examples of exercises

90-90 Hip Lift with Right Arm Reach and Balloon: This is one of the several versions of sagittal plane repositioning activities. In this activity, the patient is able to stabilize the pelvis in a neutral position, via bilateral, isometric hamstring activation, making it easier for many patients to achieve control. The addition of a balloon in any activity will promote active resistance to exhalation and concentric contraction of internal obliques and transverse abdominals. Right reaching in this activity further promotes left abdominal shortening and helps the patient to sense desired left posterior pelvic rotation (see **Figure 15**).

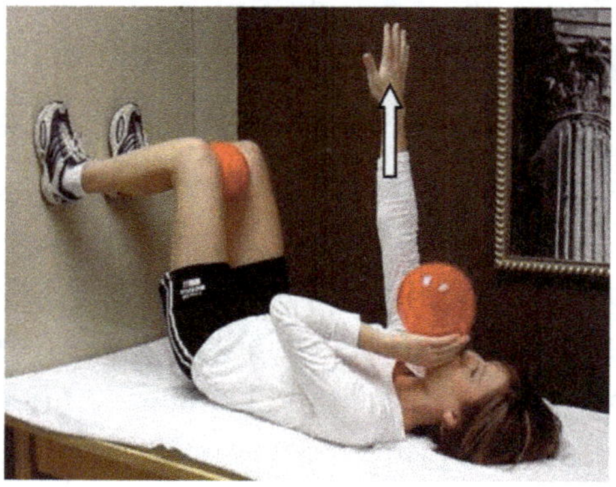

Figure 15. *90–90 hip lift with right arm reach and balloon* used with permission from the Postural Restoration Institute®. Copyright 2017, www.posturalrestoration.com

All Four Belly Lift Walk: This activity offers greater sensory awareness of position through 4 points of contact with the ground as well as movement against gravity. The patient is asked to "reach" during synchronized breathing with both hands and heels as they "walk" their feet forward, keeping knees bent. This promotes improved thoracic positioning through activation of internal obliques and transverse abdominals as well as diaphragmatic expansion and elongation of the thorax, while paraspinals are inhibited. Ankle dorsiflexion required for posterior weight shifting is an additional valuable component of this activity (see **Figure 16**).

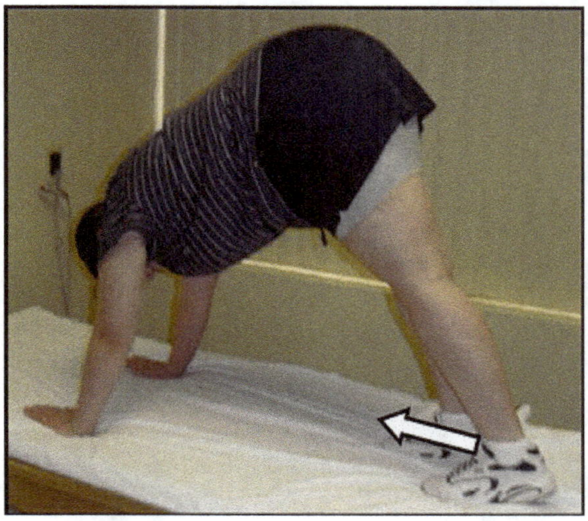

Figure 16. *All four belly lift walk* used with permission from the Postural Restoration Institute®. Copyright 2017, www.posturalrestoration.com

Left Sidelying, Left Flexed Femoral Acetabular Adduction with Right Lowered Extended Femoral Acetabular Abduction: This frontal plane sidelying exercise is a progression following the acquisition of sagittal plane neutral pelvic position. The sidelying position offers support and sensory reference to help the patient find and recruit the proper muscles. Activation of the left hip adductor helps to maintain sagittal plane neutral pelvic position. The left lateral abdominals are concomitantly activated with a right lower extremity reach to correct the left lumbar scoliosis in the frontal plane. The sidelying position offers gravitational resistance to right hip abduction, strengthening the right gluteus medius and maximus in the corrected position (see **Figure 17**).

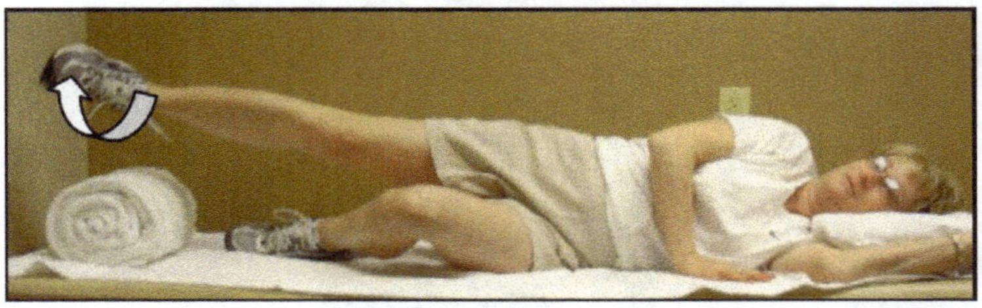

Figure 17. *Left sidelying, left flexed femoral acetabular adduction with right lowered extended femoral acetabular abduction* used with permission from the Postural Restoration Institute®. Copyright 2017, www.posturalrestoration.com

Right Sidelying Right Apical Expansion with Left Femoral Acetabular Internal Rotation (AFIR): A higher-level challenge for control of a right thoracic curvature is presented in this activity. The loaded right arm facilitates right scapular depression and retraction of the thoracic prominence toward the midline with beneficial elongation of the right lumbar spine. The left reach promotes right trunk rotation and left posterior mediastinal expansion. The pelvic position further encourages the corrective left lateral abdominals, left acetabular femoral adduction, and internal rotation (AFIR) with right acetabular femoral abduction and external rotation (AFER). Without sufficient right thoracic control, this activity can result in patients "dropping into" their thoracic curve, making this an advanced activity (see **Figure 18**).

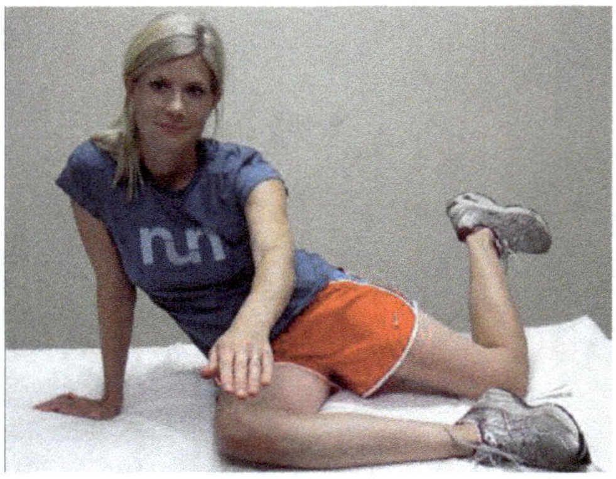

Figure 18. *Right Sidelying Right Apical Expansion with Left Femoral Acetabular Internal Rotation (AFIR)* used with permission from the Postural Restoration Institute®. Copyright 2017, www.posturalrestoration.com

Standing Supported Left Acetabular Femoral Internal Rotation (AFIR) with Right Femoral Acetabular Abduction: This frontal plane, upright, supported activity is a natural progression of a left sidelying program. For patients with left lumbar scoliosis, activation of left internal obliques and transverse abdominals creates a stabilizing triplanar force on the lumbar spine, a region clinically associated with instability in these patients. Frontal plane control of the pelvis is highlighted as the patient attempts to abduct their right leg and maintain triplanar pelvic corrections. Bringing this familiar frontal plane challenge to the upright position allows the patient to carry over sensations and control established in left sidelying to a more functional integration of postural correction (see **Figure 19**).

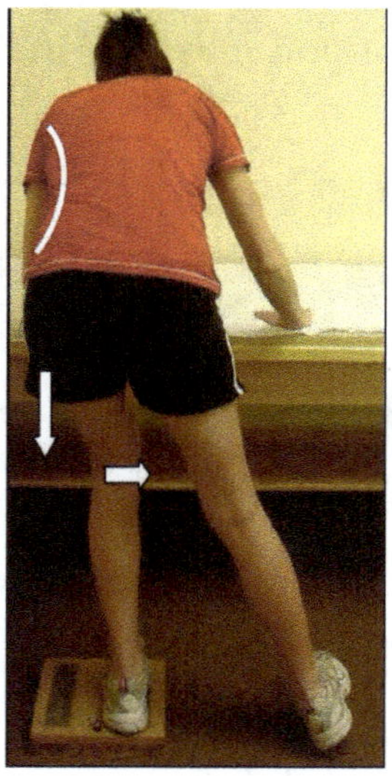

Figure 19. *Standing supported left acetabular femoral internal rotation (AFIR) with right femoral* used with permission from the Postural Restoration Institute®. Copyright 2017, www.posturalrestoration.com

Four Point Gait with Mediastinum Expansion: Efficient gait requires the pelvis to move over the stance limb with the trunk counterrotating. Patients with scoliosis are commonly challenged during left stance due to limited left pelvic rotation and right trunk counterrotation. The use of walking poles is an effective method to achieve "all 4" sensory awareness of the ground when upright. The patient is guided into a movement pattern for left pelvic orientation over the left stance limb as they simultaneously expand the left posterior mediastinum via left arm reach as they advance the left pole, promoting right trunk counterrotation (see **Figure 20**).

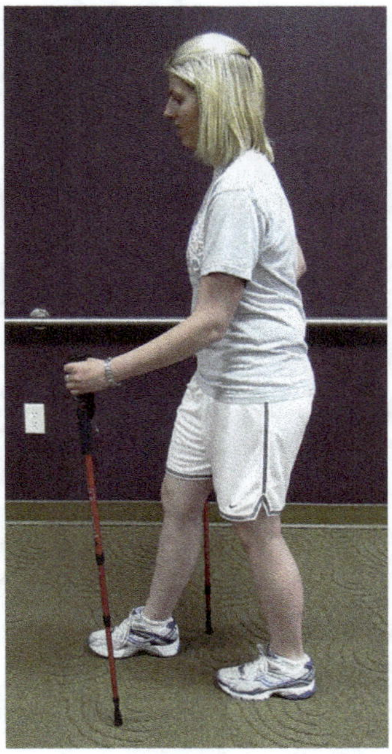

Figure 20. *Four-point gait with mediastinum expansion* used with permission from the Postural Restoration Institute®. Copyright 2017, www.posturalrestoration.com

Seated, Supported Left Acetabular Femoral Internal Rotation (AFIR) with Right Psoas and Iliacus and Right Femoral Acetabular External Rotation (AFER): In scoliosis, spinal compression is problematic because it increases spinal torsion. Sitting is likely the most common posture associated with increased spinal compression. Effective seated postural corrections are, therefore, an important skill requiring advanced, tri-planar control of the pelvis and thorax. This advanced, integrated activity positions the pelvis in left rotation with counterrotation of the thoracic spine into right trunk rotation. The lengthened right psoas is shortened and strengthened in its role as a hip flexor (see **Figure 21**).

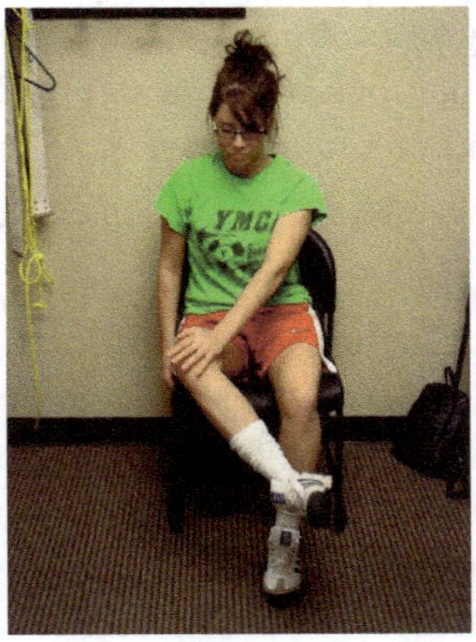

Figure 21. *Seated, supported left acetabular femoral internal rotation (AFIR) with right Psoas and iliacus and right femoral acetabular external rotation* (AFER) used with permission from the Postural Restoration Institute®. Copyright 2017, www.posturalrestoration.com

5. Case studies

5.1. Case 1

History: MD is a very active, extremely flexible, 9-year-old girl. She is passionate about ballet. She reports right hip pain and limited motion with some dance moves. Her shoulders occasionally "pop out of joint." Her mother reports numerous falls. MD was diagnosed with left thoracolumbar scoliosis at age 8, with a Cobb angle of 13°. Her doctor recommended to "wait and see." One year later, at age 9, the Cobb angle had increased to 27°. Again, her doctor recommended to "wait and see." MD's mother decided to seek conservative treatment.

Initial evaluation findings: Observation—general laxity, swayback, forward head posture, restless, constantly moving into different end-range extension positioning. Standing posture—stands on left leg, left knee hyperextension, left hip shifted to left, left pelvis positioned in swing phase (AFER), right knee bent, minimal right weight bearing. Unilateral stance—left leg 20 s, right leg 6 s. Bilateral stance (equal weight bearing)—10 s, then reverts to left stance. Forward bend—¼ range of motion, no lumbar reversal, states "my back will break." Seated hip rotation—internal: right 59°, left 45°, external: right 45°, left 45°. Spirometry (FEV)—average of three trials 1173 cc (age norm 1550 cc), weak exhale. Gait—extreme lumbar lordosis, bilateral Trendelenburg. Unable to maintain test position for ADT due to restlessness.

5.1.1. Clinical reasoning and treatment progression

MD being hypermobile demonstrated the common finding of decreased proprioception. In her physiological attempts to feel stable, she resorted to end-range positioning via hyperextension. In the sagittal plane, this lordotic posturing caused anterior pelvic rotation and anterior ribcage elevation. Chronic anterior ribcage elevation decreased diaphragmatic efficiency and resulted in the diaphragm acting as a postural extensor muscle. Due to chronic pelvic anterior rotation and overuse of her right leg, especially in dance class, right hip impingement developed. MD shifted off the right leg to avoid impingement pain. This became a strong pattern, and she could no longer maintain bilateral stance. To balance her left-sided shift, her spine migrated right. She remained in hyperextension.

Treatment began with a practice of bilateral and right stance. This was pain-free, but very challenging. *Sagittal plane*: repositioning was introduced at the second visit via the *All Four's Belly Lift Walk* (see **Figure 16**). This activity inhibited the tight paraspinals while shortening and strengthening lateral abdominals. Over the next few visits 90/90 *Hip Lift* activities were added to inhibit the paraspinal muscles in a supported position while isolating the hamstring muscles to establish pelvic neutrality. A balloon blow was added to 90/90 *Hip Lift* to increase recruitment of lateral abdominals while in a pelvic neutral position (see **Figure 15**). A sitting exercise with back supported, balloon blow, and left arm reach was added to challenge her in a more upright position. MD also practiced sitting in a chair blowing out through a straw to help her learn how to breathe diaphragmatically.

Frontal plane: Left AFIR was introduced with a hip hinge standing activity that simultaneously facilitated left posterior mediastinal (concavity) expansion.

The lateral spinal curve was eliminated in five physical therapy sessions of 1 hour each, over a 3-month period by addressing sagittal plane and respiratory dysfunction. MD's mother helped her with daily exercises. Due to her extreme hypermobility, MD is continuing physical therapy check-ins at 3–6-month intervals to maintain alignment, to stabilize, and strengthen her structure and to assure a neutral baseline. Scoliosis has not recurred. She continues her intensive ballet.

Summary: At age 9, when MD began PT, no spinal structural changes were evident, and there was no countertilt. However, her curve had progressed over a year, at Risser 0, from 13° to 27° with a rapid growth period ahead of her. Without intervention, structural change and curve progression were inevitable. This case highlights the importance of early detection and treatment. In the US, the current medical approach to juvenile and adolescent scoliosis is "wait and see." Once exaggerated curvatures in sagittal or frontal planes progress to structural change, rehabilitation is significantly more challenging and often less successful.

5.2. Case 2

History: RM is a 12-year-old female who was diagnosed with scoliosis at age 11. Her X-rays showed a right thoracic, left lumbar PRI nonpatho curve pattern, measuring 28° from T6–T12, and 21° curve from T12–L4. Her sagittal view film showed 52.4° of lumbar lordosis and 42° of thoracic kyphosis. She was told by her physician to "wait and see" and return 6 months later. New X-rays revealed progression to 38° from T6–T12 and 26° from T12–L4. She was still a Risser 0 and had not yet started menses. She was fitted for a Boston Brace, which she wore for 16–20 hours a day, for about 2½ years weaning to nights only at the beginning of her freshman year of high school and continuing. RM is an athlete playing basketball, tennis, and ultimate frisbee and more recently, doing yoga. She spends the summers at a 6-week sleep-away camp and travels internationally with her family.

Initial evaluation findings: Her starting height was 5′3″. It is speculated that she had a growth spurt from time of diagnosis over the 6-month period in which her curve progressed by roughly 10°. Standing posture—anterior pelvis, knee hyperextension left greater than right, the right medial border of scapula more prominent with the right scapula being rounded forward, protracted, and slightly elevated, her right hip is higher and shifted slightly to the right. In the sagittal view, her weight is shifted anteriorly toward her toes. Gait—arm swing was greater on the left than right, right shoulder is higher, and she lacks knee flexion at the loading response bilaterally. Her upper body stays stiff and her pelvis moves in the frontal plane more than in the transverse plane. Forward bend—visible left lumbar curve with slightly elevated right rib cage. Spirometry (FEV)—2200 cc, (age norm – 2150 cc.) Scoliometer—5° rotation to the right in mid-thoracic spine, 4° rotation to the left in mid-lumbar spine.

Clinical testing: PRI testing—*ADT* indicated left anterior hemipelvis rotation, right hemipelvis neutral position (see **Figure 12**). *HGIR* indicated bilateral ribcage elevation and external rotation, left greater than right (see **Figure 13**). *TRT*—knees go farther to the left, indicating suspected iliolumbar ligament laxity (see **Figure 14**). Both *Right Apical Chest Wall Expansion* and *Left Posterior Mediastinum (left thoracic concavity) Expansion* were limited. *Single limb stance for 60 s*—more stable in right stance, and trunk is more symmetrical in right stance than left stance. In left stance, her hip and pelvis are shifted anteriorly. Her favorite position is to stand on her right leg with her left leg crossed in front, her right hip out to the side with her right hand propping on her right hip. She was *pain-free*.

5.2.1. Treatment progression and clinical reasoning

Postural awareness and behavior changed during activities of daily living—she lightened her backpack and began to use a waist strap to redistribute weight to her pelvis from her spine. We encouraged her to sense her heels and improve standing posture. We incorporated spinal precautions (hip hinge instead of spinal flexion) due to relative anterior spinal overgrowth (RASO) and encouraged corrective postures for studying and lounging (i.e., avoiding prone on elbows and sitting in her curve pattern).

Sagittal plane: Supported supine activities to reposition pelvis were initiated by concomitant strengthening of hamstrings and lateral abdominals focusing on exhalation to bring her rib cage down anteriorly, restoring her respiratory zone of apposition. A left hip shift bias was used to help anchor her left femoral-pelvic position with her left lateral abdominals as in the *90/90 Hip Lift with Right Arm Reach and Balloon* (see **Figure 15**). Improved sagittal plane position was maintained throughout her program while addressing other planes of correction and progressing positional challenges against gravity.

Frontal plane: Exercises focusing on balancing left lumbar curve were implemented in left sidelying with a right leg reach, and by PRI left-side plank activities to lengthen her right lateral abdominals and shorten/strengthen the left. Her right thoracic curve was addressed with left sidelying activities to allow gravity to assist with centralization, as well as with positioning and muscle activation to direct air for right apical and left thoracic concavity expansion. Right upper extremity retraction/shoulder extension in external rotation was implemented to help activate her right low and middle trapezius to help reposition her right scapula toward the midline. Position was progressed from sidelying to sitting to standing. Examples of these PRI nonmanual techniques are *the Left Sidelying Left Flexed Femoral Acetabular Adduction with Right Lowered Extended Femoral Acetabular Abduction* (see **Figure 17**), and the *Standing Supported Left Acetabular Femoral Internal Rotation (AFIR) with Right Femoral Acetabular Abduction* (see **Figure 19**).

Transverse plane: Once the left respiratory zone of apposition was achieved to anchor left anterior rib flare, activities to strengthen right low trapezius and triceps were used to assist with thoracic spine derotation and rib cage balancing. Likewise, right iliacus and psoas were used for lumbar spine derotation in sitting and standing. The left serratus anterior and low trapezius were activated concomitantly to bring the left rib cage posteriorly (to expand the left thoracic concavity). Exercises were progressed from supine to seated to supported standing to freestanding, followed by the addition of resistance (dynamic stabilization) in standing for strengthening and maintenance of this correction.

Final Clinical Findings: Height—5′6 & 5/8″ (2½ years later, almost 4″ of growth), X-rays - right thoracic: T5–T12 = 35°, left lumbar: T12–L4 = 29.1°, Risser 4. Menses began summer of 2016. Her growth has stabilized, and we are hopeful to prevent progression requiring surgical correction/fixation. Spirometry (FEV)—2700 cc, which is age-appropriate. Single limb stance—more symmetrical and balanced on each leg with good observable pelvofemoral position bilaterally.

Summary: Working with teenagers can be challenging as well as rewarding due their very busy lives and neurodevelopmental immaturity to realize consequences. When trying to prevent curve progression, over a long period of time during growth, the process can become repetitive and laborious and it is easy for an adolescent to lose belief and/or motivation in the process. School and extracurricular activities can override exercise programs, especially if the patient has no pain. However, RM was diligent with her program and was able to implement concepts of correction and to perform challenging exercises while away at summer camp. Her case is an excellent example of the possibility to hold a curve that began to rapidly progress (10° in 6 months), with a starting point >25°, during a period of growth. She was able to avoid the need for surgical correction and now has a "tool bag" of exercises and positions she can use to thwart potential discomfort, as well as to maintain balanced asymmetry, throughout her lifetime. At recent follow-up, she proudly offered that she has less pain than her peers and teammates following exercise classes and games "because I now know how to take care of my spine!"

5.3. Case 3

History: JP is a 66-year-old female with primary complaint of loss of upright function for the past 10 years due to debilitating left leg sciatica. JP was able to stand and/or walk for only 10 min at a time, and this was greatly affecting her ability to participate in her choir practice and in her ability to play actively with her grandson. The patient was diagnosed with scoliosis as a teenager but was not offered any intervention. X-rays reveal right thoracic convexity between T2 and T11 (apex T8) with a Cobb angle of 26°. There is a larger, left lumbar convexity between T11 and L4 (apex L2) with a Cobb angle of 51° and clear evidence of rotary instability with moderate lateral listhesis of L4 on L5.

5.3.1. Initial evaluation findings

Standing posture—anterior translation of the pelvis. There is a notable, fixed left thoracolumbar kyphosis deformity and an associated left trunk imbalance with a right pelvic orientation in the frontal and transverse planes. JP is noted to have a flat thoracic spine and anterior rib flares bilaterally. Gait—elevated thorax with no appreciable right arm swing, the pelvis remains right-oriented throughout right and left stance phases. Clinical tests—*ADT* (see **Figure 12**) reveals the right hemipelvis is in neutral position and the left hemipelvis in anterior rotation. *HGIR* (see **Figure 13**) reveals restriction of right glenoid-humeral internal rotation due to restrictions of right apical chest expansion with elevation and external rotation of the left anterior ribcage. Palpation reveals limited expansion for both the right *Apical Chest Expansion Test* and the left *Posterior Mediastinum Expansion* Test. Spirometry (FEV) measures were 2100 cc, 1800 cc, and 1800 cc, respectively, over three trials consistent with hyperinflation and likely reduced FEV for age and gender (norms for 65-year-old woman, 2160 cc). *Functional outcome measure*—Roland

Morris Self-Report Low Back Pain Disability Questionnaire (RMDQ) was 9/24 or 37.5% self-report disability.

5.3.2. Treatment progression and clinical reasoning

Sagittal: Treatment began with sagittal plane control of pelvis and thorax to improve critical respiratory core muscle control. JP started in hooklying and supine 90–90 postures to begin activities like supine 90–90 with balloon blowing versions (see **Figure 15**). Once postural testing indicated adequate sagittal plane control, she moved to a left sidelying program.

Frontal: For this patient, the left sidelying position was felt to be best to help her begin to control frontal and transverse plane forces particularly in the region of her left lower lumbar spine, which were the most likely source of her debilitating sciatica. As JP gained control of the left abdominal wall in left sidelying and to obtain a ZOA, she began to integrate that control with combined muscular efforts culminating in left acetabular femoral internal rotation as with *Left Sidelying Left Flexed Femoral Acetabular Adduction with Right Lowered Extended Femoral Acetabular Abduction* (see **Figure 17**). JP was severely challenged with kinesthetic awareness of muscle activation and "carry over" to alternative postures. In her case, it was very helpful to have her stand up after a left sidelying activity to try to reproduce the same movement pattern in upright—her most challenging posture. Adding activities like *Standing Supported Left Acetabular Femoral Internal Rotation with Right Femoral Acetabular Abduction* (see **Figure 19**) were, therefore, quite a good challenge for improved upright control.

Transverse and alternating, reciprocating movement: As JP demonstrated further capacity for trunk control with left acetabular femoral internal rotation, we added challenges to coordinate with right trunk rotation as with gait. The use of walking poles was tremendously helpful for this patient to help with her balance, core muscle activation, kinesthetic sense of the ground and weight shifting, as well as to offer additional support for spinal elongation, a critical element in scoliosis treatment. Activities depicted like Four Point Gait with Mediastinal Expansion were further developed (see **Figure 20**).

Summary: Over the course of her last few visits (21 visits total), JP was consistently reporting dramatic and steady improvement in her function. She was playing with her grandson more than 2 hours at a time and able to stand through 3-hour choir rehearsals. Her walking progression was up to 34 min. The last RMDQ score was 3/24 or 12.5% self-report disability. All physical therapy goals were met. She was highly compliant and motivated throughout the course of her care, which no doubt, contributed to her strong outcomes.

6. Conclusion

The theoretical framework of PRI and its model of innate human asymmetry provides the clinician valuable insight into the development and progression of scoliosis and other spinal dysfunctions. This framework has the potential to redefine how clinicians evaluate and treat these conditions.

It is our experience that early detection and treatment of scoliosis and other postural disorders makes a significant difference to the success of intervention. For instance, a functional disorder resulting from an asymmetrical dominant pattern can more easily be rebalanced than one that has evolved into structural pathology. In the US, the medical approach to juvenile and adolescent scoliosis is commonly "wait and see." The PRI model recommends simple tests of balance and respiration in young people to identify those at risk. Early introduction of exercises to reestablish balanced asymmetry may effectively reduce the need for long-term rehab or surgery.

Patients of all ages and magnitude of spinal deformity can benefit from the PRI approach. Reestablishing neutrality, learning to balance tri-planar muscle activity, and optimizing respiration are among the life-long benefits of working on these exercises. Self-awareness engendered in this process is additionally empowering for many patients.

Clinical results of the application of PRI methodology have been compelling. We would like to encourage research on the many aspects of this new, innovative framework.

Acknowledgement

We are grateful to Ron Hruska MPA, PT, executive director of the Postural Restoration Institute, who formulated these concepts, developed this framework and continues to share his evolving insights.

Author details

Susan Henning*, Lisa C. Mangino and Jean Massé

*Address all correspondence to: myadvancephysicaltherapy@gmail.com

Advance Physical Therapy, Chapel Hill, NC, USA

PRI certified and Schroth Barcelona certified

References

[1] Hruska R, Anderson J. Postural Respiration: An Integrated Approach to Treatment of Patterened Thoraco-Abdominal Pathomechanics. Chapel Hill, NC: Advance Physical Therapy; 2013

[2] Hruska R, et al. Postural Restoration Institute® Advanced Intergration. Lincoln, Nebraska; 2016

[3] Hruska R, Cantrell M. Myokinematic Restoration: An Integrated Approach to Treatment of Patterned Lumbo-Pelvic-Femoral Pathomechanics. Chapel Hill, NC: Advance Physical Therapy; 2012

[4] Hruska R, Poulin J. Pelvis Restoration: An Integrated Approach to Treatment of Patterned Pubo-Sacral Pathomechanics. Cary, NC: STEPS for Recovery; 2014

[5] Figueiredo UM, James JIP. Juvenile Idiopathic Scoliosis. The Journal of Bone and Joint Surgery. 1981;**63-B**(1):61-66

[6] Ramirez N, Johnston CE, Browne RH. The Prevelance of Back Pain in Children Who Have Idiopathic Scoliosis. The Journal of Bone and Joint Surgery. 1997;**79-A**(3):364-368

[7] Wynne-Davies R. Familial (idiopathic) scoliosis. The Journal of Bone and Joint Surgery. 1968;**50-B**(1):24-30

[8] Henning S. The influence of position and breath in treatment of curvature of the spine utilizing postural restoration and Schroth methodologies. Postural Restoration Institute® Interdisciplinary Integration. Lincoln, NE; 2014

[9] Lehnert-Schroth C. Three-Dimensional Treatment for Scoliosis: A Physiotherapeutic Method for Deformities of the Spine. Martindale Press; 2000

[10] Auerbach BM, Ruff CB. Limb bone bilateral asymmetry: Variability and commonality among modern humans. Journal of Human Evolution. 2006;**50**(2):203-218

[11] Cashmore L, Uomini N, Chapelain A. The evolution of handedness in humans and great apes: A review and current issues. Journal of Anthropological Sciences. 2008;**86**:7-35

[12] Pope RE. The common compensatory pattern: Its origin and relationship to the postural model. American Academic Osteopathic Journal. 2003;**14**(4):19-40

[13] Previc FH. A general theory concerning the prenatal origins of cerebral lateralization in humans. Psychological Review. 1991;**98**(3):299-334

[14] Wolpert L. Development of the asymmetric human. European Review. 2005;**13**(2):97-103

[15] Zaidi ZF. Body asymmetries: Incidence, etiology, and clinical implications. Australian Journal of Basic and Applied Sciences. 2011;**59**(9):2157-2191

[16] Boyle KL, Olinick J, Lewis C. The value of blowing up a balloon. North American Journal of Sports Physical Therapy. 2010;**5**(3):179-188

[17] Shiel W. Webster's New World Medical Dictionary. Wiley Publishing, Inc; Hoboken, NJ. 2008

[18] Danis CG, et al. Relationship bewteen standing posture and stability. Physical Therapy. 1998;502-517

[19] Kendall FP, Kendall McCreary E, Provance PG. Muscles Testing and Function. 4th ed. Baltimore: Williams and Wilkins; 1993;**78**

[20] CliftonSmith T, Rowley J. Breathing pattern disorders and physiotherapy: Inspiration for our profession. Physical Therapy Reviews. 2011;**16**(1):75-86

[21] Sahrmann S. Diagnosis and Treatment of Movement Impairment Syndromes. In: White K, editor. St. Louis: Mosby, Inc; 2002

[22] Newton A. New conceptions of breathing anatomy and biomechanics. Part II. Rolf Lines. 1998;29-37

[23] Newton A. Breathing in the gravity field. Part I. Rolf Lines. 1997;27-33

[24] Newton A. Posture and gravity. Part III. Rolf Lines. 1998;35-38

[25] Hodges PW, et al. Contraction of the human diaphragm during rapid postural adjustments. Journal of Physiology. 1997;**505**(2):539-548

[26] Hodges PW, Heijnen I, Gandevia SC. Postural activity of the diaphragm is reduced in humans when respiratory demand increases. Journal of Physiology. 2001;**537**(3):999-1008

[27] Hodges PW, Gandevia S, Richardson CA. Contractions of specific abdominal muscles in postural tasks are affected by respiratory maneuvers. Journal of Applied Physiology. 1997;**83**(3):753-760

[28] Courtney R. The functions of breathing and its dysfunctions and their relationship. International Journal of Osteopathic Medicine. 2009;**12**:78-85

[29] Hodges PW, Richardson CA. Inefficient muscular stabilization of the lumbar spine associated with low back pain—A motor control evaluation of transversus abdominus. SPINE. 1996;**21**(22):2640-2650

[30] Lewitt K. Relation of faulty respiration to posture, with clinical implications. Journal of AOA. 1980;**79**(8):525-529

[31] Anderson J. PRI Integration for Baseball Restoring Reciprocal Performance in the Patterned Baseball Athlete. North Carolina State University; 2015

[32] Korin HW, et al. Respiratory kinematics of the upper abdominal organs: a quantitative study. Magnetic Resonance in Medicine. 1992;**23**(1):172-178

[33] Petroll W, Knight H, Rochester DF. Effect of lower rib cage expansion and diaphragm shortening on the zone of apposition. Journal of Applied Physiology. 1990;**68**(2):484-488

[34] Okumura T, Utsuno H, Kuroda J, Gittenberger E, Asami A, Matsuro K. The development and evolution of left-right asymmetry in invertebrates: Lessons from Drosophilia and snails. Developmental Dynamics. 2008;**237**(12):3497-3515

[35] Wright CVE. Mechanisms of left-right asymmetry: What's right and what's left? Developmental Cell. 2001;**1**:179-186

[36] Talasz H, et al. Phase-locked parallel movement of diaphragm and pelvic floor during breathing and coughing—A dynamic MRI investigation in healthy females. International Urogynecology Journal. 2011;**1**(22):61-68

[37] Neumann DA. Kinesiology of the hip: A focus on muscular actions. Journal of Orthopedic and Sports Physical Therapy. 2010;**40**(2):82-94

[38] Shumway-Cook A, Woolacott M. Motor Control Theory and Practical Application. Baltimore, MD: Lippincott Williams & Wilkins; 1995

[39] Lee DG. The Thorax: An Integrated Approach. Delta; 2003

[40] Mehlman CT, Araghi A, Roy DR. Hyphenated history: The Hueter-Volkmann law. American Journal of Orthopedics—Belle Mead 1997;**26**:798-800

[41] Rigo M, et al. Scoliosis intensive out-patient rehabilitation based on Schroth method. Studies in Health Technology and Informatics. 2008;**135**:208-227

[42] Guo X, et al. Relative anterior spinal overgrowth in adolescent idiopathic scoliosis. Results of disproportionate endochondral-membranous bone growth. Journal of Bone and Joint Surgery. 2003;**85**(7):1026-1031

6

Lumbar Spinal Stenosis, Clinical Presentation, Diagnosis, and Treatment

Luiz Cláudio Lacerda Rodrigues

Abstract

Lumbar spinal stenosis (LSS), a disease that mainly affects people over 50 years old, may have a dramatic presentation with pain, difficulty in walking, changes in urinary functions in addition to root symptoms, such as numbness, burning, and feeling of heaviness in the legs. The treatment is very varied with several non-surgical and surgical possibilities. With an aging population, this disease becomes increasingly preoccupant for their uncertain evolution and without a well-defined correlation with imaging tests, treatment, and outcome may be troublesome. Moreover, LSS frequently affects patients who have associated comorbidity that can hinder the treatment.

Keywords: lumbar stenosis, outcomes, degenerative disc, pathophysiology, surgical treatment, non-surgical treatment

1. Introduction

Lumbar canal stenosis was first described by Antoine Portal in 1803. However, Verbiest [1, 2] was the first to associate changes in the diameter of the vertebral canal with the clinical features and neurogenic claudication. The reduced canal diameter was only correlated to the disc degenerative process by Kirkaldy-Willis, when the authors demonstrated that disc degeneration was directly related to the changes that lead to the physiopathology of reduced vertebral canal diameter [3].

Based on a study of dissection of 50 cadavers, Kirkaldy and Willis described how changes in the zygapophyseal joints and disc degeneration may lead to root impingement and, consequently, all the set of symptoms, which will be discussed in depth later [4].

According to Farfan [5], the degenerative process starts with minor trauma, which, repeated over several years, leads to spondylosis. A few years later, Farfan et al. [6] described how each segment of the lumbar spine is composed of a complex triad: two zygapophyseal joints and the disc. Because those three joints work in tandem, any disease that affects the disc will eventually compromise the joint and vice versa. The chief lesion mechanisms are torsional forces and compression overload [7].

Farfan also describes how the degenerative process starts between the fourth and fifth lumbar vertebrae and that after that level is compromised, based on the three-joint theory, the degeneration progresses to the proximal and distal adjacent levels. Thus, it becomes a diffuse disease that affects multiple levels of the lumbar spine. The anatomic changes are described next.

The zygapophyseal joints are diarthrodial, having an articular surface, a synovial membrane, and a capsule made of collagen; they are filled with synovial fluid [8]. Their degenerative process follows a sequence described by Lewin in 1964 [9]: it starts with a synovial reaction, followed by fibrillation of the joint surface, gross degeneration of the cartilage, osteophyte formation, joint process fracture, and finally loss of the joint's natural shape, leading to instability.

The third component of this complex joint is the intervertebral disc, the largest nonvascular tissue in the human body [10], which comprises three structures: the nucleus pulposus, the annulus fibrosus, and the terminal plates [3]. Each one of these structures has its own anatomy and unique constitution, and considerable importance [10]. The annulus fibrosus is made of type I collagen, distributed in circular layers, and resistant to traction forces. The nucleus pulposus is made basically of proteoglycans, water, and type II collagen, as well as countless elastin fibers [11]. Nutrition of the disc cells occurs through diffusion, in which vessels in the subchondral space, adjacent to the terminal plate's hyaline cartilage, carry oxygen, glucose, and small molecules, thus maintaining the disc's homeostasis [12]. Such homeostasis allows the nucleus pulposus to withstand compressive forces without collapsing and forces to be homogeneously transferred to the annulus fibrosus in all spine movements [13].

Another anatomic area that may go unnoticed is the lateral region, including the intervertebral foramen. Lee et al. [14] subdivided this region into three zones: the afferent zone, located in the subarticular region, medially to the pedicles; the intermediate or middle zone, located below the pars interarticularis; and finally, the efferent zone, comprising the intervertebral foramen. The latter is very important in surgical cases, because a lack of identification may lead to incorrect decompression and persistence of symptoms after surgery [15]. The foramen is a relatively large orifice, which often contains the dorsal root ganglion, coated with a layer of fat for the protection of neural structures. It is delimited anteriorly by the posterior vertebral wall, proximally by the inferior edge of the superior pedicle, inferiorly by the superior edge of the inferior pedicle, and posteriorly by the zygapophyseal joints and the yellow ligament.

2. Historical Background

The degenerative process can also be observed in this region, where diffuse disc bulging can also be seen, associated with loss of height—all leading to a reduced diameter of the vertebral canal. The zygapophyseal joints are also directly associated with foramen stenosis, because their hypertrophy may or may not be associated with the presence of osteophytes, thus causing radicular compression. In this case, sciatica may be observed, mimicking the symptoms of disc herniation [16].

The progression of the degenerative disease still remains truly unknown [17]. However, many concepts have already been postulated. The first one concerns the definition of instability; it is defined as "excessive mobility, neural compression, or deformity." The presence of instability may be associated with a variety of clinical and anatomic manifestations [18].

Kirkaldy and Willis described the degenerative process in terms of evolution and divided it into three phases. However, the duration of each stage is unknown. The first phase was described as a dysfunction in which the disc exhibits chiefly biochemical changes. The second phase was called instability in which degenerative processes in the disc lead to an increase in the segment's motion; this is when disc herniation can occur. Finally, there is the stabilization phase in which disc height reduction, facet hypertrophy, and changes in the yellow ligament occur [18]. This phase of disc degeneration is the most important for the development of the present study, because the aforementioned changes lead to a reduction of the vertebral canal diameter and to narrow lumbar spinal canal syndrome—the disease that is the object of this study.

As was described by Kirkaldy and Willis, the cascading degeneration does not have a definite phase, but in the stabilization phase, lumbar canal stenosis can be observed. It may or may not cause symptoms, but if symptoms do occur, this is commonly observed in patients above 50 years of age. Currently, the most commonly performed type of spine surgery in patients over 65 years old in the United States is decompression of cauda equina roots [19].

Because the population is aging and life expectancy is increasing, we were motivated to conduct this project.

Narrow lumbar spinal canal syndrome comprises a number of symptoms and varied clinical features [20], which is further discussed below.

Vertebral canal stenosis, as defined by Verbiest [2], corresponds to narrowing of the vertebral canal, the lateral recess, and the intervertebral foramen, causing compression of neural elements. Vertebral canal stenosis can be divided into two main groups: congenital and acquired [21]. These main groups were further subdivided: congenital stenosis into idiopathic and achondroplasic, and acquired stenosis into degenerative, combined, spondylotic, iatrogenic, post-traumatic, and metabolic [21].

Narrow lumbar spinal canal syndrome may be confused with many other diseases. Such diseases must always be considered, and a detailed clinical examination may make all the difference. Among the conditions that should be investigated are disc herniation, vascular claudication, tumors, peripheral neuropathy, arthrosis of the hip or knee, and compressive insufficiency fractures [16].

Hall et al. [22] described symptomatic canal stenosis in detail. They described that patients complain of progressive lumbar pain, associated with an incipient pain and numbness in the distal extremities. Neurogenic claudication, the commonest symptom, is characterized by pain and weakness starting in the buttocks and thighs that becomes gradually worse in the orthostatic position and during walking, but improves after sitting down or leaning forward. Less often, one can find unilateral radiculopathy [23]. Symptoms become more acute with the disease's natural progression [24].

The progression of the disease is uncertain: according to Johnson, 70% of patients remain stable for a 4-year period, 15% improve, and 15% tend to become worse. The progression to cauda equina syndrome is extremely rare, but must always be investigated, particularly because of the possibility of other causes, but also because it is an absolute indication for urgent surgery [25].

Elderly patients may present a clinical condition very similar to neurogenic claudication, an entity called vascular claudication, associated with atherosclerosis. The pain following a walk is very similar to that in neurogenic claudication. Physical examination then becomes essential, because in a detailed examination, one can observe impotence in men, dystrophic skin, loss of hair, nail dystrophy, cyanosis, and reduced peripheral pulse. Such symptoms may be essential for the latter diagnosis [22].

3. Physical Examination

The best diagnostic test to distinguish both syndromes was described by Van Gelderen [26]. He had patients riding a stationary bicycle. Patients with lumbar canal stenosis tolerate the exercise, because the forward-leaning position causes symptoms to improve, whereas patients with vascular claudication do not tolerate the exercise, because the hypoxia caused by the underlying disease causes pain and peripheral cyanosis. Another very relevant sign in narrow canal syndrome is improvement when walking uphill and worsening when walking downhill, always associated with the flexion or extension of the trunk [27, 28]. It is postulated that the improvement associated with flexion and extension is directly related to stretching or folding of the yellow ligament. Trunk flexion causes tension in this ligament, thus increasing its diameter, whereas trunk extension causes it to fold into the spinal canal, thus further narrowing the canal that is already narrowed by the degenerative process [29, 30].

The physical examination of a patient with lumbar canal stenosis starts with the careful observation, followed by a very thorough physical examination. One must always consider the differential diagnosis from the other above-mentioned conditions; however, when compared to disc herniation, there are some subtle differences, such as age above 50 years, insidious onset, improvement with trunk flexion and worsening with its extension, and localized motor weakness. Signs of dura mater tension and muscular contraction are rarely found. Typically, a trunk flexion position is observed, due to the increased canal diameter in that position. The presence of a reduced arc of movement is associated with the joint's degenerative process and not directly with the lumbar canal stenosis. Analogous to Phalen's test, Kemp's test is described in the literature, in which the patient is kept in trunk extension for 30 s and claudication symptoms appear [31].

4. Diagnostic

Radiological diagnosis includes several examinations: common radiography, computed tomography (CT), and magnetic resonance imaging (MRI). In selected cases, myelography or myelotomography may be necessary [32].

The study of neural function and conduction speed can be performed either by electroneuromyography or by sensitive-motor evoked potentials [32].

Radiographs must be obtained in four incidences: frontal, orthostatic lateral, flexion, and extension. Then one must look for degenerative changes, such as reduced disc space, sclerosis of vertebral plateaus, sclerosis and hypertrophy of articular facets, closeness of spinous processes, and the diameter of the intervertebral foramina. In dynamic radiography, one can notice the presence of anteroposterior translation [33].

Computed tomography is a very important advance in the diagnosis of vertebral stenosis, because it shows important bone details, including the central canal, the lateral recess, the foramen, the joint facets, and their degree of degeneration [34]. CT is, however, criticized for its high rate of radiologic findings without correlation to the patient's symptoms [33].

MRI provides images of soft tissue with excellent quality, including ligaments, neural tissue, and the intervertebral discs. It is more sensitive for diagnosing lumbar stenosis than tomography. MRI findings include signal weakening at T2, with dehydration and rupture of the annulus in multiple discs; changes in terminal plates; void signal; enlarged yellow ligaments; and reduced vertebral canal [35].

For many years, myelography was the gold-standard exam for diagnosing lumbar stenosis, but although today's water-soluble contrast is less toxic, patients still have nausea, vomiting, headache, and dizziness. Myelography is an invasive exam, although it shows the dimensions of the dural sac and the neural roots in detail. Myelography findings include the partial or total interruption of contrast flow, and the dynamic examination may reveal a dynamic compression of neural structures [36]. It should be noted that electromyography is not routinely used in lumbar stenosis, because 80% of symptomatic patients have changes in one or both legs, making it necessary only for differential diagnosis, particularly to distinguish it from diseases that affect peripheral nerves [37].

The canal's diameter may be calculated by several different techniques. We used Hamanishi's technique, widely used [38], on which the calculation to determine the presence of stenosis is based. That is, Hamanishi considers a diameter of less than 100 mm^2 to define stenosis in patients with clinical symptoms and characteristic images [39].

The treatment of lumbar canal stenosis may be divided into two main types: clinical or conservative and surgical [40], each of them comprising several different modalities.

When a thorough clinical examination has been performed and there is confirmation from imaging exams, electrodiagnosis is not needed, as results are often inconclusive and, when positive, do not have an influence on either the clinical or the surgical treatment [41].

Generally, clinical treatment is preferred by over 50% of patients [42], and they mostly evolve satisfactorily. However, a small fraction suffers a more severe progression, with more unfavorable natural history and serious, limiting symptoms [43].

Many lumbar canal stenosis patients have symptoms of unilateral radiculopathy. In such cases, the most likely cause is herniation, which may affect a root in an already stenotic canal. When this happens, treatment should be more focused on the disc herniation. Despite the large number of articles in the literature, there is no consensus about when to operate such patients and, if surgery is performed, what the best technique would be [44].

5. Treatment Options

Drug treatment does not offer many possibilities. The indiscriminate and frequent use of anti-inflammatory medications for chronic lumbar pain does not have a proven satisfactory response [45] and may be associated with gastrointestinal and renal complications. Its use should be very restricted and avoided in elderly patients with narrow lumbar spinal canal syndrome [45].

Simple painkillers, muscle relaxants, and opioids may be of value. They are indicated for treating and controlling the pain but have no effect on the treatment of neurogenic claudication [45]. Gabapentin has been shown to be a safe medication; it may be taken orally and has a positive effect on patients with neurogenic claudication and the sensory alterations, which are very common in these patients [46].

Corticosteroids are also used indiscriminately. The idea is that there is an inflammatory process associated with the mechanical compression that could benefit from the medication, but this theory was not proven by Natour's study [47].

Physiotherapy, or more broadly rehabilitation, is a second non-surgical approach. Manual therapy, stretching, and muscular strengthening play an important role, in addition to the exercises. Patients who suffer from canal stenosis have, in addition to pain, a significant muscle loss, which severely limits their activities and progressively worsens their clinical condition, which leads to further impairments [48, 49].

The recommended activities include manual therapy, strengthening, and walking training, as well as exercises that improves proprioception. In addition, weight loss is important, because obese patients have been described to have a worse prognosis [47]. Cycling is a very much recommended activity, not only because patients tolerate it well, but it also allows them to improve their conditioning and does not impact other joints that may also be degenerated, such as the hip and the knee [50].

Zarife et al. [51], in a study comparing two types of conservative treatments—physiotherapy and peridural corticosteroids—concluded that, in a 6-month follow-up, both methods were effective in improving the patients' condition and ability to walk, which suggested that clinical treatment is important and effective in these delicate and active patients.

Peridural corticosteroids are another type of non-surgical treatment for narrow lumbar spinal canal syndrome, as opposed to oral corticosteroids, which were shown to be ineffective for this condition [47]. Peridural corticosteroids have some advantages, which are discussed below. There are several possibilities for their administration, with or without radioscopy, as well as several techniques: interlaminar, caudal, and transforaminal. Despite their limited benefits, their use may have lasting efficacy in many patients [52].

Cosgrove et al. [53] published an article in 2011 in which the efficacy of peridural corticosteroids was evaluated and showed that women obtained greater benefits than men and that clinical results were not related to MR findings, which was also found in Natour's study [47]. Although Cosgrove et al. [53] observed better results among women, as per the general literature, women are normally affected compared to men.

Similarly to the above-mentioned article, Charles et al. [54] showed that peridural corticosteroids produce a satisfactory response in lumbar stenosis. The results of the study showed that patients with associated radiculopathy have a better response than do patients with claudication and that 25% of patients respond more favorably up to 2 years after the procedure.

However, we also found some articles in which the use of peridural corticosteroids did not deliver the expected satisfaction, in addition to causing complications such as meningitis, arachnoiditis, aseptic meningitis, and increased serum corticosteroids [55]. Fukusaki et al. [56] compared the use of analgesics in isolation and in combination with peridural corticosteroids and reported no complications; however, the results after 3 months were unsatisfactory, with all symptoms returning.

Surgical treatment is considered the last resort for patients with treating lumbar canal stenosis. Because surgery is performed in patients over 65 years of age, there is significant morbidity and mortality, which increase with associated diseases and patient age, making it mandatory to assess the risks and benefit of the surgery [57].

Airaksinen's study [58] showed that patients over 50 years old who underwent decompression and arthrodesis evolved with a significantly reduced ability to return to work. That reduction was even greater in older patients.

There are articles that report surgical results, with conflicting results. Hurri et al. [59], in a 12-year follow-up study, did not find any differences between surgical and non-surgical results, showing that regardless of surgery, the outcome is the same. Another study comparing operated and non-operated patients was the Maine Lumbar Spine Study [60, 61], in which operated patients were followed up for a period from 4 to 10 years. Results showed that operated patients had better postoperative results than non-operated patients, with an average of 72% satisfaction among the former and 52% among the latter at 4 years of follow-up. The same comparison made at 10 years showed inferior results, but operated patients still had a perception of improvement.

Turner et al. [62] performed a meta-analysis and found that 64% of patients showed good results after surgical treatment, for a period varying from 3 to 6 years.

Surgical treatment is indicated when clinical treatment fails or neurological symptoms worsen [63]. Today, there are several different surgical techniques. The classical technique is laminectomy, performed by an incision along the midline followed by decompression, removing up to 50% of facets. In addition, there are minimally invasive techniques, such as opening and decompressing only one side of the lamina, which is called recalibration [64]. Interspinous spacers have been recently included in the surgical arsenal for canal stenosis, but studies are still under way, and there are no studies yet evaluating for an adequate follow-up period. For this reason, the actual benefit of this kind of surgery is not yet well established. However, it is known that it does offer some advantages, such as short hospitalization periods and limited bleeding. Its indication takes into account that by tensioning the yellow ligament, the canal diameter is increased [65].

The median approach with broad exposure of the spine has the advantage of satisfactorily exposing the spinal canal, which allows the intervertebral foramina to be viewed, broad decompression to happen up to the efferent zone with direct view, and roots to be evaluated. However, care must be taken to preserve half of the facets; otherwise, postoperative instability will occur as an iatrogenic complication that may compromise the results for the patient. The main problem with this broad approach is blood loss, which may be large or even catastrophic in some cases, because muscular lesion leads to large arterial and venous bleeding [63].

The indication for instrumentation and fusion varies in the literature, with some authors indicating fusion in the presence of degenerative spondylolisthesis or if there is a translation greater than 5 mm in dynamic X-rays. Instrumentation may also be indicated in cases of degenerative scoliosis in which the neural foramen is compressed on the concave side of the curvature and resection of more than 50% of the articular facet is needed in order to decompress the root stuck inside [66, 67].

The minimally invasive approach in spinal canal stenosis associated with foraminal stenosis may be indicated for patients with lumbar and radicular pain associated with stenosis in imaging exams, but its main contraindication is the presence of instability in X-rays, associated with a scoliosis of more than 10° in X-rays, in the orthostatic position. The main complication is recurring symptoms, in approximately 20% of cases, with reoperation being necessary, with broad exposure of the spine [68].

Interspinous spacers are a new generation of implants. Their mechanism of action is by blocking extension, as well as tensioning the stenosis level, which theoretically increases the spinal canal diameter. Studies have shown that such an increase may reach 20% of the initial diameter [69], but these studies are questioned due to the possibility of commercial interests. They are indicated for lumbar canal stenosis patients with two levels of stenosis, but they are not used in the L5-S1 level and are contraindicated for patients with degenerative spondylolisthesis or radiological signs of instability [70].

Postoperative care of lumbar canal stenosis patients may vary slightly, but basically, patients are instructed to walk on the first day after surgery. Longer rest is indicated for patients with incidental durotomy, in which case the recommendation is at least 2 days rest. Deambulation with the aid and training by a physiotherapist is very important [71]. Rehabilitation exercises must include stretching the posterior muscles of the thighs and legs, training trunk flexibility, and strengthening the abdominal and paravertebral muscles. Improving cardiopulmonary capacity is also a target of rehabilitation, always respecting the patients' limits [72].

The need for orthesis is very much relative. Their use is generally not indicated. In osteoporotic patients, when there is the risk of an acute failure of implants, their use may be indicated for a period of up to 6 weeks, but overall, the literature is highly controversial about this subject [73].

The complications observed in surgery for lumbar canal stenosis may be divided into complications in the operated area and systemic complications. The most commonly observed systemic complications are urinary retention, worsening of heart failure in previously affected patients, delirium, and thoracic pain. Such symptoms are usually temporary, but they increase hospitalization time [74].

Surgical complications vary according to the series. Jolles et al. [75] report sensorial and motor deficit, dura mater lesions with cerebrospinal fluid fistula, surgical site hematoma, and superficial and deep infection.

Epidemiologically, surgery for lumbar canal stenosis has the same incidence of complications as knee arthroplasties, but greater than hip arthroplasties [76]. Mortality is currently at an average of 10%, but it increases with patient age. Clinical complications vary from 3 to 31% [77]. However, the most common complication observed in lumbar canal stenosis surgery is incidental durotomy, with an average incidence of 16%, increasing in case of reoperation [78]. Cerebrospinal fluid fistula, with leakage of cerebrospinal fluid, is the chief cause of reoperation in the first 2 days after surgery [79].

6. Conclusion

In conclusion, lumbar canal stenosis is a complex syndrome, which comprises degenerative processes in the lumbar spine. This degeneration may lead to a painful and limiting clinical condition, which must always be investigated through an exhaustive study of imaging examinations. Even though treatment is varied, with a large number of possibilities found in the literature, studies usually compare different techniques, either surgical or conservative, to find the most effective one. Apparently, the surgical approach with decompression, either associated with arthrodesis or not, has provided not only the best clinical results but also a greater incidence of complications and mortality, which must always be weighed together with the patient before surgery.

Author details

Luiz Cláudio Lacerda Rodrigues

Address all correspondence to: luizclaudiolacerdarodrigues@gmail.com

1 Santa Marcelina Medical School, São Paulo, Brazil

2 Oswaldo Cruz German Hospital, Rua Treze de Maio, São Paulo - SP, Brazil

References

[1] Verbiest H. A radicular syndrome from developmental narrowing of the lumbar vertebral canal. J Bone Joint Surg Br;36:230–237, 1954.

[2] Verbiest H. The significance and principles of computerized axial tomography in idiopathic developmental stenosis of the bony lumbar vertebral canal. Spine;4:369–378, 1979.

[3] Kirkaldy-Willis WH, Paine KW, Cauchoix J, Mclvor G. Lumbar spinal stenosis. Clin Orthop;99:30–50, 1974.

[4] Kirkaly-Willis WH, Wedge JH, Yong-Hing K, Reilly J. Pathology and pathogenesis of lumbar spondylosis and stenosis. Spine;3(4):319–328, 1978.

[5] Farfan HF. Effects of torsion on the intervertebral joints. Can J Surg;12:336–341, 1969.

[6] Farfan HF, Sulivan JB. The relation of facet orientation to intervertebral disc failure. Can J Surg;10:179–18, 1967.

[7] Yong-Hing K, Reilly J, Kirkald-Willis WH. The ligamentun flavum. Spine;1:226–234, 1976.

[8] Sullivan JD, Farfan HF, Kahn DS. Pathological changes with intervertebral joint rotational instability in the rabbit. Can J Surg;13:71–79, 1971.

[9] Lewin T. Osteoartrits in lumbar synovial joints. Acta Orthop Scand Suple;73:1–112, 1964.

[10] Yong-soo C. Pathophysiology of degenerative disc disease. Asian Spine J;3(1):39–44, 2009.

[11] Borgesen SE, Vang PS. Herniation of the lumbar intervertebral disk in children and adolescents. Acta Orthop Scand;45:540–549, 1974.

[12] Key JA. Intervertebral disc lesions in children and adolescents. J Bone Joint Surg Am; 32:97–102, 1950.

[13] Parisini P, Di Silvestre M, Greggi T, Miglietta A, Paderni S. Lumbar disc excision in children and adolescents. Spine;26:1997–2000, 2001.

[14] Lee CX, Ranching W, Glenn W. Lateral lumbar spinal canal stenosis. Classification, pathology anatomy and surgical decompression. Spine;13:313–320, 1980.

[15] Haward S, Glover MJ. Lumbar spinal stenosis: historical perspectives, classification, and pathoanatomy. Semin Spine Surg;6(2):69–77, 1994.

[16] Thomas SA. Spinal stenosis: history and physical examination. Phys Med Rehabil Clin N Am;14:29–39, 2003.

[17] Inoue Nozomu MD, Orias AE. Biomechanics of interverebral disc degeneration. Orthop Clin North Am;42(4):487–499, 2011.

[18] Kirkaldy-Willis WH, Farfan HF. Instability of the lumbar spine. Clin Orthop Relat Res. 1982 May;(165):110-23.

[19] Deyo RA, Gray DT, Kreuter W et al. United States trends in lumbar fusion surgery for degenerative conditions. Spine;30:1441–1445, 2005.

[20] Epstein NE, Maldonado VC, Cusik JF. Symptomatic lumbar spinal stenosis. Surg Neurol;50:3–10, 1998.

[21] Arnoldi CC, Brodsky AE, Cauchoix J et al. Lumbar spinal stenosis and nerve root entrapment: syndromes, definition and classification. Clin Orthop;115:4–5, 1976.

[22] Hall S, Bartleson JD, Onoforio BM et al. Lumbar spinal stenosis. Clinical features, diagnostic procedures and results of surgical treatment in 68 patients. Ann Intern Med; 103(2):271–275, 1985.

[23] Naylor A. Factors in the development of the spina stenosis syndrome. J Bone Joint Surg Br;61(3):319–328, 1978

[24] Blau JN, Logue V. Intermittent claudication of the cauda equina. Lancet;1:1081–1086, 1961.

[25] Johnsson KE, Rosen I, Uden A. The natural course of lumbar spinal stenosis. Clin Orthop;279:82–86, 1992.

[26] Dyck P, Doyle JB. Bicycle test of Van Gelderen in diagnosis of intermittent cauda equina compression syndrome. J Neurosurg;46:667–670, 1997.

[27] Denn HG, Zimmerman RS, Lyons MK et al. Measurement of exercise tolerance on the treadmill test in patients with symptomatic lumbar spinal stenosis: a useful indicator of functional status and surgical outcome. J Neurosurg;83:27–30, 1995.

[28] Fritz JM, Erhard RE, Delitto A et al. Preliminary results of the two-stage treadmill test as a clinical diagnostic tool in the differential diagnosis of the lumbar spinal stenosis. J Spinal Disord;10:410–416, 1997.

[29] Olszewski AD, Yaszemski MJ, White AA III. The anatomy of the human lumbar ligamentum flavum: new observations and their surgical importance. Spine;21:2307–2312, 1996.

[30] Sairyo K, Biyani A, Goel V et al. Pathomechanism of ligamentum flavum hypertrophy: a multidisciplinary investigation based on clinical, biomechanical, histologic, and biologic assessments. Spine;23:2649–2656, 2005.

[31] Katz JN, Dagas M, Stucki G et al. Degenerative lumbar spinal stenosis: diagnostic value of the history and physical examination. Arthrit Rheum;38(9):1236–1241, 1995.

[32] Spengler DM. Current concepts review. Degenerative stenosis of the lumbar spine. J Bone Joint Surg;69-A:305–308, 1987.

[33] Dyck P, Doyle JP Jr. "Bicycle Test" of Van Gelderen in diagnosis of intermittent cauda equina compression syndrome. Case Report/Neurosurgery;46:667–670, 1977.

[34] Arnoldi CC, Brodsky AE, Cauchoix J, et al. Lumbar spinal stenosis and nerve root entrapment syndromes. Definition and classification. Clin Orthop Relat Res. 1976 Mar-Apr;(115):4–5.

[35] Frymoyer JW, Newberg A, Pope MH, Wilder DG, Clements J, Macpherson B. Spine radiographs in patients with low-back pain. An epidemiological study in men. J Bone Joint Surg Am;66(7):1048–1055, 1984.

[36] Herkowitz HN, Garfin SR, Bell GR, Bumphrey F, Rothman RH. The use of computerized tomography in evaluating non-visualized vertebral levels caudad to a complete block on a lumbar myelogram. A review of thirty-two cases. J Bone Joint Surg Am;69(2): 218–224, 1987.

[37] Czervionke LF. Lumbar intervertebral disc disease. Neuroimaging Clin N Am;3:465–485, 1993.

[38] Hamanishi C, Matukura N, Fujita M, Tomihara M, Tanaka S. Crosssectional area of the stenotic lumbar dural tube measured from the transverse views of MRI. J Spinal Dis; 7:388–393, 1994.

[39] Owlia MB, Salimzadeh A, Alishiri G, Haghighi A. Comparison of two doses of corticosteroid in epidural steroid injection for lumbar radicular pain. Singapore Med J; 48(3):241–245, 2007.

[40] Amundsen T, Weber H, NOrdal HJ, Magnaes B et al. Lumbar spinal stenosis: conservative or surgical management? A prospective 10 year study. Spine;25(11):1424–1435, 2000.

[41] Haig AJ, Tong HC, Yamakawa KS, Quint DJ et al. The sensitivity and specificity of eletrodiagnostic testing for the clinical syndrome of lumbar stenosis. Spine;30(23): 2667–2676, 2005.

[42] Atlas SJ, Kelle RB, Wu YA et al. Long-term outcomes of surgical and nonsurgical management of lumbar spinal stenosis: 8 to 10 years results from the Maine Lumbar Spine Study. Spine;30(8):936–943, 2005.

[43] Waters WC, Bono CM, Gilbert TJ et al. An evidence based clinical guideline for the diagnosis and treatment of degenerative lumbar spondylolisthesies. Spine J;8(2):305–310, 2008.

[44] Chou R, Qasemm A, Snow V et al. Diagnosis and treatment of low back pain: a joint clinical practice guideline from the American college of physicians and the American Pain Society. Ann Intern Med;147(7):478–491, 2007 Oct 2.

[45] Stephane G, Steven JA . Lumbar spinal stenosis. Best Pract Res Clin Rheumatol;24(2): 253–265, 2010 April.

[46] Yaksi A, Ozgonenel L, Ozgonenel B. The efficiency of gabapentin in patients with lumbar spinal stenosis. Spine;32(9):939–942, 2007.

[47] Rodrigues LC, Natour J. A double-blind, randomized controlled, prospective trial assessing the effectiveness of oral corticoids in the treatment of symptomatic lumbar canal stenosis. J Negat Results Bioemed;13:13, 2014.

[48] Rittemberg JD, Ross AE. Functional rehabilitation for degenerative lumbar spina stenosis. Phys Med Rehabil Clin N Am (14);111–120, 2003.

[49] Whtiman JM. Flyn TW, Frotz JM. Nonsurgical management of patients with lumbar spine stenosis: a literature review and a case series of three patients managed with physical therapy. Phys Med Rehabil Clin N Am;14(1):77–101, 2003.

[50] Whitman JM, Flym TW, Chids JD, Wainer RS et al. A comparassion between two physical therapy treatment programs for patients with lumbar spinal stenosis: a randomized clinical trial. Spine;31(2):2541–2549, 2006.

[51] Zarife K, Suheda O, Kncuy S et al. Effectiveness of physical therapy and epidural steroid injections in lumbar spinal stenosis. Spine;34(10):985–989, 2009.

[52] Parr AT, Diwan S, Adbdi S. Lumbar interlaminar epidural injections in managing chronic low back and lower extremity pain: a systematic review. Pain Physician;12(1): 163–188, 2009 Jan–Feb.

[53] Cosgrove JL, Berlote M, Chase SL et al. Epidural steroid injections in the treatement of lumbar spinal stenosis efficacy and predictability of successful response. Am J Phys Med Reabil;90:1050–1055, 2011.

[54] Charles DR, Neil K, Ralph B, Kathy V. A retrospective analysis of the efficacy of epidural steroid injections. Clin Orthopaed Relat Res;228;270–273, 1998.

[55] Cuckler JM, Bernini PA, Wiesel SW et al. The use of epidural steroids in the treatment of lumbar radicular pain. J Bone Joint Surg Am;67:63–66, 1995.

[56] Fukusaki M, Kobayashi I, Tetsuya H Sumikawa K. Symptoms of spinal stenosis do not improve after epidural steroid injection. Clin J Pain;14:148–151, 1988.

[57] Shabat S, Arizon Z, Folman Y et al. Long-term outcomes of decompressive surgery for lumbar spinal stenosis in octogenarians. Eur Spine J;17:193–198, 2008.

[58] Airaksinen O, Hermo A, Saari T. Surgical treatment of lumbar spinal stenosis: patients postoperative disability and working capacity. Eur Spine J;3;261–264, 1994.

[59] Hurri H, Slatis P, Soini J et al. Lumbar spinal stenosis: assemtment of long-term outcome 12 years after operative and conservative treatment. J Spinal Disord;11:110–115, 1998.

[60] Atlas SJ, Keller RB, Robson D et al. Surgical and nossurgical manangement of lumbar spinal stenosis: four-years outcomes from the Maine lumbar spine study. Spine;25:556–562, 2000.

[61] Atlas SJ, Keller RB, Wu YA et al. Long-term outcomes of surgical and nonsurgical management of lumbar spine study. Spine;30:936–943, 2005.

[62] Turner JA, Ersek M, Herron L, Deyo R. Surgery for spinal stenosis: attempt meta-analysis of the literature. Spine;17:1–8, 1992.

[63] Ra'kerry KR, Douglas DN, Daniel EG, Kornelis AP, Steven CL. Lumbar spinal stenosis. Curr Orthop Pract;19(4):351–356, 2008.

[64] Asgarzadie F, Khoo LT. Minimally invasive operative management for lumbar spinal stenosis: overview of early and long-term outcomes. Orthop Clin N Am;38:387–399, 2007.

[65] Zucherman JF, Hsu KY, Hartjen CA, et al. A prospective randomized multicenter study for the treatment of lumbar spinal stenosis with the X stop interspinous implant: 1-year results. Eur Spine J;13:22–31, 2004.

[66] Deburg A, Bex M, Lassale B, Bitan F. Technique chirurgicale dans le traitement des Stenoses du canal Lombaire. Acta Orthop Belg;53:412–419, 1987.

[67] Spinavak J. Degenerative lumbar spinal stenosis. J Bone Joint Surg (Am);80-A:1053–1066, 1998.

[68] Yamada K, Matsuda H, Nabeta M et al. Clinical outcomes of microscopic decompression for degenerative lumbar foraminal stenosis: a comparison between patients with and without degenerative lumbar scoliosis. Eur Spine J;20:947–953, 2011.

[69] Richards JC, Manjubar S, Lindsey DP. The treatment mechanism of an interspinous process implant for lumbar neurogenic intermittent claudication. Spine;30:744–749, 2005.

[70] Siddiqui M, Nicol M, Karadimas E et al. The positional magnetic resonance imaging changes in the lumbar spine following insertion of a novel interspinous process distraction device. Spine;30:2677–2682, 2005.

[71] Turner J, Ersek M, Herron L et al. Patient outcomes after lumbar spinal fussions. JAMA; 268:907–911, 1992.

[72] Fairbank J. Frost H, Macdonald W, Yu L et al. Randomised controled trial to compare surgical stabilization of the lumbar spine with an intensive rehabilitation programme for patients with chronico low back pain: the MRC spine stabilization trial. Br Med J. 2005 May 28;1–7 330(7502): 1233.

[73] Herkowitz HN, Garfin SR. Indications and surgical results of arthrodesis following spinal stenosis Spinal Stenosis. Philadelphia: Ed. Sauders. The Spine 1999;p. 806M-T. 132.

[74] Fredmann B, Arizon Z, Zohar E et al. Observations on the safety and efficacy of surgical decompression for lumbar spinal stenosis in geriatric patients. Eur Spine J;11:571–574, 2002.

[75] Jolles BM, Porchet F, Theumann N. Surgical treatment of lumbar spinal stenosis. J Bone Joint Surg (Br);83:949–953, 2001.

[76] Alto TJ, Mallmivaara A, Kovacs F et al. Preoperative predictors for postoperative clinical outcome in lumbar spinal stenosis: systematic review. Spine;31(18):E648–E663, 2006.

[77] Genevay S, Atlas SJ. Lumbar spinal stenosis. Best Pract Res Clin Rheumatol;24(2);253–265, 2010.

[78] Eismont FJ, Wiesel SW, Rothman RH. Treatment of dural tears associated with spinal surgery. J Bone Joint Surg Am;63:1132–1136, 1981.

[79] Sin AH, Caldito G, Smith D et al. Predictive factors for dural tear and cerebrospinal leakage in patients undergoing lumbar surgery. J Neurosurg Spine;5:224–227, 2006.

7

A Pilot Study on the Effect of Outpatient Schroth Exercises on Thoracolumbar and Lumbar Curves in Adult Scoliosis Patients

Shu-Yan Ng, Wing-Yan Chan, Tsz-Ki Ho and Yin-Ling Ng

Abstract

Study design: This is a pilot prospective cohort study.

Objectives: To investigate if outpatient Schroth exercises (SBP) affect thoracolumbar or lumbar curves in adult scoliosis patients.

Background: Adult scoliosis tends to progress and is associated with an increased prevalence of low back pain. The outcome of conservative treatment is not satisfactory, as treatment is not directed towards spinal deformity. This study investigates if SBP influences the thoracolumbar and lumbar curves in patients with adult scoliosis.

Materials and methods: Adult patients with thoracolumbar and lumbar curves ≥ 20° were taught SBP exercises once weekly for 4 weeks. They then performed the exercises at home three times a week, for 9 months. Baseline measurements included Cobb angles, coronal offset, sagittal vertical axis (SVA), T4-12 kyphosis, L1-S1 lordosis, sacral slope, pelvic incidence and pelvic tilt. They were compared to post-intervention measurements, using paired t tests.

Results: SBP exercises statistically significantly decreased the Cobb angle ($p = 0.0032$), improved the ATR ($p = 0.012$), increased the sacral slope ($p = 0.03$), decreased the pelvic tilt ($p = 0.0032$) and the SVA ($p = 0.032$).

Conclusion: The SBP exercises improved the Cobb angles and SVA in adult scoliosis patients with thoracolumbar and lumbar curves.

Keywords: adult scoliosis, adult idiopathic scoliosis, degenerative lumbar scoliosis, Schroth exercises, physiotherapeutic scoliosis specific exercises, scoliosis rehabilitation

1. Introduction

Scoliosis is a three-dimensional spinal deformity with a lateral curvature in excess of 10°. Adult scoliosis refers to scoliosis after skeletal maturity. It can arise from a wide range of conditions, including neuromuscular diseases, metabolic diseases, trauma, etc. Most commonly, the condition includes adult idiopathic scoliosis and degenerative lumbar scoliosis (DLS) [1–3], which are discrete conditions. Sometimes they coexist and are difficult to distinguish.

Adult scoliosis is increasing in importance in recent years, as its prevalence is increasing, as a result of increased life expectancy of the population [2, 3]. Adult scoliosis with thoracolumbar and lumbar curves is associated with a higher prevalence of low back pain. Also, they tend to progress. Many adult AIS patients consult because of the progression of their curves or of symptoms that decrease their quality of life inducing functional impairment [4]. Thoracolumbar curves receive the highest percentage of surgical treatment among adult coronal deformities; it accounted for 32.6% of all surgeries for adult scoliosis [5].

Apart from causing low back pain, thoracolumbar and lumbar curves tend to progress. Weinstein and Ponseti showed that 68% of the AIS curves progressed after skeletal maturity, especially when the Cobb angle exceeds 30° [6, 7]. In a retrospective study on progression of adult scoliosis, Marty-Poumarat et al. found that curves in adult AIS as well as DLS patients' progress, irrespective of the initial Cobb angle [8]. The rate of progression for lumbar or thoracolumbar single curve was 0.82°/year (0.34–1.65°) for adult AIS patients and 1.64°/year (0.77–3.82°) for DLS patients, respectively. Similarly, Iida et al. reported that AIS patients with thoracolumbar and lumbar curves (Lenke 5C) with a Cobb angle over 30° have a high risk of progression [9].

Symptomatic adult scoliosis patients are generally treated conservatively by NSAIDs, analgesics, manipulation, acupuncture, and electrotherapy [10]. These conservative treatments have not been found to be effective [11]. Everett and Patel found a low level of evidence in support of conservative treatment. They identified level IV evidence for physical therapy, chiropractic care, and bracing and level III evidence for steroid injections [11]. Similarly, Glassman et al. assessed the cost associated with nonsurgical treatment of adult scoliosis and found that despite the substantial mean cost of US$10,815 per patient, there was no improvement in any HRQOL (Health-Related Quality of Life) measure over 2-year follow-up [12].

The unsatisfactory outcome of the treatment approach is possibly due to the fact that it targets at the symptoms of the adult scoliosis, but not the spinal deformities which are the one of the causes of the symptoms. The present study attempts to investigate whether Schroth best practice (SBP) exercises, which have been found to improve curves in AIS patients [13–18], do affect thoracolumbar and lumbar curves in adult scoliosis patients.

2. Materials and methods

2.1. Patient selection

Adult scoliosis patients with AIS and degenerative lumbar scoliosis of either sex, who were aged 20–70 years and were seen in the Wanchai Chiropractic Clinic were included. Patients with lumbar spondylolisthesis, congenital scoliosis, syndromic scoliosis, functional scoliosis due to leg length discrepancy and secondary scoliosis due to antalgia, and compression fractures were excluded.

2.2. Procedures

Consecutive adult scoliosis patients consulted for low back pain between January 2014 and October 2015 in the Wanchai Chiropractic Clinic, with signs of thoracolumbar or lumbar scoliosis were referred for standing postero-anterior (PA) full spine radiographs. When the Cobb angle was ≥20° and the apex of the curve lied in the thoracolumbar or lumbar area, the subject would be asked for consent to participate in the study and was then referred for standing full spine lateral radiograph.

The angle of trunk rotation (ATR) of the patients was measured. The subjects then completed the Chinese version of the SRS-22 which has been found to have satisfactory internal consistency and excellent reproducibility [19]. They were then instructed to perform the SBP exercises [20, 21], which essentially involve holding the lumbar spine in lordosis and horizontally translating the trunk to the side of the lumbar convexity, whilst simultaneously lowering the contralateral pelvis to deflex the lumbar spine. The subjects then breathed into the areas of concavities [22] and exhaled forcefully with isometric contraction of all the trunk muscles [22]. The breathing method is termed "rotational angular breathing (RAB)"and is an inherent part of the Schroth exercise approach [22]. Corrective postures to be undertaken during daily activities [21, 23, 24] were also taught by a certified SBP therapist.

The subjects took four weekly classes. They then performed the exercises at home for at least three times a week and adopted corrective postures basing on their curve types [21, 23] and the side of the curves during daily activities. They had to mark on their log book the dates they did the exercises. They returned quarterly for assessment to see if they had been performing the exercises correctly.

The subjects were advised not to take up any sports or activities that they did not do prior to the intervention nor engage in any therapy and/or treatments targeted to the spinal deformities, as these might confound the outcome.

After 9 months, PA and lateral full spine X-rays of the patients were again taken and the ATR measured. The patient filled in the Chinese version of SRS-22 again.

2.3. Measurement of radiographs

All the radiographs were scanned, masked, and coded before being measured by an independent radiologist at the end of the study to avoid measurement bias. The Surgimap software was used for measurement, as it had been found to have good to excellent inter and intraobserver reliability [25].

The coronal Cobb angle, coronal offset, T4-T12 kyphosis, T10-L2 kyphosis, L1-S1 lordosis, sacral slope, pelvic tilt, pelvic incidence [26, 27], and C7-S1 sagittal vertical axis (SVA) [28, 29] were measured (**Figure 1**). The coronal offset, which is the distance from the center of C7 to the vertical line drawn from the center of the sacrum (central sacral line CSL), was also

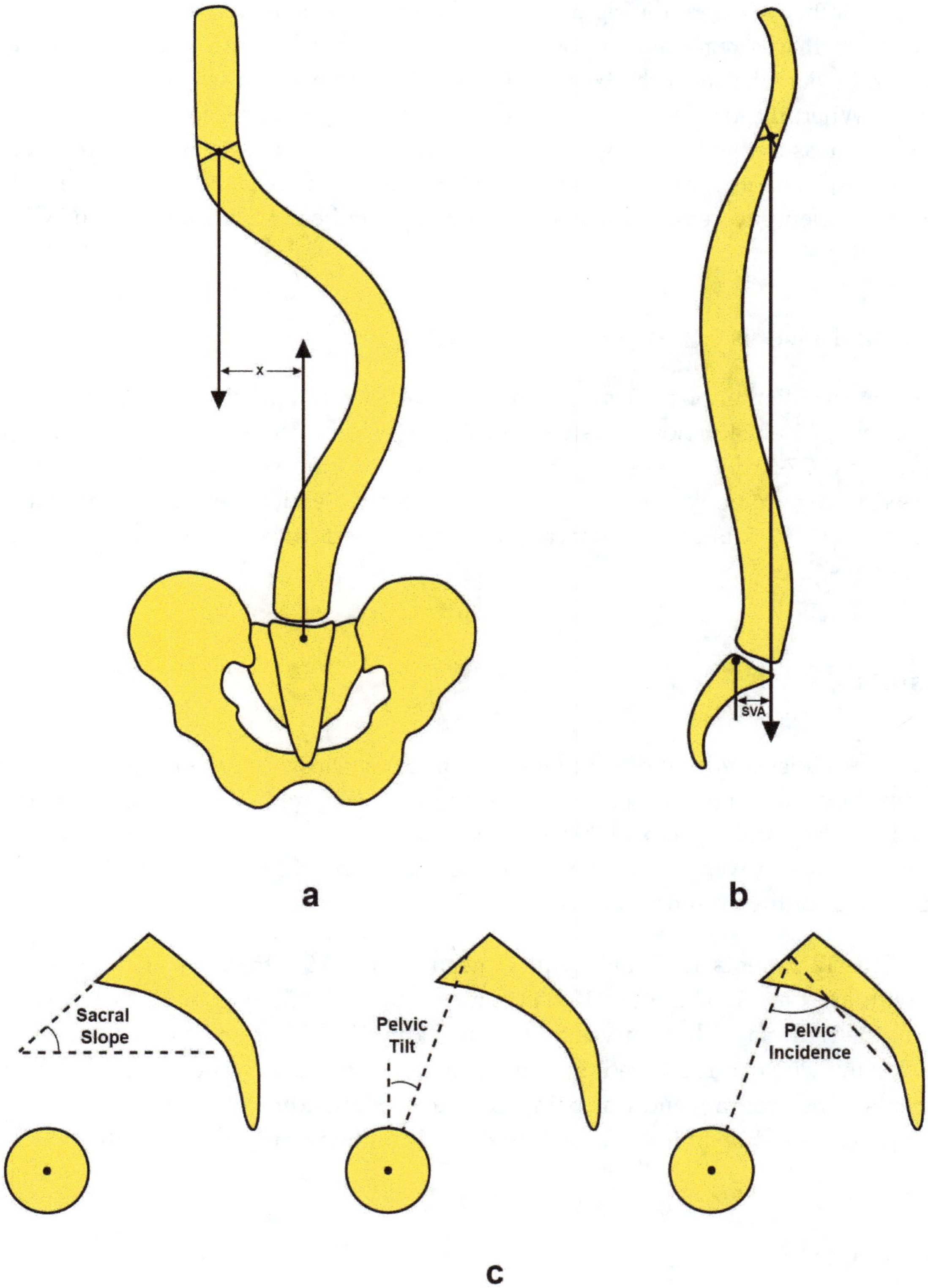

Figure 1. Measurements of the radiographic parameters. (a) "x" stands for the coronal offset. It is the distance between the center of the body of C7 and a perpendicular line from the center of sacrum (CSL). When C7 is situated to the right of CSL, the measurement was designated at "−;" otherwise it was regarded as "+." (b) SVA stands for sagittal vertebral axis. It is the distance between a perpendicular line from the center of the body of C7 to the superoposterior corner of S1. When the line is in front of the superoposterior corner of S1, the measurement was regarded as "+;" otherwise it was regarded as "−." (c) The measurements of other spinopelvic parameters.

determined. When C7 is to the right of CSL, the measurement was designated as negative "-;" otherwise it was regarded as positive "+." The SVA, which was the distance between the perpendicular line from the body of C7 to the superoposterior corner of sacrum, was measured. When the perpendicular dropped in front of the superoposterior corner of the sacrum, the measurement was regarded as positive "+," otherwise it was regarded as negative "-". Measurements of spinopelvic parameters which included the sacral slope, pelvic tilt and pelvic incidence were performed as previously described by Schwab et al. and Glassman et al. [28, 29].

2.4. Statistical analysis

The post-intervention Cobb angles, the coronal offset, sacral slope, pelvic tilt, pelvic incidence, L1-S1 lordosis, T10-L2 kyphosis, T4-12 kyphosis, the pelvic incidence-lumbar lordosis (PI-LL) mismatch, and C7-S1 SVA were compared to the baseline measurements. Paired t tests were conducted to determine whether the post- and pre-intervention difference was statistically significant at $p < 0.05$. Similar statistical analysis was performed for ATR as well as SRS-22 domain scores.

3. Results

Twenty-three patients with thoracolumbar or lumbar scoliosis were enrolled into the study. Six dropped out soon after consent for various reasons (**Figure 2**). This left 17 patients. All of them followed the study protocol. Near the end of the study, five patients went overseas for study and work and were not available for final assessment. Finally, only 12 patients' data were collected for the present analysis.

Eleven of the 12 patients are female, with a mean age of 45.9 ± 15.0. Two had thoracolumbar curve, with apex at L1. The other 10 had lumbar curves, with apex at L2 or L3. Three had curves to the right and 9 had curves to the left (**Table 1**). All but one complained of chronic low back pain. One had recovered from an acute low back pain episode three weeks prior to enrolment on the program and was pain-free at the commencement of the study. Nine of the patients had adult idiopathic scoliosis, one had adult idiopathic scoliosis with DLS and two had DLS.

3.1. Cobb angle

The mean baseline Cobb angle was 31.2 ± 9.6°, which dropped to 27 ± 7.4° after 9 months. Based on the criterion that a reduction of 6° Cobb angle represents improvement [30], four subjects had improvement of the curves. The improvement rate is thus 33.3%. Pre- and post-intervention paired t test showed that $p = 0.0032$, which was statistically very significant (**Table 2**).

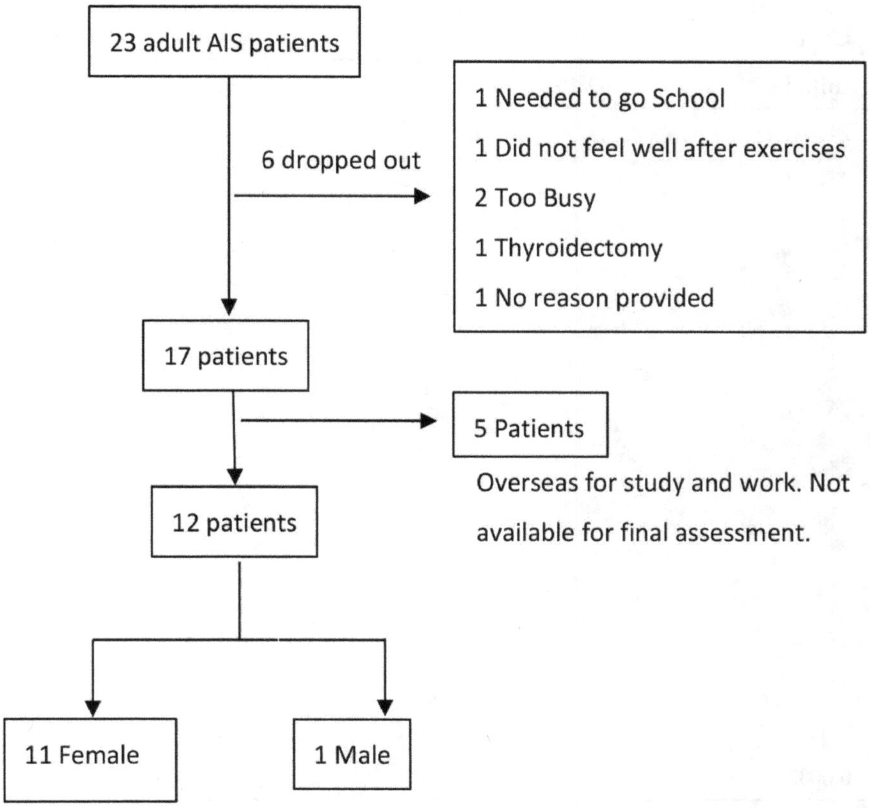

Figure 2. The flowchart of adult scoliosis patients.

Patient	Age	Sex	S/C	Range of curve		Apex		Types of scoliosis
				Initial	9 months	Initial	9 months	
1	24	F	L	T11-L4	T10-L4	L2	L2	AIS
2	56	F	L	L1-L4	L1-L4	L3	L3	AIS+DLS
3	51	F	L	L2-L5	L1-L4	L3	L2	AIS
4	58	F	L	T12-L4	L1-L4	L2	L2-L3	DLS
5	41	F	L	L1-L4	L1-L4	L3	L3	AIS
6	61	F	L	T12-L4	T12-L4	L2	L2	AIS
7	70	F	R	T12-L3	T12-L4	L2	L2	DLS
8	43	F	R	T10-L4	T10-L4	L2	L1	AIS
9	31	F	L	T11-L4	T10-L4	L1	T12	AIS
10	24	M	L	L1-L4	L1-L4	L3	L3	AIS
11	37	F	R	T12-L4	T12-L4	L1	L1	AIS
12	55	F	L	T12-L4	T12-L4	L2	L2	AIS
Mean	45.9							
SD	15							

S/C, side of convexity; AIS, adult idiopathic scoliosis; DLS, degenerative lumbar scoliosis.

Table 1. The age, sex, and the curve characteristics of the subjects.

Subjects	Cobb angle (°)			Coronal offset (mm)	
	Initial	9 months	Change	Initial	9 months
1	24	23	−1	6.8	3.6
2	43	33	−10	−8.8	−10.8
3	24	23.5	−0.5	2.3	3.8
4	43	31.5	−11.5	1.9	−7.6
5	28	24	−4	7.1	6
6	21	20	−1	−1	−1.4
7	26	23	−3	−2.7	−4.6
8	42	36	−6	−10.5	−11.7
9	42	37	−5	7.2	9.1
10	27	20	−7	4.1	−0.5
11	17	16	−1	−2.8	−2.3
12	37	37	0	11.6	10
Mean	31.17	27	−4.17	5.57	4.6
SD	9.58	7.4	3.84	3.58	5.5
P-value	0.0032*			0.35	

* Statistical significance.

Table 2. The Cobb angle and the coronal offset (the distance between the centre of C7 from the central sacral line) at baseline and conclusion of the study .

3.2. Coronal offset

Seven curves had C7 offset to the left of CSL and 5 had offset to the right at baseline. After 9 months, four subjects in the former group had reduced coronal imbalance and three had increased coronal imbalance (**Figure 3**). For the latter group, four had an increase in coronal imbalance and only one had an improved coronal balance. The change in coronal offset, however, was not statistically significant (**Table 2**).

3.3. ATR measurement

Ten subjects had improvement of ATR after the program. Statistically, there was a significant difference between the baseline and post-intervention measurements (p = 0.0115) (**Table 3**).

The reduction of ATR during RAB in a forward bending position was more marked, at 2.08 ± 1.83° after the 9 months of training (**Table 3**). The difference was statistically very significant, with p = 0.0023.

3.4. T4-12 kyphosis, L1-S1 lumbar lordosis, T10-L2 kyphosis

In general, there was a trend toward a reduction in thoracic kyphosis. The change in lumbar lordosis and thoracolumbar kyphosis was not statistically significant (**Table 4**).

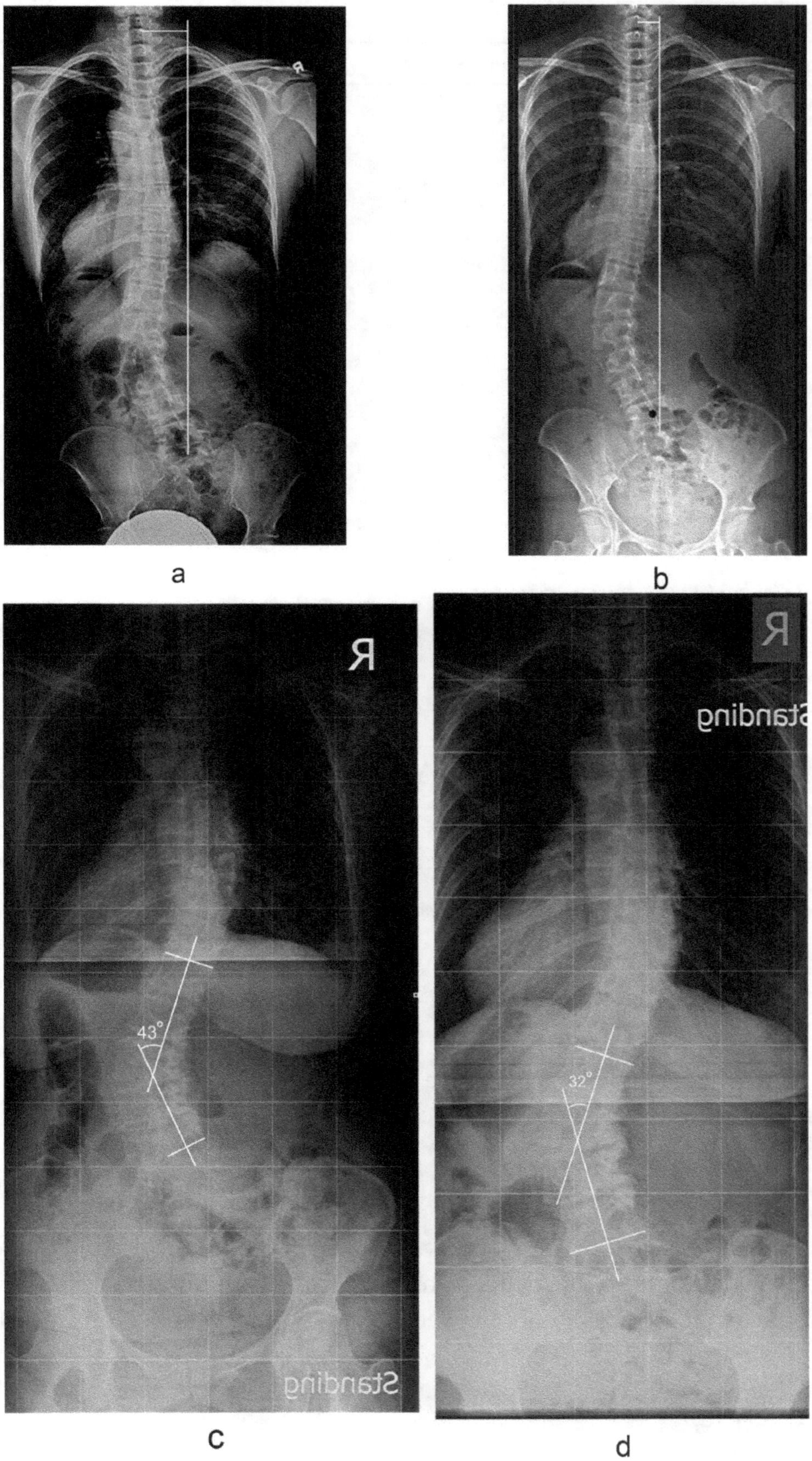

Figure 3. Posteroanterior full spine X-rays of a patient pre-intervention (a) and (b) post-intervention. It is noteworthy that her coronal balance improved. (c and d) The pre- and post-intervention X-rays of another patient, and the improvement of Cobb angle was noted.

	ATR°		ATR° in rotational angular breathing	
	Baseline	**9 months**	**Baseline**	**9 months**
1	7	5	4	0
2	21	21	19	15
3	11	10	8	5
4	13	9	10	6
5	10	9	7	6
6	9	11	6	7
7	12	11	9	7
8	16	13	9	9
9	21	19	18	17
10	6	4	2	2
11	5	1	4	0
12	23	15	16	13
Mean	12.83	10.67	9.33	7.25
SD	6.15	5.85	5.6	5.5
P-value		0.0115*		0.0023*

*Statistical significance.

Table 3. Angle of trunk rotation (ATR) in normal and rotational angular breathing at baseline and conclusion of the study.

3.5. Sacral slope

Interestingly, 9 of 12 patients had an increase in sacral slope (**Table 4**). The post- and pre-intervention difference was statistically significant with $p < 0.030$.

3.6. Pelvic tilt

As the sacral slope increased, the extent of pelvic tilt would reduce, as the sum of sacral slope and pelvic tilt is equal to pelvic incidence, which is a constant (**Table 4**). Nine patients had a reduction in pelvic tilt. The difference between post- and pre-intervention was statistically very significant at $p < 0.0032$.

3.7. Sagittal vertical axis

After 9 months, the global sagittal balance of the spine improved, with reduction of the antero-posterior truncal shift toward a more neutral position. The post- and pre-intervention difference was statistically significant at $p < 0.032$ (**Table 4**).

Patient	T4-12 kyphosis°		L1-5 lordosis°		T10-L2 kyphosis°		SS°		SVA (mm)		PI°		PT°		PI-LL°	
	B	9 months	B	9 months	B	9 months	B	9 months	B	9 months	B	9 months	B	9 months	B	9 months
1	45	41	45	46	6	4	23	25	−45	−42.5	42	40	19	15	−3	−6
2	8	1	4	12	51	55	17	23	108.7	67.3	62	64	45	41	58	52
3	42	41	28	28	30	31	15	18	85.3	26.3	33	32	18	14	5	4
4	11	25	32	43	−22	−21	21	33	−8.3	−6.1	44	47	23	14	12	4
5	17	6	33	32	12	7	36	45	30	−14	62	65	26	20	29	33
6	60	37	48	47	1	2	31	32	−12	−11.3	52	54	21	22	4	7
7	32	19	10	24	20	27	17	22	23.5	0	35	32	18	10	25	8
8	42	39	48	54	−16	−19	20	25	−46	−42.4	33	31	13	6	−15	−23
9	32	27	42	36	16	30	23	30	−32.8	−61.9	42	45	19	15	0	9
10	49	46	40	39	15	20	35	32	−22.1	0	52	48	17	16	12	9
11	13	18	48	50	−38	−18	38	33	2.7	−4.8	54	52	16	19	6	2
12	32	22	33	36	11	19	28	28	38	0	33	30	5	2	0	−6
Mean	31.9	26.8	34.3	37.3	7.2	11.4	25.3	28.8	10.2	−7.5	45.3	45.0	20.0	16.2	11.1	7.8
SD	16.6	14.4	14.5	12	23.8	23.4	8	7	49.2	33.5	10.9	12.4	9.4	9.7	1.9	1.9
p	0.083		0.097		0.066		0.03*		0.032*		0.68		0.0032*		0.114	

Subj, subjects; B, baseline; SS, sacral slope; SVA, sagittal vertical axis; PI, pelvic incidence; PT, pelvic tilt; PI-LL, pelvic incidence minus lumbar lordosis. Except for SVA, all measurements were in degrees.

* Statistical significance.

Table 4. The pre- and post-intervention spinopelvic and global sagittal balance measurements .

Domains	Period	Subjects												Mean	SD	P-value
		1	2	3	4	5	6	7	8	9	10	11	12			
Function	Initial	4.4	3.6	4	3.8	3.6	3.6	4.2	4.4	4.4	4.6	4	4.2	4.07	0.36	0.49
	9 mths	4.6	2.8	4.6	3.8	4	3.8	4	5	5	4.8	4.2	4.4	4.17	0.61	
Pain	Initial	4.2	2.6	3	4	3.2	3.8	5	4.2	4.2	4.8	3.4	3.3	3.81	0.73	0.19
	9 mths	4.4	2.5	4.4	4.4	3.6	3.5	4.6	4.4	5	4	3.6	4.3	4.06	0.67	
Self-image	Initial	3.2	2.6	2.6	3	2.8	3	3.8	3.2	3.2	3	3.2	2.6	3.02	0.35	0.001*
	9 mths	3.6	2.4	4.2	4	3	3.4	4.2	3.6	3.8	3.8	3.6	3.4	3.58	0.51	
Mental health	Initial	4.2	3	3.4	4	3.2	4	4.4	3.8	3.6	4.4	4	2.6	3.72	0.57	0.04*
	9 mths	4.2	3	4.6	4.4	4	4	4.8	4.6	4.6	4.6	4.4	1.8	4.08	0.86	
Satisfaction/ dissatisfaction	Initial	4.5	4.5	4.5	3	4.5	3.5	4	3.5	4	4	3	2	3.42	1.33	0.018*
	9 mths	4.5	4.5	5	4.5	4	4.5	4.5	4	4	4.5	4.5	4.5	4.42	0.29	
Total score	Initial	4	3.1	3.4	3.6	3.3	3.6	4.1	3.9	3.9	4.2	3.6	3.1	3.65	0.38	0.0016*
	9 mths	4.2	2.9	4.5	4.2	3.7	3.8	4.4	4.4	4.5	4.3	4	3.5	4.03	0.48	

Mths, months.

* Statistical significance

Table 5. The SRS-22 Score of the subjects pre- and post-intervention.

3.8. SRS-22

Comparing the baseline and the results at 9th month showed that there was no significant difference of scores in the function and pain domains (**Table 5**). There were, however, significant difference of scores for the self-image ($p = 0.001$), mental health ($p = 0.004$), and satisfaction/dissatisfaction domains (0.018). The difference in SRS-22 total score was also statistically different ($p = 0.0016$).

4. Discussion

Overall, 9 months of home-based Schroth exercises significantly improved the Cobb angle, the ATR, the ATR during RAB, the sacral slope, the pelvic tilt, the sagittal vertical axis as well as SRS-22 scores.

4.1. Cobb angle

The SBP exercise improved the Cobb angle very significantly. This is consistent with previous findings [17, 20, 21, 31, 32] in AIS patients. Curves of adult AIS patients can be reduced through multi-modal rehabilitation approaches [13, 14, 16]. SEAS (Scientific Exercise Approach to Scoliosis Exercises) [15, 17], Schroth [18] and side shift exercises [31] have been reported to reduce curve severity in adult AIS patients. Negrini et al. reported an adult AIS female, aged 25 with a double curve, treated by SEAS for 1 year. The main lumbar curve reduced from 47 to 28.5° [15]. Similarly, Yang et al. reported an AIS adult female with thoracic Cobb angle of 20.51°, treated by stretching, SBP, and strengthening exercises. In 8 weeks, the Cobb angle reduced to 16.35° [18]. Side shift exercises were also reported to reduce the Cobb angle of 69 patients with a mean age of 16.3 years. After an average follow up of 4.2 years, the mean Cobb angle reduced from 31.5 to 30.3° [31]. A retrospective cohort study also showed that curves of adult AIS patients can be reduced through SEAS. After 2 years of intervention, 68% experienced an improvement which averaged 4.6°. On average, the thoracolumbar curve reduced by 3° and the lumbar curve reduced by 3.6°. The improvement, however, was not statistically significant [17]. In comparison, our results showed that the improvement rate was 33.3%, when 6° curve reduction was regarded as an improvement. The average improvement was 4.2°. The findings closely matched that of the study by Negrini et al. [17]. It has, however, to be noted that not all of the patients in the present study had adult AIS.

Interestingly, nonscoliosis specific exercises have also been found to improve the Cobb angle in AIS and DLS patients [32]. Fishman et al. found that performing side plank yoga pose with the curve convexity facing downwards, for as long as possible once daily for 3–22 months resulted in an improvement of the Cobb angle [32]. The side plank yoga pose improved the Cobb angle in the 12 patients with DLS, from an average of 50.4–33.1° [32]. Yet, the study has a number of weaknesses and limitations. The study included patients with Cobb angle as small as 6°. Strictly speaking, these patients should not be regarded as suffering from scoliosis. Also, a reduction of 3° Cobb was regarded as improvement, though curve improvement is defined as a reduction of 6° Cobb angle [30].

4.2. Coronal offset

Glassman et al., in a study in 2005, showed that a coronal imbalance of 4 cm is associated with deterioration of pain and function scores in unoperated patients [12]. Similarly, Ploumis et al. showed that a coronal imbalance of 5cm is associated with a reduction in functionality [33]. Also, trunk shift is a predictor of surgery for patients with thoracolumbar and lumbar curvatures [34]. Lafage et al., however, showed no correlation between clinical outcomes and coronal global balance [35]. The magnitude of the coronal deformity did not impact pain and disability [35].

In the present cohort, the largest coronal offset was only 11.6 mm at baseline (**Table 2**). At ninth month, seven patients had an increase in coronal imbalance but five had an improvement. Yet, the change was small and was possibly clinically insignificant. The worsening of the coronal imbalance in some of the subjects is believed to be a result of the compensation to realign the spine by reducing the Cobb angle. The increase did not reach statistical significance.

4.3. Angle of trunk rotation

The change in ATR was statistically significant. On average, the reduction was only 2.2°. This is less than that previously reported in AIS patients, which averaged 3–4° [20, 36]. The difference between our study and others may be related to the fact that their subjects were adolescents and had better spinal flexibility than the present cohort.

The difference in ATR when performing RAB in forward flexion between baseline and at ninth month was statistically very significant ($p = 0.0023$). After 9 months of home-based training, the ATR during RAB reduced from a mean of 9.3–7.3°. The decrease of 2° is consistent with the findings by Borysov and Borysov in much younger patients [20].

We are not aware of any study that measured the ATR changes in adult scoliosis patients after performing PSSE and are therefore unable to make any comparison.

4.4. Sagittal balance and alignment

In recent years, the spinopelvic parameters and sagittal spinal balance have been found to be more important than the coronal curves in relation to clinical outcomes [26, 37–39]. Glassman et al. evaluated the relationships between radiographic parameters and health status. They found that the severity of symptoms is linearly related to the extent of sagittal spinal imbalance [29]. Anterior translation of the trunk, with the SVA in excess of 7 cm is associated with an increase in clinical symptoms [29]. Similarly, Lafage et al. showed a correlation between the SVA and Scoliosis Research Society (SRS) total scores and Oswestry Disability Index (ODI) [35]. Schwab et al. found that a SVA in excess of 47 mm, in combination with a pelvic tilt in excess of 22° and pelvic incidence-lumbar lordosis (PI-LL) mismatch in excess of 11° was closely correlated with disability [40].

The present study showed that SBP exercises did not impact the thoracic kyphosis and lumbar lordosis significantly. The findings concurred with previous findings [41, 42] in AIS patients. Weiss and Klein found that the Physio-logic® program did not improve the thoracic kyphosis [42] and Noh et al. found that Schroth exercises did not improve the thoracic kyphosis and lumbar lordosis [41]. The findings are not unexpected, in view of the fact that the spine of adult scoliosis patients is generally more rigid than that of AIS patients and improvement of curves is less likely.

Yet, the present study found that SBP exercises increased the sacral slope, decreased the pelvic tilt, and improved the SVA significantly (**Table 4**). It is noteworthy that the improvement involved two of the three key radiographic parameters correlated with disabilities [40]. At baseline, the mean sacral slope was 25.3°, which is lower than the mean sacral slope of 39 and 40.9° reported in normal volunteers by Troyanovich et al. and Duval-Beaupere et al., respectively [43, 44]. Our results, however, compared well with the results reported by Iida et al. in adult scoliosis patients. They reported a sacral slope of 26.6° of the DLS patients group and 27.5° for the adult AIS group, respectively [9]. Yang et al. reported a mean sacral slope of 32° in the 99 adult patients with spinal deformities (ASD) with a median age of 67 years [45]. The difference between our data and that of other studies may be related to the magnitude of the scoliosis [9, 45], as progression of lumbar scoliosis has been found to reduce the sacral slope [35, 46].

Duval-Beaupere et al. suggested that a reduction in sacral slope reduced the stability of the pelvis [47]. At the conclusion of the study, the sacral slope increased significantly from a mean of 25.3–28.8°, suggesting that the intervention may improve the stability of the pelvis requiring less hip extensor activity to maintain balance [47].

The pelvic tilt reduced from 20 to 16.2° post intervention. The difference was statistically significant. A study has shown that a pelvic tilt angle of above 22° correlated with disability [43]. Similarly, a number of studies have shown that a large pelvic tit is associated with increased pain and decreased function [35, 38]. A study which analyzed the pre and post-operative differences in spinopelvic parameters and their relationship to postoperative pain showed that patients with a larger postoperative pelvic tilt were likely to have postoperative residual pain than patients with a smaller postoperative pelvic tilt [38]. Similarly, Lafage et al. showed clear evidence that an increased pelvic tilt was associated with increased pain and decreased function [35]. Thus, the reduction of pelvic tilt after intervention may be associated with a better clinical outcome.

PI-LL mismatch has also been found to strongly correlate with disability [40]. A mismatch suggests that the lumbar lordosis does not compensate adequately [40]. The mismatch is clinically significant when it is in excess of 10°. At baseline, 5 had PI-LL mismatch, whereas after 9 months, only 2 had any significant PI-LL mismatch. Yet, the pre- and post-intervention differences were not statistically significant.

Positive sagittal spinal imbalance has also been found to correlate with the severity of symptoms and disability [29, 40]. Duval-Beaupere et al. showed that an anterior translation of the center of gravity in excess of 30 mm in front of the coxofemoral joints require the contraction of the hip extensors for balance [44]. This may be related to the increase in symptoms in patients with positive sagittal spinal imbalance. In the present study, it was shown that the SVA reduced significantly after intervention, suggesting that the patients had an improved global sagittal spinal balance. This may be clinically significant as Schwab et al. showed that a SVA in excess of 47 mm correlated with disability [40].

4.5. SRS-22

Glassman et al. showed that patients with thoracolumbar and lumbar curves tended to have a lower pain and function scores as compared to those with thoracic curves [12, 29]. The present study showed that the exercises tended to increase the SRS pain domain scores, but the pre- and post-intervention difference was not statistically significant. This might be due to the fact that most of the patients did not have marked pain at baseline. It was possible that most of the subjects had adult idiopathic scoliosis, which was not as disabling or painful as those with DLS [45].

The SRS-22 self-image ($p = 0.001$) and mental health ($p = 0.04$) scores, however significantly improved after the 9 months of scoliosis pattern specific exercises. The improvement in self-image is unlikely to be a result of the change of the subject's perspective [48] as the study spanned over a few months. The improvement in self-image is important as studies [48, 49] have shown that operated AIS patients and adult patients with thoracolumbar and lumbar curves had lower SRS-22 self-image scores, as compared to nonoperated group [48]. Pizones et al. found that the surgical cohort had worse SRS-22 scores in all domains with mean values under 3.1 points (range = 2.4–3.1), as compared to the conservatively treated cohort [4]. In our study, there was a significant improvement in the scores in the self-image domain. Seven subjects had scores below 3.1 points before the intervention, but after the program, only two had scores below 3.1 points. Also, the improvement of SRS-22 self-image and satisfaction scores exceeded 0.4, which is regarded as the minimal clinical important difference relating to SRS-22r (refined) in surgically treated adults with spinal deformity [50]. Improvement of the self-image may reduce the drive for surgical intervention.

4.6. Clinical implications

This preliminary study showed that SBP exercises improved the Cobb angles, sagittal spinal balance, and some SRS-22 domain scores in adult patients with thoracolumbar and lumbar curves. In view of the fact that curves of ASD and DLS progress and that the present nonoperative treatments addressing adult scoliosis patients with low back pain are not effective, the authors believe it is worthwhile implementing SBP exercises in conjunction with standard medical or physiotherapeutic treatments on adult scoliosis patients with risk of progression, particularly when the patients have lumbar curves in excess of 30°, AVR ≥ 33%,, thoracolumbar kyphosis, and positive sagittal spinal imbalance [29, 40]. A low intercristal line is also a risk factor [6]. When the line joining both iliac crests lies below the L4/5 level, L4 is more mobile and prone to instability and translation.

4.7. Limitations

The study has a number of weaknesses. The small sample size reduced the statistical power of the study. Also, the group was not homogeneous, with different degrees of degenerative changes in the lumbar spine. This would confound the outcome, as subjects with more flexible spines are expected to have better improvement. Also, it was difficult to ensure that patients followed the exercises protocol strictly at home.

Further studies are required to elucidate whether SBP positively influences the thoracolum bar and lumbar curves in adult scoliosis patients, particularly those with curves that are susceptible to progression and whether SBP when combined with the standard conservative treatments improve their effectiveness.

5. Conclusion

The study showed that out-patient Schroth Best Practice© exercises statistically significantly improved the Cobb angles, the sacral slope, the pelvic tilt, and SVA as well as the SRS-22 self-image and mental health domain scores in adult scoliosis patients with thoracolumbar and lumbar curves. Yet, in view of the small sample size and the weak power of the study, it is suggested that further studies be conducted to investigate whether SBP exercises are effective for the treatment of adult scoliosis patients with thoracolumbar and lumbar curves.

Acknowledgements

All the authors are grateful to Professor Josette Bettany-Saltikov for her review and construc tive comments of the manuscript.

Author details

Shu-Yan Ng[1]*, Wing-Yan Chan[2], Tsz-Ki Ho[2] and Yin-Ling Ng[2]

*Address all correspondence to: ngshuyanhcc@gmail.com

1 Wanchai Chiropractic Clinic, Wanchai, Hong Kong

2 Spine Technology Ltd, Wanchai, Hong Kong

References

[1] Hong JY, Suh SW, Modi HN, Hur CY, Song HR, Park JH. The prevalence and radiological findings in 1347 elderly patients with scoliosis. J Bone Joint Surg Br. 2010; **92**(7):980.

[2] Urrutia J, Diaz-Ledezma C, Espinosa J, Berven SH. Lumbar scoliosis in postmenopausal women: Prevalence and relationship with bone density, age, and body mass index. Spine (Phila Pa 1976). 2011 Apr 20; **36**(9):737-40.

[3] Jimbo S, Kobayashi T, Aono K, Atsuta Y, Matsuno T. Epidemiology of degenerative lumbar scoliosis: A community-based cohort study. Spine (Phila Pa 1976). 2012 Sep 15; **37**(20):1763-70.

[4] Pizones J, Martin-Buitrago MP, Perez-Gruesco JS et al. Function and clinical symptoms are main factors that motivate thoracolumbar adult scoliosis patients to pursue surgery. Spine 2017; **42**(1);E31-E36.

[5] Schwab F, Farcy JP, Bridwell K et al. A clinical impact classification of scoliosis in the adult. Spine. 2006; **3**:2109-2114.

[6] Weinstein SL, Ponseti IV: Curve progression in idiopathic scoliosis. J Bone Joint Surg Am. 1983; **65**(4): 447-455.

[7] Ascani E, Bartolozzi P, Logroscino CA, et al: Natural history of untreated idiopathic scoliosis after skeletal maturity. Spine (Phila, Pa, 1976). 1986; **11**(8):784-789.

[8] Marty-Poumarat C, Scattin L, Marpeau M, Garreau de Loubresse C, Aegerter P. Natural history of progressive adult scoliosis. Spine. 2007; **32**(11):1227-1234.

[9] Iida T, Ohyama Y, Katayanagi J, Ato A, Mine K, Matsumoto K et al. Differences between pre-existing type and de novo type left convex thoracolumbar/lumbar scoliosis. Scoliosis. 2015; **10**(2):S6.

[10] Kluba T, Dikmenli G, Dietz K, Giehl JP, Niemeyer T. Comparison of surgical and conservative treatment for degenerative lumbar scoliosis. Arch Orthop Trauma Surg. 2009; **129**:1-5.

[11] Everett CR, Patel RK. A systematic literature review of nonsurgical treatment in adult scoliosis. Spine (Phila PA 1976). 2007; **32**(19); S130–S134.

[12] Glassman SD, Berven S, Bridwell K, Horton W, Dimar JR. Correlation of radiographic parameters and clinical symptoms in adult scoliosis. Spine. 2005; **30**:682-688.

[13] Morningstar MW, Woggon D, Lawrence G. Scoliosis treatment sing a combination of manipulative and rehabilitative therapy: A retrospective case series. BMC Musculoskelet Disord. 2004; **5**:32.

[14] Morningstar MW, Joy T. Scoliosis treatment using spinal manipulation and the Pettibon Weighting System™: A summary of 3 atypical presentations. Chiropr Osteopathy. 2006; **14**:1.

[15] Negrini A, Parzini S, Negrini MG, Romano M, Atanasio S, Zaina F, Negrini S. Adult scoliosis can be reduced through specific SEAS exercises: A case report. Scoliosis. 2008; **3**:20.

[16] Morningstar MW. Outcomes for adult scoliosis patients receiving chiropractic rehabilitation: A 24-month retrospective analysis. J Chiropr Med. 2011; **10**:179-184.

[17] Negrini A, Negrini MG, Donzelli S, Romano M, Zaina F, Negrini S. Scoliosis-Specific exercises can reduce the progression of severe curves in adult idiopathic scoliosis: A long-term cohort study. Scoliosis. 2015 Jul 11; **10**:20.

[18] Yang JM, Lee JH, Lee DH. Effects of consecutive application of stretching, Schroth, and strengthening exercises on Cobb's angle and the rib hump in an adult with idiopathic scoliosis. J Phys Ther Sci. 2015 Aug; **27**(8):2667-2669.

[19] Cheung KM, Senkoylu A, Alanay A, Genc Y, Lau S, Luk KD. Reliability and concurrent validity of the adapted Chinese version of Scoliosis Research Society-22 (SRS-22) questionnaire. Spine (Phila Pa 1976). 2007 May 1; **32**(10):1141-1145.

[20] Borysov M, Borysov A. Scoliosis short-term rehabilitation (SSTR) according to 'Best Practice' standards—are the results repeatable? Scoliosis. 2012 Jan 17; **7**(1):1

[21] Weiss HR, Lehnert-Schroth C, Moramarco M. Schroth Therapy: Advancements in Conservative Scoliosis Treatment. Lambert Publication, Saarbrucken, Germany 2015.

[22] Lehnert-Schroth C. Three dimensional Treatment for Scoliosis. Physiotherapeutic Method for Deformities of the Spine. Martindale Press, California; 2007.

[23] Monticone M, Ambrosini E, Cazzaniga D. Active self-correction and task-oriented exercises reduce spinal deformity and improve quality of life in subjects with mild adolescent idiopathic scoliosis. Results of a randomised controlled trial. Eur Spine J. 2014; **23**:1204-1214.

[24] Weiss HR, Moramarco MM, Borysov M, Ng SY, Lee SG, Nan X, Moramarco KA. Postural rehabilitation for adolescent idiopathic scoliosis during growth. Asian Spine J. 2016; **10**(3):570-581.

[25] Lafage R, Ferrero E, Henry JK, Challier V, Diebo D et al. Validation of a new computer-assisted tool to measure spino-pelvic parameters. Spine J. 2015; **15**(12):2493-2502.

[26] Mac-Thiong JM, Labelle H, Charlebois M, Huot MP, de Guise JA. Sagittal plane analysis of the spine and pelvis in adolescent idiopathic scoliosis according to the coronal curve type. Spine. 2003; **28**:1404-1409.

[27] Roussouly P, Gollogly S, Berthonnaud E, Dimnet J. Classification of the normal variation in the sagittal alignment of the human lumbar spine and pelvis in the standing position. Spine. 2005; **30**:346-353.

[28] Schwab F, el-Fegoun AB, Gamez L, Goodman H, Farcy JP. A lumbar classification of scoliosis in the adult patient: preliminary approach. Spine. 2005; **30**(14):1670-1673.

[29] Glassman SD, Bridwell K, Dimar JR, Horton W, Berven S, Schwab F. The impact of positive sagittal balance in adult spinal deformity. Spine. 2005; **30**(18):2024-2029.

[30] Negrini S, Atanasio S, Fusco C, Zaina F. Effectiveness of complete conservative treatment for adolescent idiopathic scoliosis (bracing and exercises) based on SOSORT management criteria: results according to the SRS criteria for bracing studies—SOSORT Award 2009 Winner. Scoliosis. 2009; **4**:19.

[31] Maruyama T, Kitagawal T, Takeshita K, Nakainura K. Side shift exercise for idiopathic scoliosis after skeletal maturity. Stud Health Technol Inform. 2002; **91**:361-364.

[32] Fishman LM, Groessl EJ,Sherman KJ. Serial case reporting yoga for idiopathic and degenerative scoliosis. Global Adv Health Med. 2014; **3**(5):16-21.

[33] Ploumis A, Liu H, Mehbod AA, et al. A correlation of radiographic and functional measurements in adult degenerative scoliosis. Spine. 2009; **34**:1581-1584.

[34] Smorgick Y, Mirovsky Y, Baker KC, Gelfer Y, Avisar E, Anekstein Y. Predictors of back pain in adolescent idiopathic scoliosis surgical candidates. J Pediatr Orthop. 2013; **33**(3):289-292.

[35] Lafage V, Schwab F, Patel A et al. Pelvic tilt and truncal inclination: two key radiographic parameters in the setting of adults with spinal deformity. Spine (Phila Pa 1976). 2009; **34**: E599-606.

[36] Moramarco M, Fadzan M, Moramarco K, Heller A, Righter S. The influence of short-term scoliosis-specific exercise rehabilitation on pulmonary function in patients with AIS. Curr Pediatr Rev. 2016; **12**:17-23.

[37] Li WS, Li G, Chen ZQ, et al. Sagittal plane analysis of the spine and pelvis in adult idiopathic scoliosis. Chin Med J. 2010; **123**:2978-2982.

[38] Savage JW, Patel AA. Fixed sagittal plane imbalance. Global Spine J. 2014; **4**:287-296.

[39] Lazennec JY, Ramare S, Arafati N, et al. Sagittal alignment in lumbosacral fusion: relations between radiological parameters and pain. Eur Spine J. 2000; **9**:47-55.

[40] Schwab F, Ungar B, Blondel B, et al. Scoliosis Research Society-Schwab adult spinal deformity classification: A validation study. Spine. 2012; **37**:1077-1082.

[41] Noh DK, You JH, Koh JH, Kim H, Kim D, Ko SM, Shin JY. Effects of novel corrective spinal technique on adolescent idiopathic scoliosis as assessed by radiographic imaging. J Back Musculoskelet Rehabil. 2014; **27**:331-338.

[42] Weiss HR, Klein R. Improving excellence in scoliosis rehabilitation: A controlled study of matched pairs. Pediatr Rehabil. 2006; **9**(3):190-200.

[43] Schwab FJ, Blondel B, Bess S, Hostin R, Shaffrey CI et al. Radiographical spinopelvic parameters and disability in the setting of adult spinal deformity: A prospective multicenter analysis. Spine (Phila Pa 1976). 2013 Jun 1; **38**(13):E803-12.

[44] Troyanovich SJ, Cailliet R, Janik TJ, Harrison DD, Harrison DE. Radiographic mensuration characteristics of the sagittal lumbar spine from a normal population with a method to synthesize prior studies of lordosis. J Spinal Disord. 1997; **10**(5):380-386.

[45] Duval-Beaupére G, Schmidt C, Cosson P. A barycentremetric study of the sagittal shape of spine and pelvis: The conditions required for an economic standing position. Ann Biomed Eng. 1992; **20**:451-462.

[46] Yang C, Yang M, Chen Y, Wei X, Ni H et al. Radiographic parameters in adult degenerative scoliosis and different parameters between sagittal balanced and imbalanced ADS patients. Medicine (Baltimore). 2015; **94**(29):1198.

[47] Wang H, Ma L, Yang DL, Ding WY, Shen Y et al. Radiological analysis of degenerative lumbar scoliosis in relation to pelvic incidence. Int J Clin Exp Med. 2015 Dec 15; **8**(12):22345-22351.

[48] Duval-Beaupere G, Marty C, Barthel F, Boiseaubert B, Boulay Ch et al. Sagittal profile of the spine prominent part of the pelvis. Stud Health Technol Inform. 2002; **88**:47-64.

[49] Souder C, Newton PO, Shah SA, Lonner BS et al. Factors in surgical decision making for thoracolumbar/lumbar AIS: It's about more than just the curve magnitude. J Pediatr J. 2016 Mar 3.

[50] Crawford CH, Glassman SD, Bridwell KH, Berven SH, Carreon LY. The minimum clinically important difference in SRS-22R total score, appearance, activity and pain domains after surgical treatment of adult spinal deformity. Spine (Phila Pa 1976). 2015 Mar 15; **40**(6):377-381.

8

The Principles and Biomechanics of the Rigo Chêneau Type Brace

Grant I. Wood and Manuel Rigo

Abstract

All scoliosis braces bearing the name "Chêneau" as part or all of their designation share a common history, originating in 1979 with the Chêneau Toulouse Munster (CTM) brace, developed by Dr. Jacques Chêneau and Professor Matthias of Munster. Since then, several variations of this brace have evolved to enhance support/correction of scoliosis in three dimensions. Design features based on the Rigo classification of scoliosis and further modifications by the co-author led to the Rigo Chêneau type brace. This is a dynamic brace, with expansion rooms to accommodate tissue migration, growth and breathing movements. The brace by the authors is hand-made and customized to the curve pattern, skeletal maturity, flexibility and structural component of each individual. It applies both de-torsional forces and three-point pressure systems to improve spinal alignment in all three planes. It is also designed to work synergistically with Schroth physiotherapeutic scoliosis specific exercises to optimize effectiveness of a conservative approach.

Keywords: scoliosis bracing, Wood Chêneau Rigo (WCR) brace, Schroth physical therapy, Rigo Chêneau type brace, Rigo classification of scoliosis and brace design

1. Introduction

The purpose of this chapter is to share with scoliosis professionals the biomechanics and design of the Rigo Chêneau brace. A historical background of the Rigo Chêneau brace is provided to show the evolution and improvements in it over the last three decades, particularly changes outlined since 2005, which have led to good fit and function. Equally important to the end result is good patient follow-up care and brace quality control by the referring MD, physical therapist and orthotist.

The original brace was called the Chêneau Toulouse Munster (CTM) brace after Dr. Jacques Chêneau of Toulouse, France and Professor Matthias of Münster, Germany who first presented it in 1979. Later, the brace came to be known as the Chêneau brace. In 1996, Dr. Chêneau outlined the hand-casting procedures and discussed the three-curve and four-curve Chêneau brace types, outlines in his manual named "Orthese de Scoliose" [1, 6] which outlined the hand-casting procedures and discussed the three-curve and four-curve Chêneau brace types (**Figure 1**).

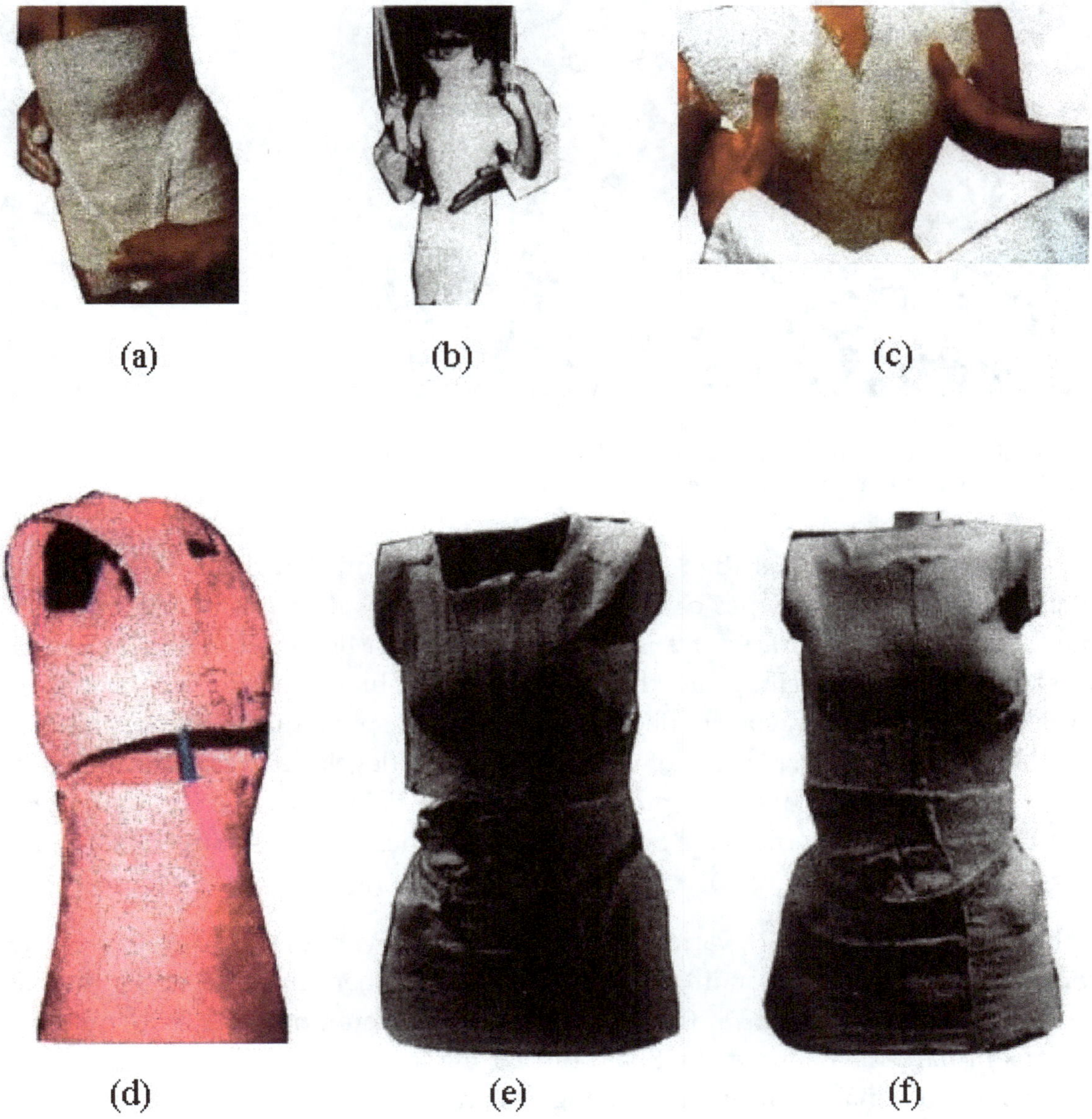

(a) (b) (c) (d) (e) (f)

Figure 1. The three-curve and four-curve casting technique for providing optimal fit at the iliac crests in (a) and (b). The orthotist elongates the patient by applying an extension force at the axillas in (c). The negative cast cut-and-position technique of correction and alignment of the Chêneau brace in (d)–(f) [6].

The original Chêneau brace had two brace designs. These were based on the curve classification from Katharina Schroth, which treated scoliosis as a three-curve pattern or four-curve pattern. Therefore, we had a three-curve Chêneau brace and the four-curve Chêneau brace (**Figure 2**).

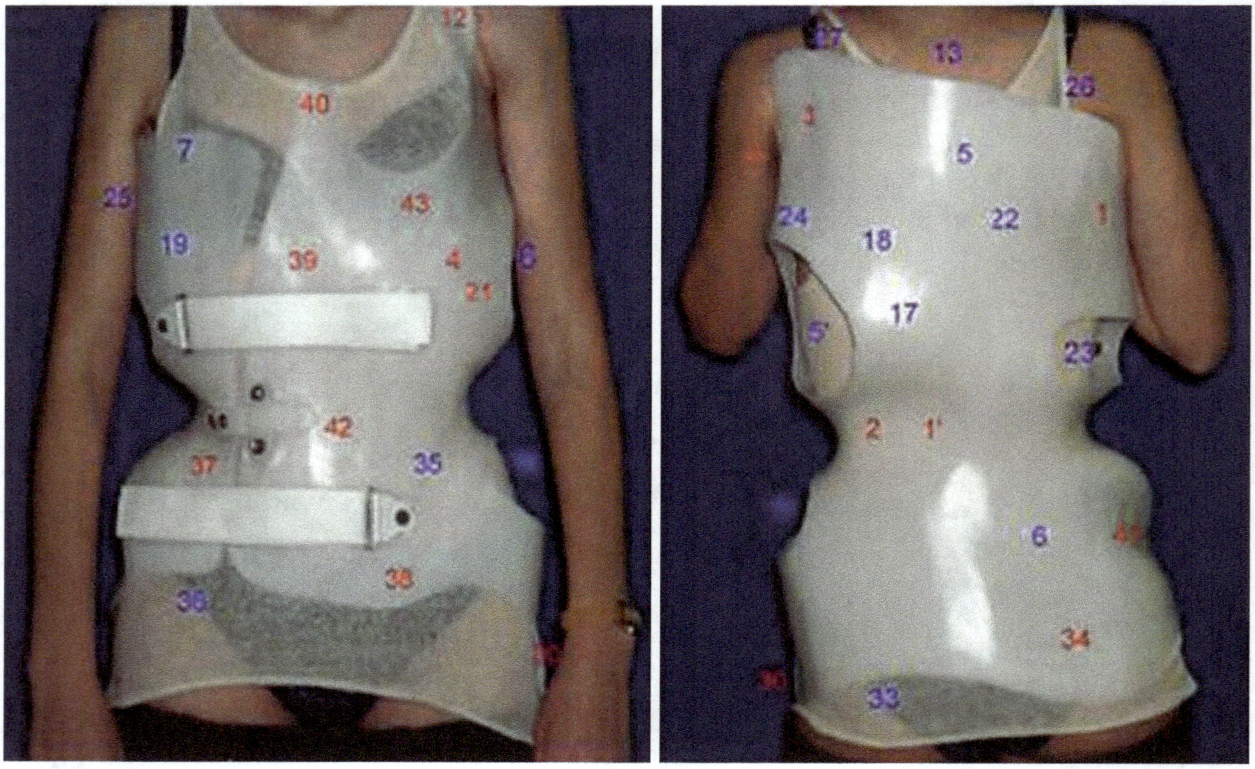

Figure 2. An old style, four-curve handmade Chêneau brace from 1999, Malaga, Spain. A numbering system was utilized by Dr. Chêneau to identify all the pressure and expansion areas [2].

In the late 1990s, Dr. Manuel Rigo (MR) of Barcelona found that these two designs were insufficient for the distinct types of curve patterns. As a result, the King classification was adapted for the Chêneau brace for a few years. However, MR found that there were brace failures with the King classification when it was used for brace design. The King classification was developed for surgeons to decide on the level of spinal fusion during surgery, and not specifically for bracing. Because of these failures, MR developed a classification to guide the brace design [3], which was first presented by MR et al. in 2010. This was presented later by Grant Wood at the International Society for Prosthetics and Orthotics (ISPO) of 2010 in Leipzig, Germany [4].

Since the original brace in 1979, various Chêneau brace derivatives were developed. The first author of this paper, GW, began in 1995 with the original Chêneau brace, under the training and teachings of Dr. Chêneau. Dr. Chêneau and Dr. Rigo were providing brace modification workshops in Barcelona and Sevilla Spain during the late 1990s. During these workshops, the shape of the original Chêneau brace changed significantly, mainly through modifications suggested by MR, including significant increases in the size and locations of plaster expansion zones and pressure areas. These modifications led to the familiar large flowing and asymmetrical shapes that are more commonly seen today.

In 2012, due to the wide range of brace standards and various levels of quality of Chêneau braces using the Rigo principles, GW, the main author, named his brace according to his own methodology and hand modifications aimed at addressing the complexities of the original design, and named the brace Wood Chêneau Rigo (WCR) brace.

The WCR brace evolved from the original Chêneau brace (1995), which was subsequently refined using the Rigo classification of scoliosis, and hand modifications aimed at addressing the complexities of the original design.

The WCR brace incorporated the best of modern CAD CAM and "old school" hand modifications. Generally speaking, technical advances in brace design and production have increased productivity, albeit at the cost of individualization to each patient's anatomy, curve pattern, and preferences, the lack of which can degrade the brace's fit and function. For this reason, the WCR brace has, since its inception in 1995, applied the most critical patient modifications by hand.

The differences between the original Chêneau brace and the author's Chêneau-Rigo handmade type brace are the following:

1. The brace was designed using the Rigo classification of scoliosis and brace design, incorporating many significant changes from the original Chêneau brace.
2. The new Chêneau brace follows the current design shapes taught by MR. Thus, it is a Chêneau-Rigo modern CAD CAM design brace in combination with handmade modifications.
3. The Wood Chêneau Rigo (WCR) brace is the author's personal version of the Chêneau-Rigo brace, and it represents the natural evolution of the original Chêneau brace.

In 2017, due to the multiplicity of versions and variations in the quality of the Rigo Chêneau type brace, Dr. Rigo, Grant Wood and Luke Stikeleather founded the Association of Rigo-Chêneau specialists (ARCS), which has the goal of maintaining and providing a standard of quality and education for orthotists who have practiced these principles.

The Rigo Chêneau type brace is a corrective orthotic device which must be individualized to each patient's specific curve pattern and other unique body characteristics.

It is not an orthopedic product but rather a corrective concept for the specific use in the conservative treatment of scoliosis.

A 3D scan or handmade cast is used to capture the patients exact body shape and anatomy. The scan or cast then produces a positive mold that is rectified to provide a 3D corrected positive mold, which in turn is used to adapt the thermoplastic to provide the finished brace.

Using the handmade original tech, a 3D corrected positive mold is created to provide specific pressure areas or pads of contact, and expansion areas or rooms. These pressure areas or pads have specific levels, orientations, depths and shapes. The pressure areas are generally located on the convexities and prominences of the scoliosis body. Contacts or pads are individually oriented in space and shaped to provide 3D correction (**Figure 3**).

The expansion areas, or rooms, are not windows where a simple hole is cut out of the plastic, but instead, actual buildups of significant space created in the original positive mold. They are generally located in the concavities and prominences of the scoliotic body. Expansion rooms are for tissue migration, growth and breathing movements, thus converting a rigid brace into a dynamic brace [5].

The Rigo Chêneau type brace is a thermoplastic brace with a ventral opening and Velcro closures. It follows many of the original 3D concepts of Dr Chêneau, and utilizes the Rigo classification of scoliosis and brace design.

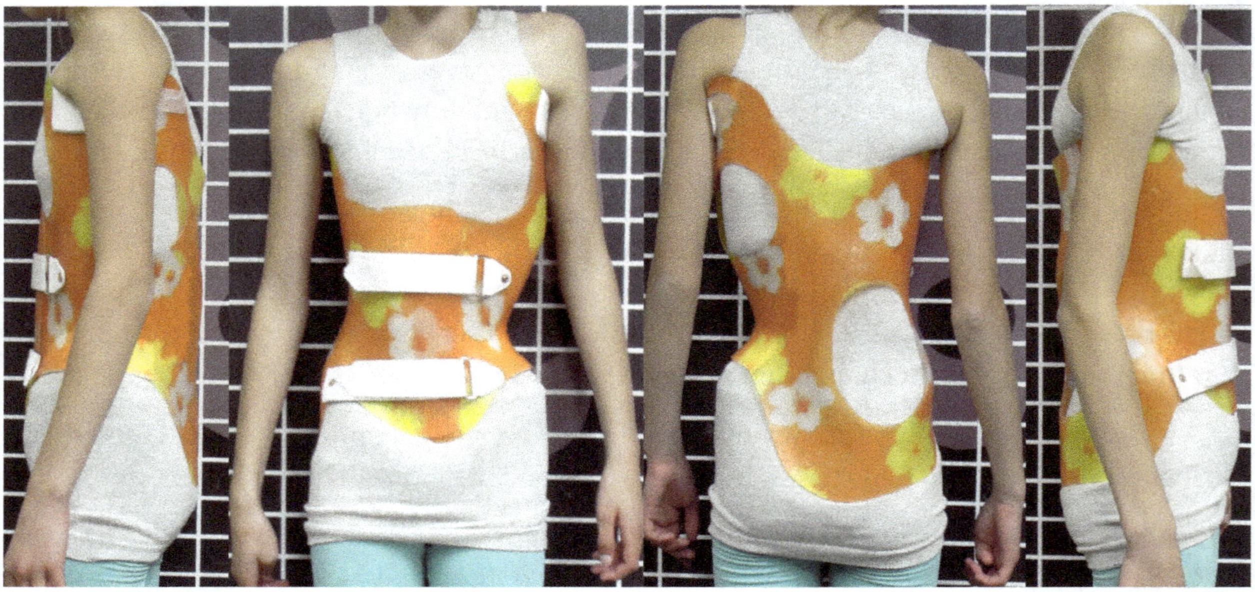

Figure 3. A WCR brace modified and fit by the main author, shows the left lateral, anterior, posterior and right lateral views of the patient with 3D correction in a C2 type brace using the Rigo classification of scoliosis [3].

2. Design and methods

This chapter reviews the biomechanics and breathomechanics of all three planes of the body. The transverse thoracic section demonstrates improvement of the thoracic hypokyphosis. The diagram of patient elongation describes how specific pressure points simultaneously provide for elongation, derotation and lateral curve correction. The pelvis and trunk translations are described, and shown to outline how the Rigo Chêneau brace overcorrects body posture to allow an improved clinical presentation for A-type, B-type, C-type and E-type Rigo classification brace types (**Figure 4**).

2.1. In-brace correction

There is a perception that the in-brace Cobb angle correction must be 50% to be considered acceptable. This is often true and it is also true that the Cobb angle, which is easily assessed, has been the gold standard of measurement for brace quality. However, not all patients can and/or should be corrected to 50% in-brace correction. In some cases, a 25% in-brace correction coupled with good 3D correction is acceptable and sufficient to prevent scoliosis progression, when greater Cobb angle correction would cause negative compensations. Overall, some patients are best served by targeting a low in-brace correction, whereas for others an 80% in-brace correction is both achievable and desirable (**Figure 5**).

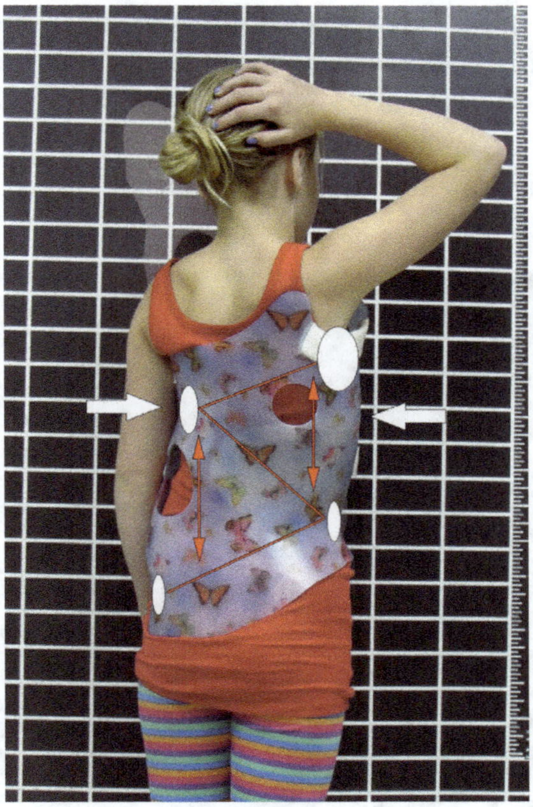

Figure 4. In-brace correction of the Cobb angle has been the gold standard for the measurement of successful bracing. This patient's curvature was reduced from pre-brace 21° Cobb angle to an in-brace Cobb angle of less than 5° in a Rigo Chêneau type brace. The pre-brace X-ray shows the pelvis translated to the left and the trunk to the right. The in-brace X-ray shows the pelvis corrected to the right and the trunk balance to the left.

These high and low targets for in-brace corrections depend on several factors, including the Rigo classification brace type, curve pattern, skeletal maturity, flexibility, and the structural component of the scoliosis, which limits correctability. This last factor is particularly important to the effectiveness of the Rigo Chêneau brace which is supposed to work through the detorsional forces and the amount of the mechanical torsion.

3D correction is defined.

1. Regional and local derotation in the transverse plane.
2. Three-point pressure systems for the best possible alignment and balance in the frontal plane (See **Figure 6**).
3. The best possible alignment and balance in the sagittal plane.
4. Reactive breathing mechanics to restore physiological thoracic kyphosis.

The expansion is noticeable and the volume depends on the body morphology. Expansion areas or rooms are not just to be there to be filled at the time but to define the orientation and shape of the contacts. An essential function of the brace design is to produce the right body reaction during breathing (**Figures 6** and **7**).

The orientation of the dorsal and ventral pads is different. The ventral pad is a little more frontally oriented compared with the dorsal pad which is a little more sagittal orientated. The two main forces can be combined into one main force vector. These vectors act as a pair of forces for derotation. The ventral component is always the major one, and the dorsal is the minor one. That way, the ribs and coupled spine will derotate and translate backwards (**Figure 8**).

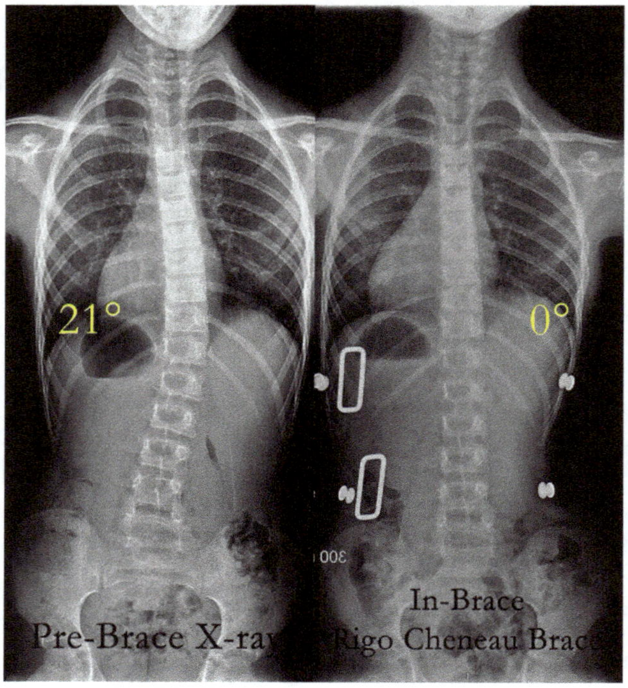

Figure 5. The transverse view of a Rigo Chêneau type brace, which was made for right thoracic and left lumbar curves. The light-colored line represents the thoracic expansion areas and the darker line represents the lumbar expansion areas.

2.2. Breathomechanics

The sagittal diameter increases during rotation, bringing the spine out, rounding the back, thus improving the morphological flatback.

The two forces need to be at the same transversal level to be effective. Ventral and dorsal prominences are for different transversal levels. Pushing on them is not enough to get correction.

The intention is to produce a better physiological shape, where the physiological shape in the sagittal plane is more or less pronounced, depending on the pelvic structure (i.e. the pelvic incidence) (**Figure 9**). The normalization of the sagittal configuration of the spine is not possible in most cases due to structural lordotization, and any kyphotizaton of the main thoracic region at the expense of spinal flexion will just increase the proximal and distal compensatory kyphosis.

With 3D corrections, the priorities are; first, to reduce the Cobb angle, second, to reduce rotation, and third, to reduce morphological flatback.

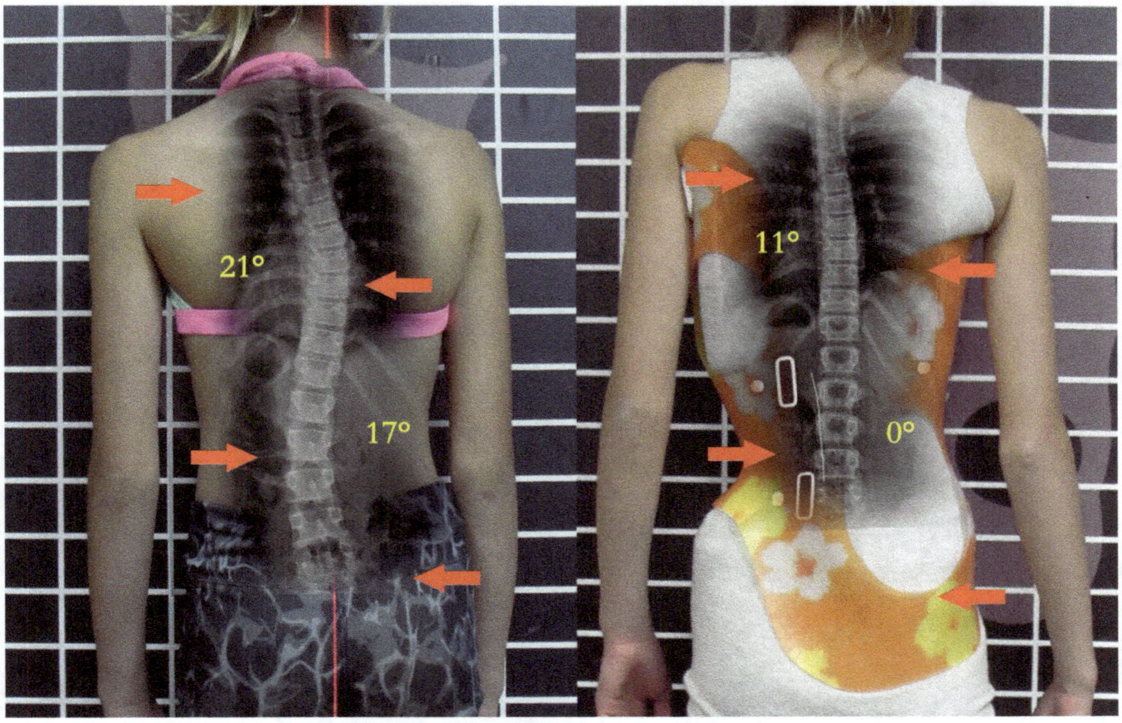

Figure 6. The transverse thoracic view of the thoracic section of a Rigo Chêneau type brace. Derotation of the spine at the thoracic level helps to achieve a more normal physiological sagittal profile of the spine to reduce flatback.

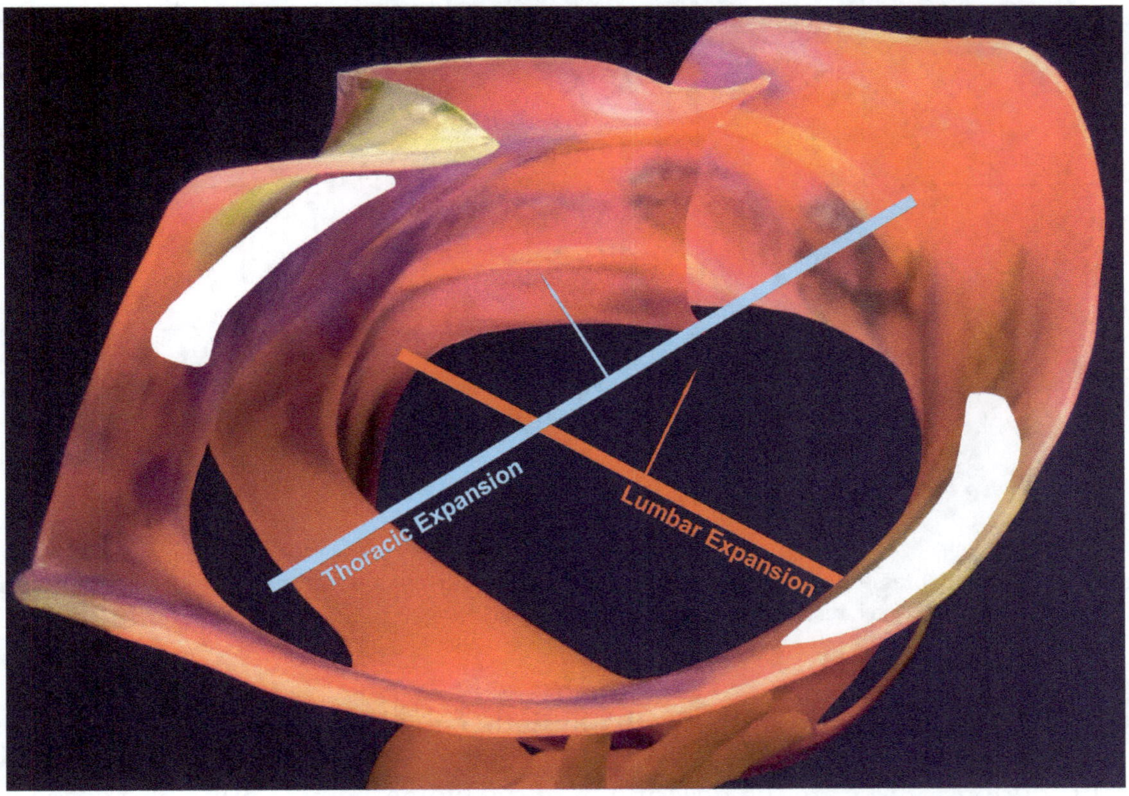

Figure 7. These forces are needed to bring the patient into optimal coronal plane correction through a corrective three-point pressure system and to bring the anterior prominence to a higher level.

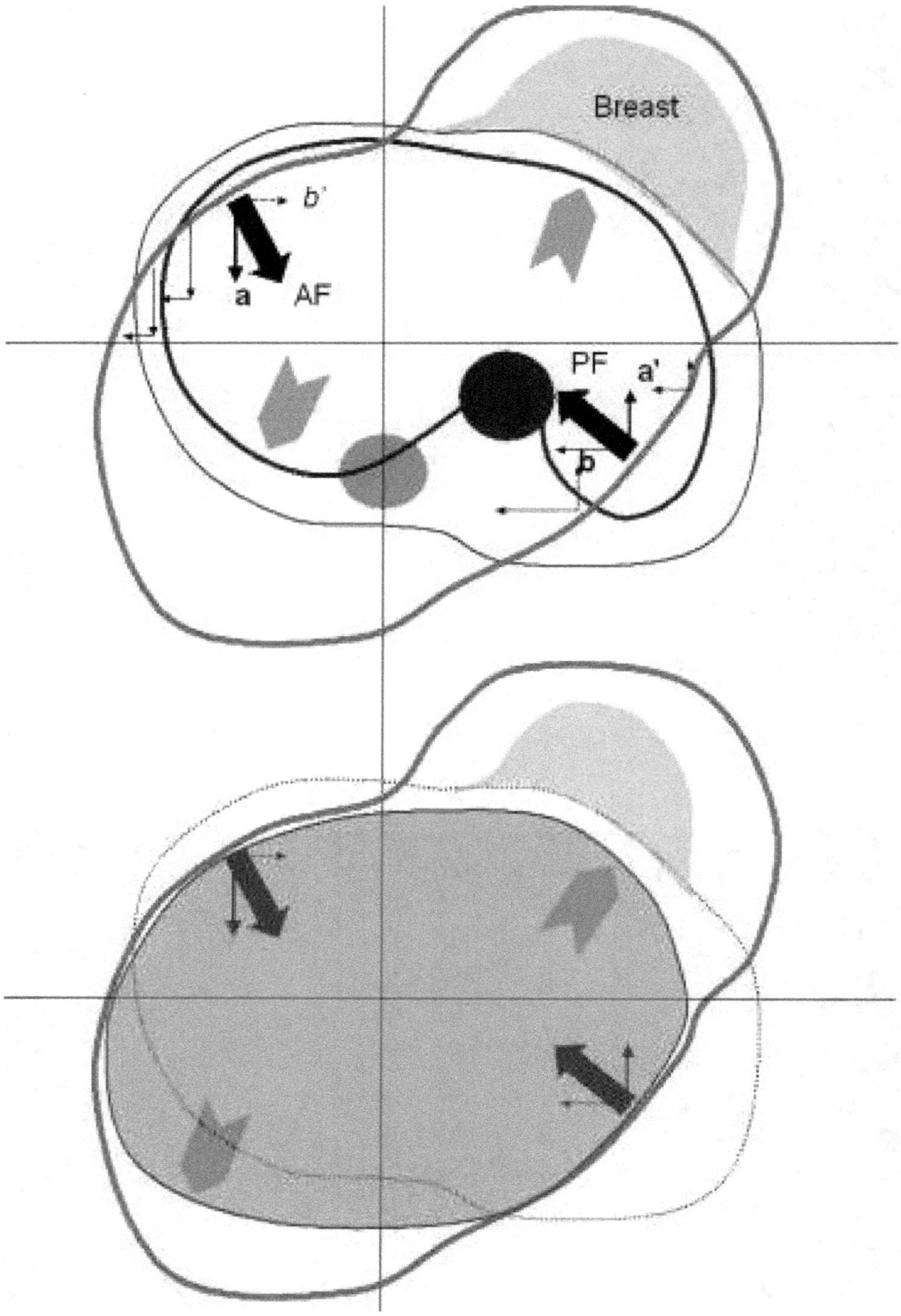

Figure 8. The three-point pressure system allows better frontal plane correction, improves collapse of ribs, and brings the ventral rib hump to higher level, resulting in elongation of the spine.

2.3. Rigo Chêneau type brace and Schroth physiotherapeutic scoliosis specific exercises

The contributions of MR are the description of the biomechanical principles of the brace design and a creation of the specific scoliosis classification developed to help to standardize the brace design and construction. This classification also correlates with Schroth

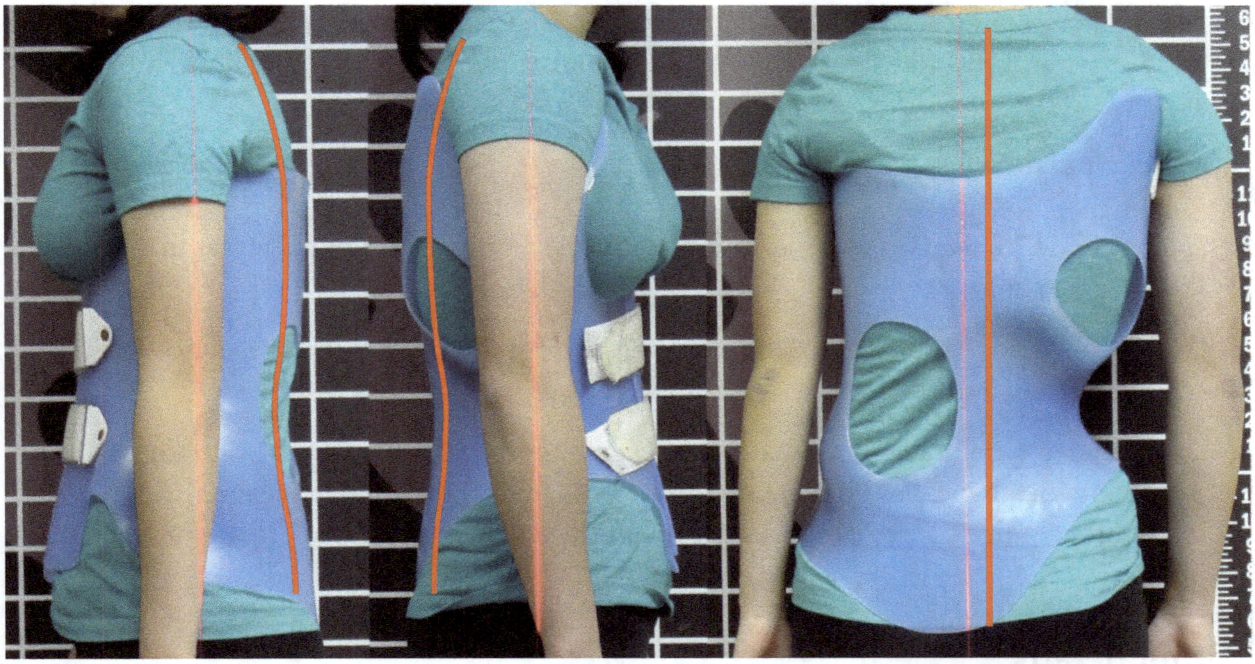

Figure 9. This figure shows the same patient on her left and right sides, with two different sagittal plane shapes on each side. The patient is wearing a WCR brace for the treatment of a left thoracic and right lumbar B1 type scoliosis [3].

physiotherapeutic scoliosis specific exercises (PSSE) both according to the Barcelona School (BSPTS) as well as the original German Schroth school according to Katharina Schroth [5].

The Rigo-Chêneau type brace and the Schroth PSSE address the 3D biomechanics of the deformity in the similar way. The increased expansions in the brace correspond to the Schroth PSSE so-called de-rotational breathing mechanics, which strive to expand the collapsed areas of the trunk affected by scoliosis, aiming at correcting the horizontal (axial) plane of the body. Specific pressure areas in the brace and Schroth PSSE principles work hand in hand to correct the frontal and sagittal planes of the body. That is why the Rigo Chêneau type brace and Schroth PSSE are considered to be a 3D conservative treatment of scoliosis.

This three-dimensional correction cannot be achieved using classic braces, commonly used to treat scoliosis for decades, because their biomechanical design generally does not address the rotational aspect of scoliosis.

3. Conclusion

The Rigo classification of scoliosis and brace design is intended to categorize scoliosis curve patterns. The objectives of the Rigo Chêneau type braces are to improve the clinical presentation of the patient and to improve or prevent progression of the scoliosis. Rigo Chêneau type braces, including the Wood-Chêneau-Rigo braces, were outlined in this chapter. An orthotist must provide optimal fit and function of the brace prescribed by the referring physician. Adherence to certain basic design principles and close follow up by the orthotist—especially during growth spurts—are critical to its effectiveness.

The optimal results in treatment of scoliosis are achieved when modern Chêneau type braces that address the three-dimensional aspects of scoliosis are used in conjunction with Schroth PSSE.

It was concluded that:

1. The original Chêneau brace, when fabricated with a proper design, provides the necessary 3D brace design.
2. The Chêneau type brace is not an orthopedic product, but a corrective concept. Specific knowledge and experience is necessary to produce the expected results.
3. The Chêneau type brace should be used in conjunction with Schroth PSSE to treat scoliosis from "outside" by applying the corrective forces imposed by the brace and from "inside" by using the muscle force produced by the corrective Schroth PSSE.

Author details

Grant I. Wood[1*] and Manuel Rigo[2]

*Address all correspondence to: gwood@align-clinic.com

1 Align Clinic, San Mateo, California, USA

2 Institute Elena Salvá, Barcelona, Spain

References

[1] Chêneau J. Orthese de Scoliose, 2nd ed. In: [Unpublished Manual], Chêneau J, editor. Saint Orens; 1996

[2] Wood GI. Comparison of Surface Topography and Radiograph Values During Idiopathic Scoliosis Treatment Using the Chêneau Brace (the Chêneau System). England: University of Salford; 2003

[3] Rigo MD, Villagrasa M, Gallo D. A specific scoliosis classification correlating with brace treatment: Description and reliability. Scoliosis 2010;**5**:1-11

[4] Wood GI. Specific Scoliosis Classification Correlating with Brace Treatment: Description and Reliability of Rigo Classification. Proceedings of the International Society of Prosthetists and Orthotists World Congress 2010 (ISPO'10); 10-15th May 2010; Leipzig, Germany; 2010

[5] Rigo M, Jelacic M. Brace technology thematic series: The 3D Rigo Chêneau-type brace. Scoliosis and Spinal Disorders. 2017;**12**:10. DOI: 10.1186/s13013-017-0114-2

[6] Chêneau J. Orthese de Scoliose, 1st ed. In: [Unpublished Manual], Chêneau J, editor. Saint Orens; 1990

9

A 3D Spine and Full Skeleton Model for Opto-Electronic Stereo-Photogrammetric Multi-Sensor Biomechanical Analysis in Posture and Gait

Moreno D'Amico, Edyta Kinel,
Gabriele D'Amico and Piero Roncoletta

Abstract

Quantitative functional evaluation of spine is highly desirable in posture and movement analysis. Given the complexity of the spine biomechanical system, very few studies outline the behaviour of the spine in posture and movement analysis. During a research lasting 25 years, a complete three-dimensional (3D) parametric biomechanical skeleton model including a 3D full spine model based on the measurements of the positions of suitable body landmarks labelled by passive markers has been implemented. Around this model, a fully dedicated 3D opto-electronic stereo-photogrammetric system named Global Opto-electronic Approach for Locomotion and Spine (GOALS) has been developed. Depending on different analysis purposes, the model can work at different stages of complexity. The model can integrate seamlessly data deriving from multiple measurement devices, such as 3D stereo-photogrammetric systems, force platforms, surface electro-myography and foot pressure maps. In addition to single-trial analysis, the possibility to assess and to extract mean behaviours either for posture or for cyclical tasks (e.g. multiple strides in gait) has been included. The aim of this paper is to describe the current level of development of the GOALS system and its versatility as a clinical tool. To this purpose, examples of multi-factorial quantitative functional descriptions of paradigmatic cases are presented.

Keywords: stereo-photogrammetry, posture, 3D spine, skeleton model, movement and gait analysis, surface electro-myography

1. Introduction

The interest in spinal- and postural-related pathologies and the evaluation of their related functional impairment is widely represented in both biomechanical and clinical research literature. The need for quantitative posture and spine shape analysis is recognized as crucial for clinical assessments in physical medicine and rehabilitation [1] and very important in designing and developing treatment programmes, planning of orthopaedic surgical procedures [2], and monitoring the progression of pathology and/or treatment outcomes [3, 4].

Posture, that is, the attitude in the space of the body whilst sitting, walking or standing, is a dynamic event, even in relation to the simple neutral-standing-erect position. In fact, even for the neutral erect standing, which is usually considered as a static posture, we know that, in reality, the body is continuously oscillating. So, the standing posture could be characterized by an 'equilibrium status' (i.e. the mean standing position) together with the intrinsic variability in terms of oscillations around this status (i.e. the standard deviation associated to the mean). In an analogous way, also cyclical-repetitive movements such as gait, in which the lower limbs move in an alternating cyclic way, can be described by an 'equilibrium status' (i.e. the mean gait cycle) together with the associated variability. It is very well-known that posture (i.e. equilibrium status and associated variability) is strictly related to any given mental and/or physiological status (healthy, pathological, voluntarily maintained, fatigued, under physical and/or psychological stress etc.). Further, different factors can affect one's postural demeanour including familial physical aspects, anatomical structural impairments, postural habits and work activities.

In this way, from a neurophysiological point of view, by analysing this mean status and connected variability it is possible to derive important information about the functional status of a human body system as well as the related control mechanisms provided by the central nervous system (CNS) [5, 6].

The quantification of such functional evaluation in an unobtrusive and innocuous but complete way is a big challenge from an instrumental point of view.

This is particularly true when the analysis of the full-skeletal posture, including the three-dimensional (3D) shape of the spine, is considered. In fact, although in the last decades, a real enhancement in the diagnostic technologies based on image processing (e.g. digital X-ray, digital 3D stereo X-ray reconstruction, computed axial tomography (CAT) scans and magnetic resonance imaging (MRI)) has led to a significant improvement in accurate and detailed information, in the evaluation of skeletal anatomical structures and spine-related pathologies. However, except for dynamic X-ray and the very recent dynamic MRI, no single one of these techniques is able to provide information about the functional state of the vertebral column and related patient posture [7, 8].

Indeed, two-dimensional (2D) X-ray-based images with their potentially harmful ionizing effects and their 'single-shot' nature are still commonly used in clinical examination. Moreover, they are not free from technical limitations such as the presence of image noise, distinctive characteristics of imaging techniques and the variable positioning of the patient during image acquisition, which represent a major source of variability and create the risk of evaluation errors that may conceal the actual geometrical relationship between anatomical structures [9].

Many efforts have been made in recent years to develop non-invasive techniques to overcome such X-ray-based shortcomings. Unfortunately, many of these new approaches still embody certain limitations. Namely, they are either able to provide only partial measurements or alternatively are unable to perform simultaneous 3D measurements throughout the whole spinal column. In some cases, they require that the subject maintain a specific and restricted postural demeanour, which significantly affects the outcomes, as occurs for both electro-goniometric and/or flexicurve devices [1, 10, 11]. More recently, some interesting low-cost photographic methods have appeared in the literature. However, even if these new methods present promising results they still exhibit significant intrinsic limitations: the single-shot approach, lack of genuinely instantaneous 3D posture measurement (the coronal and sagittal planes are not recorded simultaneously) together with weak calibration procedures, all of which limit their use to follow-up monitoring [12–15].

Furthermore, even the more commonly available rastereography back-surface measurement technique raises questions and doubts that require further clarification. Curiously, even if it has been introduced for the evaluation and follow-up of scoliosis, particular concern is related to discrepancies found in spine shape with respect to X-ray techniques in the coronal plane [10, 16].

Given the restrictions above, it has been demonstrated that, in this context, a technique, named opto-electronic stereo-photogrammetry, offers a significant solution for the capture of functional information necessary for addressing clinical problems in rehabilitation medicine and is increasingly being reported in the literature for use in exploring different original approaches [1, 6–8, 17–30]. Basically, this approach is reliant on the possibility of obtaining 3D measurement of points in space using a number of calibrated TV cameras (at least two) using stereo-vision principles. With this technique, the measurement is restricted to few specific body landmarks, labelled by retro-reflective or active markers, neglecting other information such as the back surface of the trunk (as in rastereography) to lower the computational effort allowing very fast measurements (hundreds per second).

So, for a static-erect posture both the 'equilibrium status' (averaged shape measurement) and the intrinsic variability (standard deviation around the mean) in term of oscillations around this status can be easily obtained. Additionally, the analysis can be expanded to quantitatively document the kinematics of the full skeleton during movement. Given that this method has no harmful effects, it provides a 'natural' approach for both the capturing and monitoring of the progression of pathology and/or treatment outcomes.

Among the various 3D opto-electronic stereo-photogrammetric original approaches presented in the literature [6–8, 18–30], we focus here on a new recently proposed integrated stereo-photogrammetric opto-electronic system named GOALS[1] (Global Opto-electronic

[1]Bioengineering & Biomedicine Company Srl Pescara, Italy.

Approach for Locomotion and Spine based on Optitrack[2] hardware) fully founded on the protocol and procedural techniques formerly presented by D'Amico et al. [7] together with the subsequent development and upgrading of the system [6–8, 17, 27–30].

The actual implementation of the GOALS system and related biomechanical skeleton model allows for the analysis of the full human skeleton 3D posture and movement taking into account the 3D spine shape considering each vertebral level as well as the postural attitude of the head, the trunk, the pelvis, the legs and when necessary the upper limbs. It is able to perform a multi-sensor approach, fully integrating data deriving from force platforms, surface electro-myography (SEMG) and foot pressure maps. In addition to kinematic measurements, depending on the specific analysis requirements to be fulfilled, this can also include the measurement of the forces, torques and electro-muscular activity of participants or patients. By means of data fusion and optimization procedures, all these inputs can be used in the skeleton model to assess internal joint forces, torques and muscular effort. This allows for the correlation of the full-functional evaluation of subjects with their morphological characteristics.

The possibility of assessing and extracting mean behaviours for cyclic or repetitive tasks (such as multiple strides in gait) has been included as well [8, 27, 28, 31].

The applications and the valued contribution in clinical-functional diagnoses of different classes of posture, locomotion and spine-related pathologies using the GOALS system together with its original biomechanical approach have been presented in literature [6–8, 27–31]. Thousands of patients are currently analysed and followed up with this methodology.

The highly sophisticated and demanding computing tasks to acquire data and to solve the whole skeleton model's equations and algorithms can be approached even on relatively low-cost powerful PC workstations. Examples of multi-sensor quantitative functional descriptions of pathological cases are presented to describe the actual level of development of the GOALS system/skeleton model and the actual capability to use them as a clinical tool.

2. Materials and methods

As described in Section 1, the GOALS system has been specifically developed for the use of an opto-electronic stereo-photogrammetric measurement approach within a clinical environment. This project stems from over 25 years of biomechanical-clinical research conducted by our research group having in mind the following three specific 'GOALS':

(1) Find a way to use stereo-photogrammetry to measure the posture and/or movement to achieve the greatest possible number of clinically relevant parameters.

(2) Include in the measurements, a detailed description of the 3D shape of the spinal column in relation to the description of the whole-body posture, to appropriately study the disorders of the spine.

[2]NaturalPoint Inc., OR, USA.

(3) Represent the results in clinical and intuitive manner, with strict biomechanical principles, but at the same time hiding the weight of complex mathematical methods involved.

To meet the above points, we have developed an adjustable body skeleton model, which automatically adapts to the measures of the subject. To allow the use of this method in a simple and quick way in daily clinical practice, the model was designed with the intention to maintain the smallest possible number of body landmarks.

2.1. Hardware configurations

The GOALS system can present different configurations depending on the requirements necessary to be fulfilled for the specific analysis that needs to be performed. In general, for the analysis of erect standing posture coupled to measurements of lateral and forward bending movements to evaluate the functional mobility of the spine, a configuration with six specially designed infrared TV cameras (IR TVC) (0.3 Mpix resolution) is sufficient to have a fully automated measurement process. When more complex movements such as gait, running, jumping, cycling, and so on are of interest, a 12–16 IR TVCs (1.3 Mpix at 120 fps) configuration has been found to be appropriate. For some very special advanced motor tasks related to sports activities such as those in artistic/rhythmic gymnastics, in which large acquisition volumes are required and fast jumps and rotations are performed, the GOALS system allows configurations that can employ IR cameras with a resolution of 1.7 Mpix at 360 fps or even up to 4.1 MPix at 180 fps in an arrangement that can easily reach 100 or even more IR TVCs (**Figure 1**).

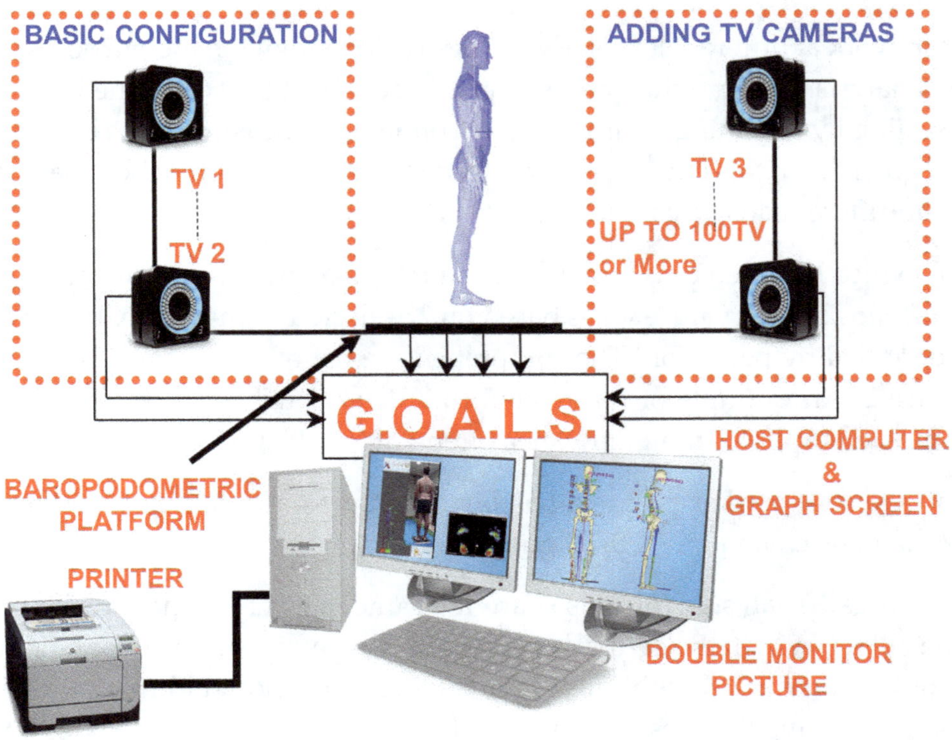

Figure 1. A general schematic configuration of GOALS system.

For posture evaluation (six IR TVCs at 0.3 Mpix resolution), the usual acquisition volume (i.e. the physical calibrated volume of the room, inside which the subject can be measured with known accuracy and precision) is in general somewhat like 3-m wide by 3-m deep by 2-m high. With such a configuration, the usual final mean 3D stereo-photogrammetric error is limited to a range of 0.3–0.4 mm throughout the entire working volume. If higher resolution IR TVCs are used, the 3D stereo-photogrammetric error is even lower. The whole calibration phase takes less than 5 min. This calibration step is needed only when the cameras are initially installed or when they are moved to a new position. When the installation is fixed in a research laboratory, the calibration is performed only occasionally to maintain an accurate calibration level.

2.2. Model configurations and associated protocols

As mentioned above, in order to analyse the full human skeleton posture and movement, our group started a project in the mid-1990s to create a complete and accurate 3D biomechanical model of the human skeleton, with particular attention to the accurate reproduction of spinal detail. This was achieved by merging different segmental biomechanical models presented in the literature [7].

The accuracy and precision of the model rely on anatomical findings (cadaver dissections, in vivo X-ray and gamma ray measurements parametric regression equations) [32–35] as well as a variety of signal-processing procedures and optimization methods described in the literature [6–8, 27–31]. The model was conceived in an adjustable form in order to enable the scaling of the individual characteristics of any subject. This was achieved by fitting the 3D anthropometric size of a given skeletal segment, to 3D opto-electronic measurements of the corresponding body landmarks labelled by passive retro-reflective markers [7].

The model can work at different levels of complexity depending on the purposes and requirements of the analysis. In fact, when necessary, it is possible to increase the level of detail for parametric scaling by obtaining additional anthropometric measurements relative to specific anatomical segments. To this end, various protocols involving different body labels have been established for different analytical purposes [6–8, 27–31].

The protocol, which has been developed for the analysis of human posture and spine-related pathologies (scoliosis, back pain, etc.), is based on 27 selected human body bony prominences accurately identified by palpation. The comprehensive list of these anatomical landmarks is given in **Figure 2**. An example of the related full 3D skeleton reconstruction, obtained via opto-electronic stereo-photogrammetric measurement, can be found in **Figure 3**.

For gait analysis, a 49-marker protocol has been set-up to appropriately define the pelvis-lower limb kinematic chain [8, 27, 28] (**Figure 4**).

The posture and gait analysis protocols share the same landmarks that are set for the head, trunk and the pelvis. Within the 49-marker protocol, the pelvis-lower limb apparatus is modelled by a 9-link chain model, with the pelvis, thigh, shank and foot links joined by ball and socket joints representing the hips, the knees and the ankles, respectively. At least three markers per each segment have been used, in particular: for the pelvis: (as above) bilateral anterior and posterior superior iliac spine (ASIS and PSIS) bony landmarks; femur: great trochanter

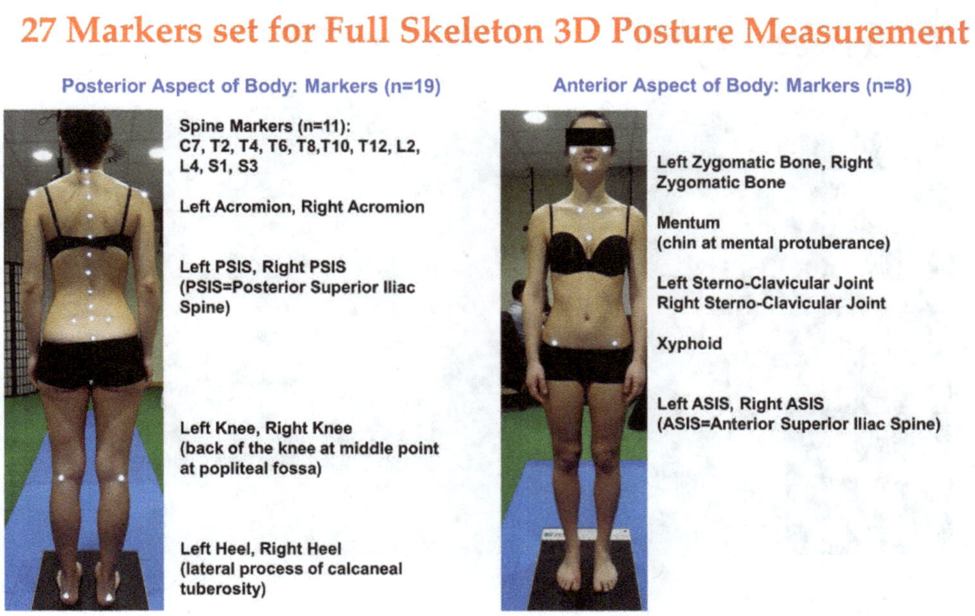

Figure 2. Protocol for 3D posture analysis: list of 27 anatomical landmarks identified by palpation.

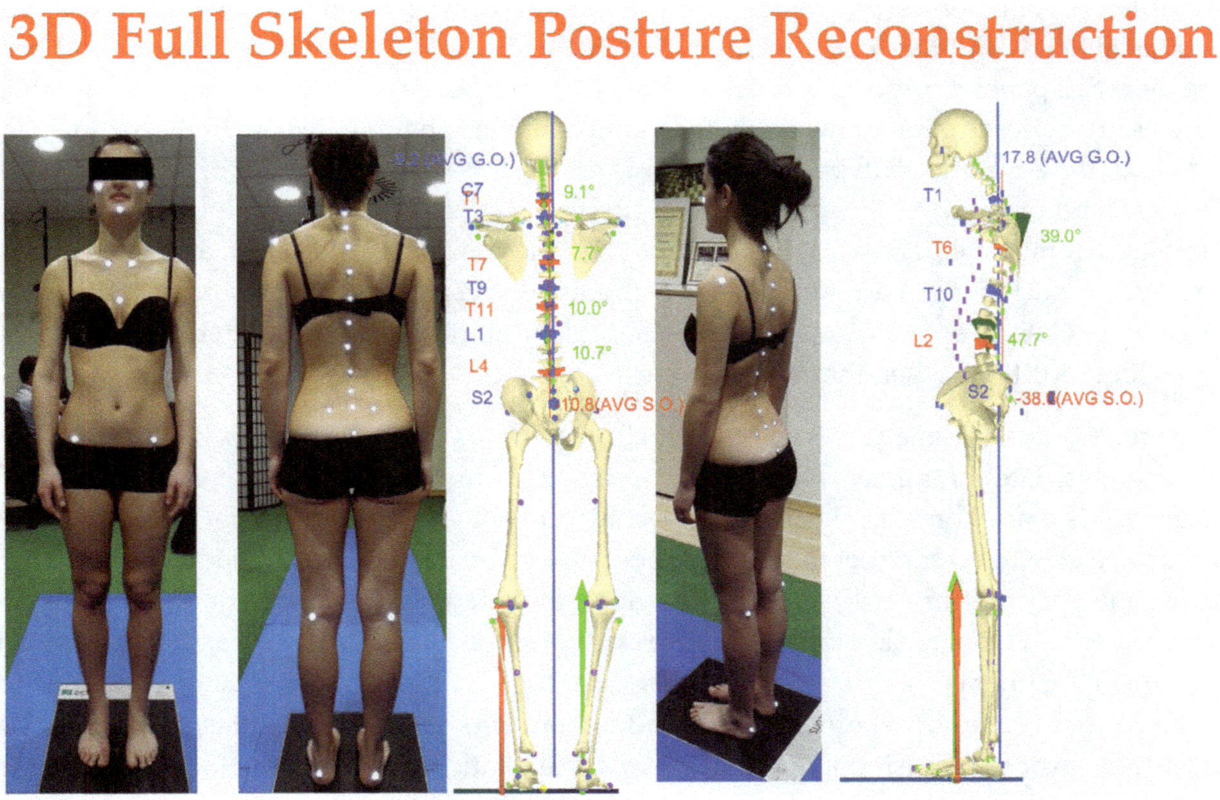

Figure 3. Subject's pictures and assessed full 3D skeleton reconstruction.

middle thigh and lateral and medial femoral epicondyles; shank: head of fibula, tibial tuberosity, middle shank, lateral and medial malleoli; foot: heel (calcaneus process), the first and fifth metatarsal heads, distal big toe end point (**Figure 4**).

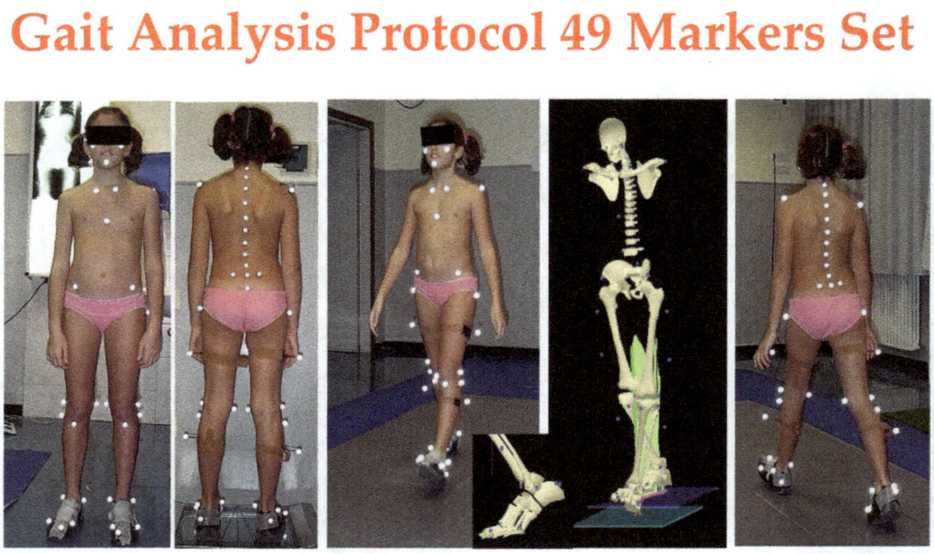

Figure 4. Protocol for 3D gait analysis includes a set of 49 identified anatomical landmarks.

The foot marker set in particular allows for the modelling of the foot and is subdivided into two different rigid bony segments: fingers-forefoot segment identified by big toe first and fifth metatarsal heads and rear-mid-foot identified by the first and fifth metatarsal heads and heel (see the small panel representing the flexed forefoot in **Figure 4**). This latter choice allows for a more accurate description of the ankle-foot complex biomechanics. By using regression equations [32], the ASIS and PSIS positions provide the basis for the assessment of hip joint centre positions and of pelvis width. The knee joint centre is taken as the mid-point of the segment linking the femur medial and lateral epicondyles, and the ankle joint centre as the mid-point of the segment joining the two malleoli. A modified version of this latter protocol (adding the humerus lateral epicondyle and ulnar styloid landmarks) allows the determination of the upper limb positions when they are of interest.

When the focus of the analysis is on neck and back pain, specific test batteries have been established to evaluate the related postural and spinal dysfunction. In this case, a further three-marker set is placed on a head band and are added to either the 27- or 49-marker protocols in order to be able to reconstruct the head and neck even during a forward-bending test. In fact, during the patient's forward-bending execution the three markers placed on the face (zygomatic bones and chin needed to measure the skull position and orientation) usually disappear from the TV-cameras' field of view. In this case, the skull landmarks cannot be identified anymore. To overcome this problem, three added markers are placed on a head band: during orthostatic posture acquisition, the rigid geometrical relationship occurring between the head band markers and the anatomical skull markers ones is established.

Afterwards, during forward bending, the markers on the head band always remain visible to the cameras, thus allowing the skull and neck position and orientation reconstruction alongside all the movement measurements. In the same way, head axial rotations can also be evaluated for neck pain patients. In addition to the 3D kinematic measurements, the GOALS system capability can be expanded, when necessary, by gathering additional biomechanical data (forces, pressures, electromyographic signals, etc.) measured simultaneously by different sensors, allowing to perform what is defined in the literature as a 'multi-factorial approach' [36] (**Figure 5**).

The 'multi-factorial approach' means the capability to fully integrate all these measurement data into a unified approach to correlate and combine all the morphological-kinematic characteristics measured in order to achieve a full-functional evaluation with the aim of using the results of such measurement for clinical purposes and objectives.

By using the multi-factorial approach, additional useful functional information is available. In particular, by using ground reaction forces and the segmental inertial and gravitational contributions derived from the skeleton/body model, it is possible to assess the joint net forces and torques at each lower limb joint and even at each spine inter-vertebral level by using a model derived from Liu and Wickstrom in 1973 [35].

Baropodometric platforms and/or baropodometric in-shoe insole system allow to measure the underfoot pressure distribution maps. These latter are very useful when a better description of the foot-floor interaction is needed to proceed to plantar foot orthoses custom design.

When of interest, SEMG is recorded by a telemetric system following the SENIAM European project recommendations [37]. In gait analysis, the activity of lower limb muscles is recorded to investigate motor co-ordination/dysfunction. In low back pain (LBP), the multifidus (MF) and erector spinae-longissimus dorsi (ESLD) activities are bilaterally collected to study the flexion-relaxation phenomenon (FRP) (see case n. 4 in Section 3 for a detailed explanation) [38]. In neck pain patients, SEMG is generally recorded bilaterally on the upper trapezius and sternocleidomastoid muscles.

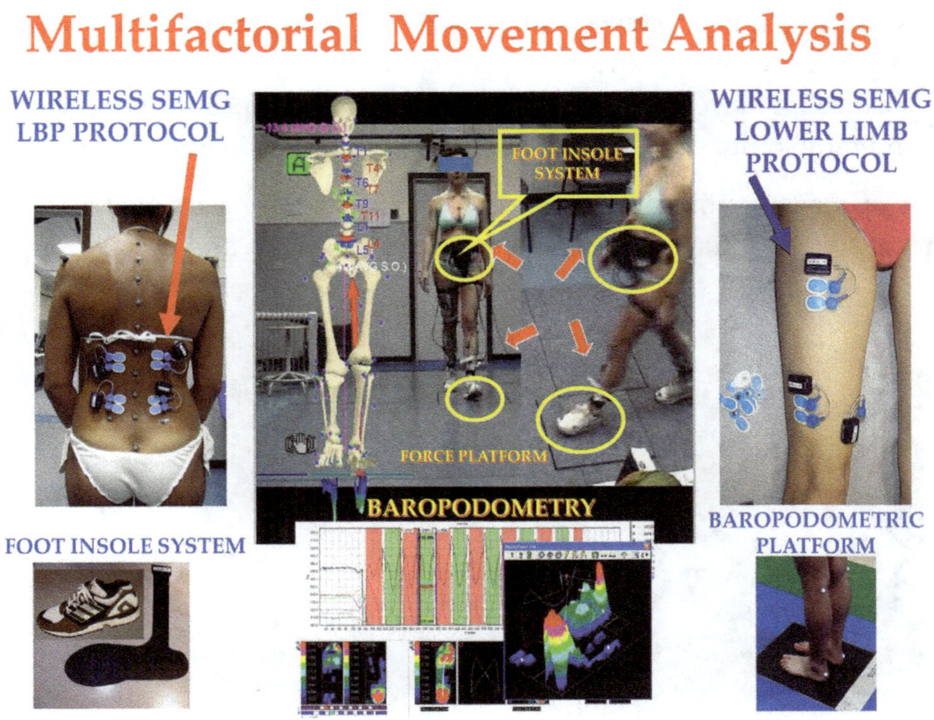

Figure 5. General 'multi-factorial-multi-sensors' experimental set-up for GOALS system for 3D posture and movement analysis.

2.3. Biomechanical data acquisition and measurement processing

The standard trial session aims to completely define the subject's posture both in the orthostatic position and in simple or complex dynamic conditions. Each static postural attitude is considered correctly recorded when at least five, 2-s lasting, acquisitions are performed. Given the GOALS system data acquisition rate depending on the hardware configuration, we can have rates starting from 100 up to 360 Hz); this means that a minimum of 1000 measurements are averaged per each static postural stance [6–8, 27–31]. Before averaging, an amount of pre-processing is needed on the acquired 3D raw data in order to comply with clinical analysis requirements.

Once the 3D skeleton reconstruction is obtained, it is possible to compute, on the derived model, all the clinical parameters that are generally calculated on the radiographic image and used for the correct description and biomechanical characterization of spinal pathology (i.e. Cobb and kypho-lordotic angles).

Moreover, a set of significant biomechanical variables describing the three-dimensional nature of body posture are obtained. To describe trunk and global unbalancing, spinal offset and global offset (i.e. displacements of each spine markers with respect to the vertical line passing through the S3 vertebra and with respect to the vertical line passing through the middle point between the heels, respectively) are used [6–8, 27–31]. Both global and spinal offset values are finally averaged to obtain descriptive data that summarize these parameters (**Figure 6**).

Other parameters include pelvis frontal and sagittal inclinations, pelvis torsion, shoulder-to-pelvis, pelvis-to-heels and shoulder-to-heels horizontal rotations (**Figure 7**), joint forces, joint torques and several more. The 49 markers set can be used not only for gait or movement measurements but it can be very useful when deeper information about lower limbs segmental posture is sought (intra-extra rotations, ab-adductions flexion-extension). In fact, in this way the posture measurements are complemented by the pose of each lower limb chain segment enlightening joint adaptations, anomalies and/or weakness.

Our studies as well as our clinical experience led us to identify a set of static attitudes (such as indifferent orthostasis—that is, neutral erect standing—with and/or without an underfoot

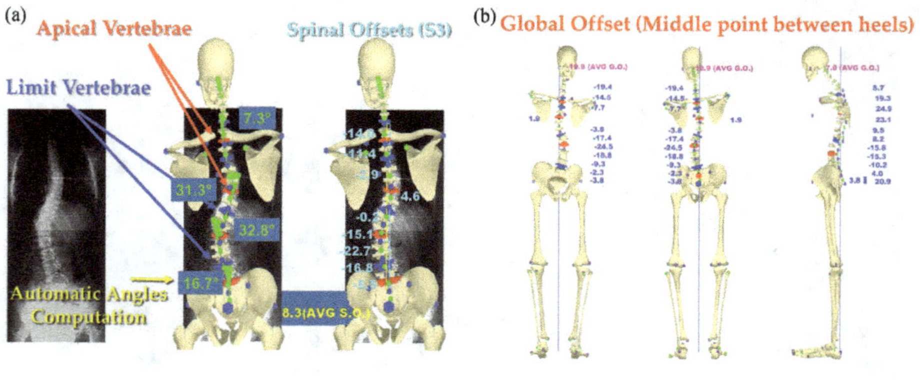

Figure 6. (a) From left to right: automatic identification of frontal plane spinal curves, related Cobb angular values and spinal offsets with respect to the vertical line passing through S3; (b) full 3D skeleton posture reconstruction (frontal and sagittal views), including global offsets computation and visualization.

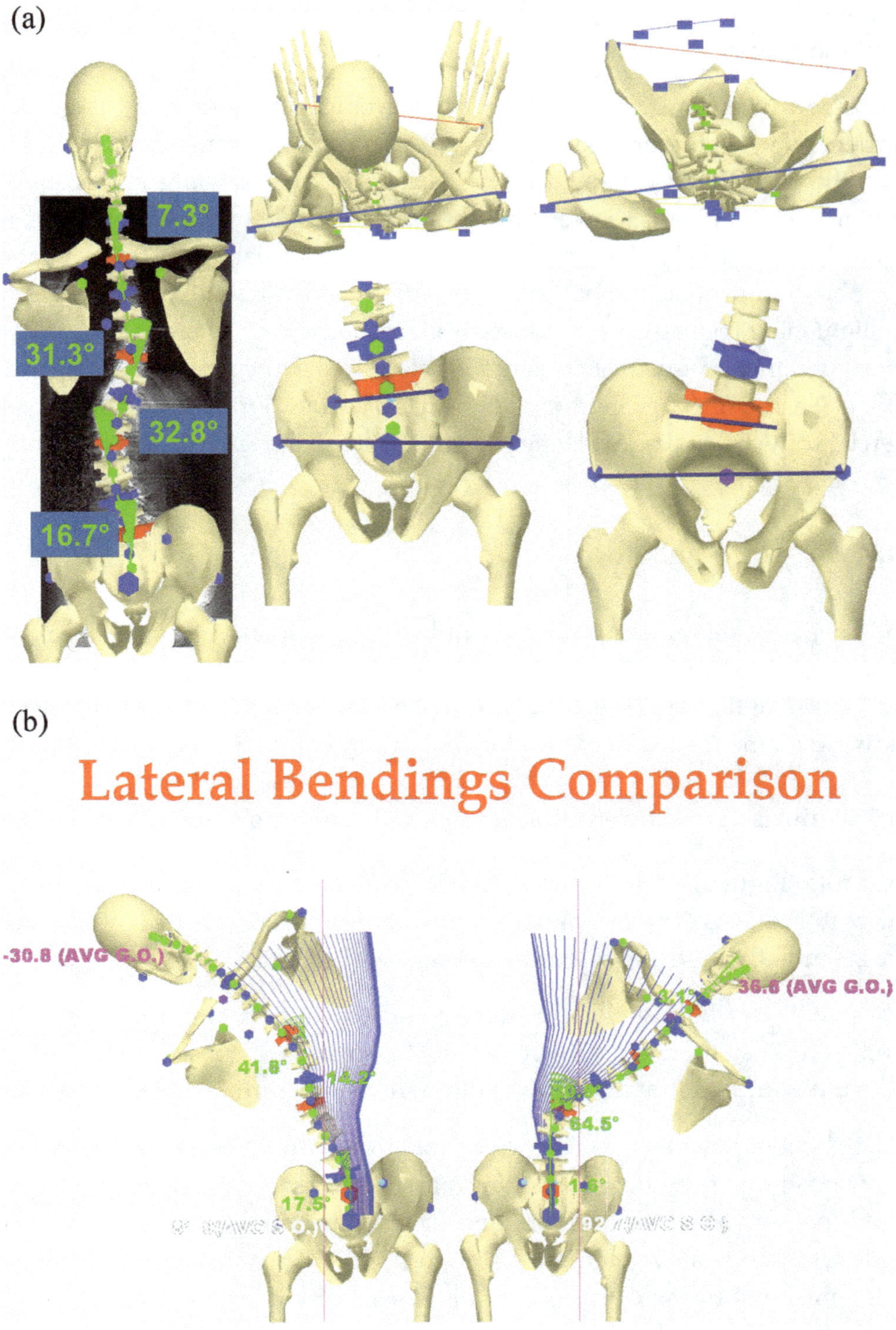

Figure 7. (a) Frontal spinal angles, pelvis orientation and torsion as derived by the relative position of PSIS and ASIS landmarks; (b) leftward and rightward lateral-bending tasks performed by a scoliotic subject.

wedge, self-corrected manoeuvres, ante-retroversion static postural exercises and sitting posture), which can provide a complete documentation of subject postural, balancing and morphological characteristics. As for static posture, also for gait the possibility to extract the mean gait cycle characteristics has been considered and developed.

The mathematical details for the optimization of the procedure as well as the average gait cycle computation are beyond the limits of this chapter [8, 27, 28].

The final outcome is the mean gait cycle in which the average time course and associated standard deviation is defined per each variable of interest [8, 27, 28, 31]. Two main advantages can be enumerated with the possibility to extract the mean characteristics of both static posture and cyclic motor task (gait): first, it allows to overcome the single measurements analysis limits by taking into account the ensemble behaviour improving the statistical reliability of the evaluation; second, it permits to obtain information about the repeatability and variability of the performed motor task, thus enlightening the subject's motor control capability. For the graphical representation as well as clinical parameter visualization and enlightening, a software package (named ASAP 3D Skeleton Model©) based on 3D graphic modelling has been developed. This latter is now available as a commercial software package (Bioengineering & Biomedicine Company S.r.l. Italy).

3. Results

Several studies are currently being carried out by our group about spine and posture disorders with the described methodology. A few examples are summarized below in order to show the capability of this multi-factorial approach to process many different measurements, thereby allowing all the results to be combined in a unified view.

3.1. Case n.1 scoliosis 3D posture static and dynamic analysis versus X-ray measurement

The first example (**Figures 6** and **7**) represents the outcome of the procedure for the analysis of a patient with scoliosis. The left panel shows the description of the spinal deformity that shows full agreement with the X-ray measurement which is displayed.

On the right panel, a full 3D skeletal posture reconstruction in both the frontal and sagittal planes is depicted. The end and apical vertebrae, Cobb angle values as well as the spinal and global offset values and their averages are automatically identified and computed.

In **Figure 7a**, the pelvis orientation is described together with the associated torsion as derived by the relative position of PSIS and ASIS landmarks (left panel); in addition, the relative rotations of shoulder-pelvis-feet on the horizontal plane are represented (a second illustration without skull and feet is also given on a side to highlight trunk torsion). In **Figure 7b**, the dissimilarities in the stiffness of different spinal segments along the vertebral column are depicted, due to position and magnitude of scoliotic curves, describing hyper/hypomobility during the performance of lateral bending tasks.

3.2. Case n.2 scoliosis and leg length discrepancy: multi-factorial static and gait analysis first evaluation versus control

This describes a 13-year-old patient with scoliosis and leg length discrepancy (LLD). The LLD is corrected during measurements at the first evaluation by placing an underfoot wedge—the optimal value of which (10 mm under left foot) was determined as the one producing the best global posture outcome considering all the combined spine deformities and postural parameters. In addition, the analysis of underfoot pressure distributions suggested the use of customized foot orthoses to reduce ankle pronation at both feet, complemented by the wedge correction under the left foot. The patient was measured after a period of 6 months during which she was wearing the recommended foot orthoses.

In **Figure 8**, the within-sessions comparison (both at first evaluation and at control measurement session after 6 months) between a neutral-standing posture and an underfoot wedge-corrected neutral-standing posture (upper row panels) is presented. At the control session, for the wedge-corrected standing position, instead of a simple heel rise the patient was measured with her customized foot orthoses. A cross-session comparison between neutral orthostasis at first evaluation and wedge-corrected neutral orthostasis at control is also displayed in the bottom-row panels.

The model is able to indicate and explain the almost perfect realignment of the spine and trunk balance induced by foot orthoses/wedge correction worn during a 6-month period, with a dramatic reduction of spine deformities in the frontal plane.

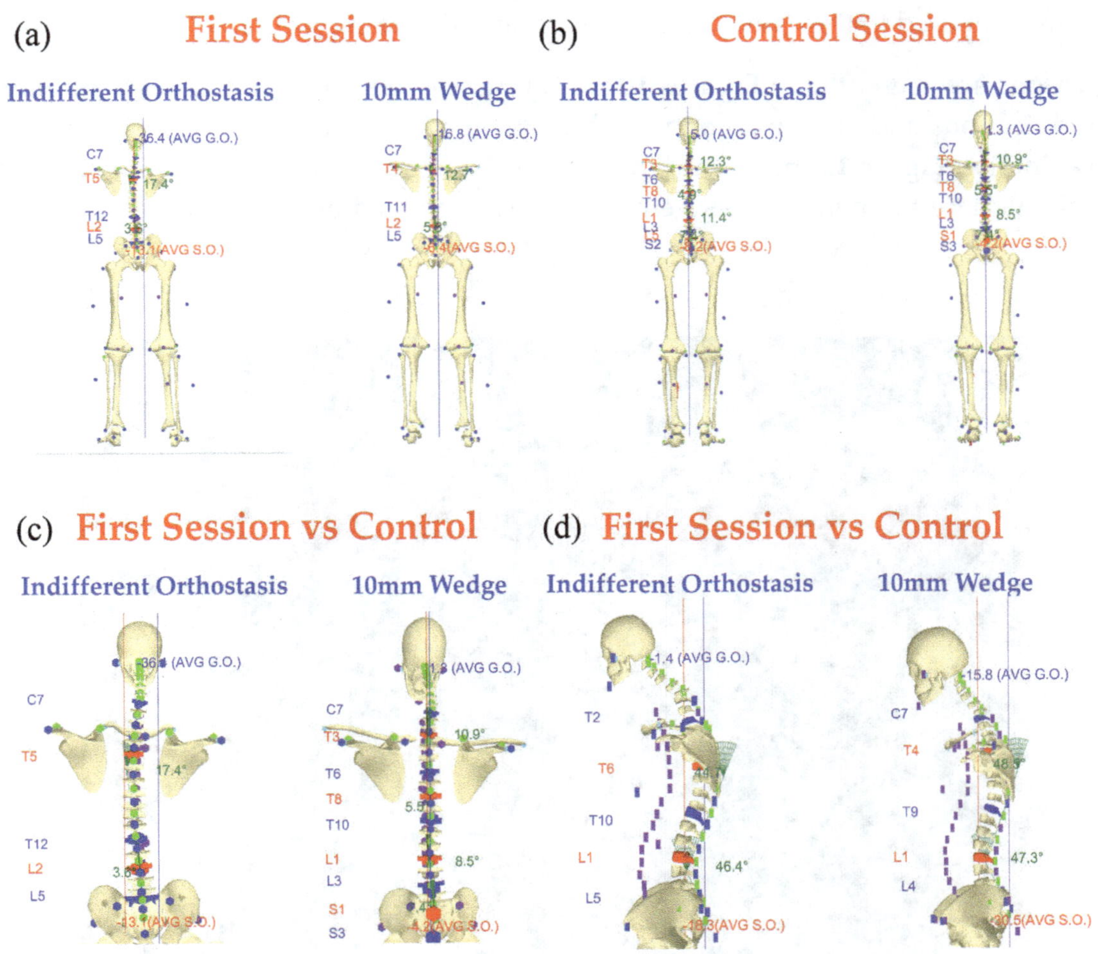

Figure 8. Composite figures representing comparison of posture, and related balance and spine morphology changes in the frontal and sagittal planes between indifferent (i.e. neutral) orthostasis (left side of a,b,c,d panels) and wedge-corrected neutral orthostasis (right side of a,b,c,d panels), of a 13-year-old patient presenting with a leg length discrepancy (LLD), when 10-mm heel rise was positioned under left foot. The same patient underwent a gait analysis test at both first and follow-up (after about 6-month) sessions.

For this patient, the study of gait biomechanics was also performed. **Figure 9** shows the mean gait cycle computed over 10 different strides. The mean trajectories of each considered landmark together with the associated frame-by-frame standard deviations are represented. Each trajectory is depicted by a time series of spheres, each one being centred in the frame-by-frame computed mean 3D co-ordinate and having radius given by the magnitude of the assessed standard deviation. In addition, the mean patterns of ground reaction forces are displayed.

It is interesting to note how the standard deviations of the trunk-spine landmark trajectories are significantly smaller than those of the head and lower limb landmarks (as shown by the different dimensions of spheres). Such findings demonstrate, from a biomechanical standpoint, that the patient was preserving her mechanical energy and minimizing oscillations. The patient also had a very strict repetitive motor pattern for the trunk (where most of the body mass is amassed), while she was releasing more variability in the distal segments. Our group is currently conducting studies to further explore this phenomenon on a wider population.

In this case, the model allowed the investigators to also assess the ROMs of the spinal deformity angles as well as the variation of stresses acting on the spine during gait. Such outcomes have been compared to the values assessed during orthostasis.

Comparisons are presented in **Figures 10** and **11**, where the effects of LLD on both morphology modifications and stresses acting on the patient's spine during orthostasis and gait are put on evidence. **Figure 10** shows the cross-session comparison between neutral orthostasis at first evaluation (left panel) and wedge-corrected (customized orthoses) neutral orthostasis at

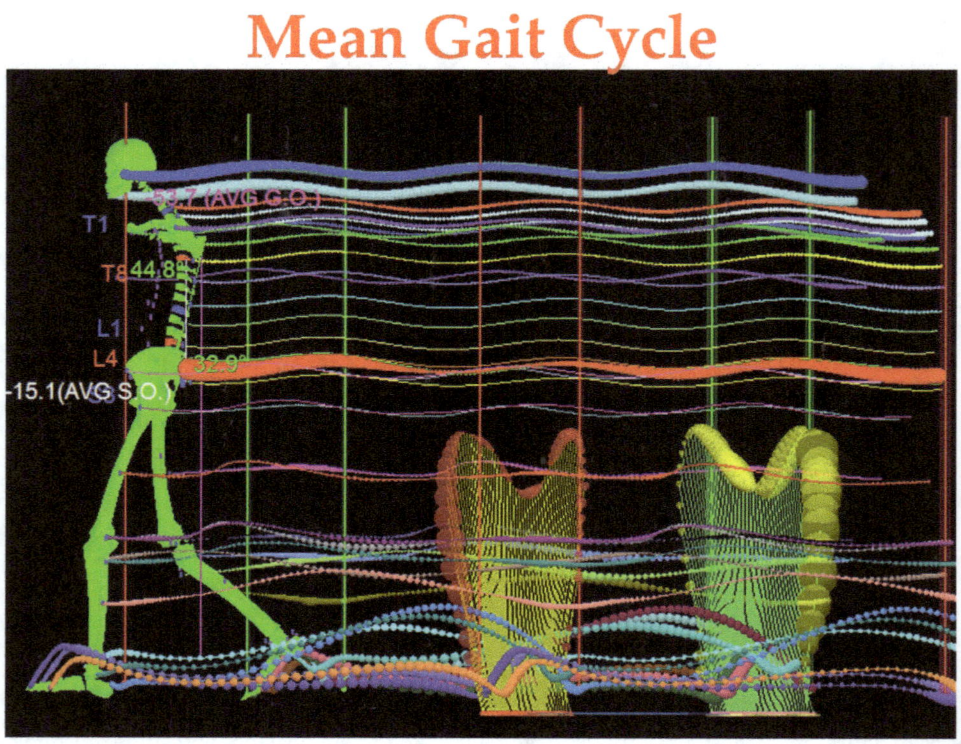

Figure 9. The mean gait cycle. Averaged 3D trajectories of each considered landmark and of ground reaction forces patterns, together with the associated frame-by-frame standard deviations (3D radius of each depicted sphere).

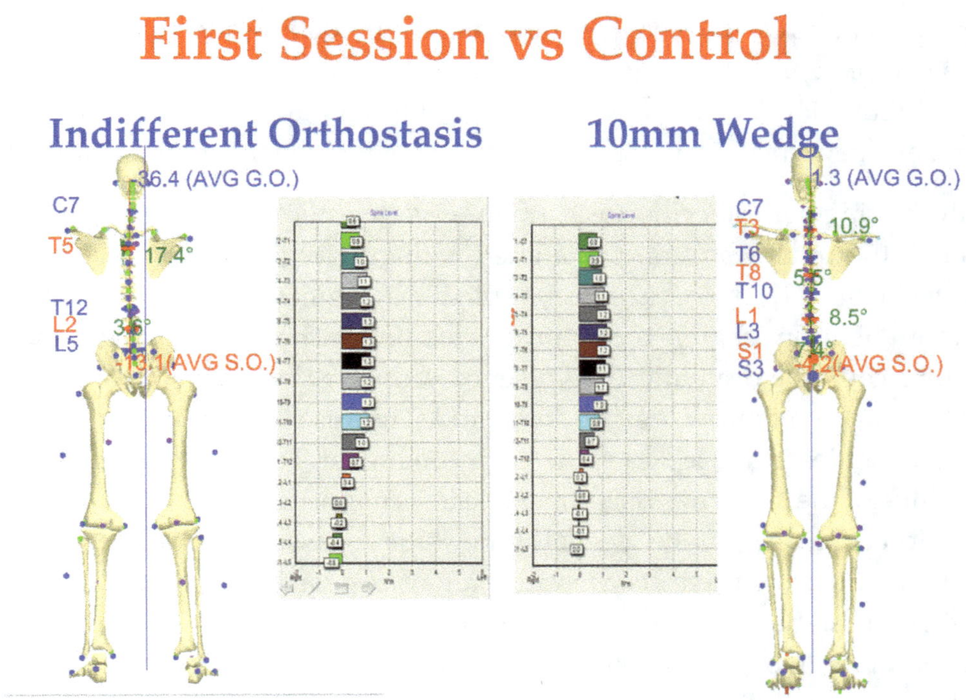

Figure 10. Composite figures representing comparison of posture, spine morphology and related spine torques in frontal plane between neutral orthostasis (left panels) and orthostasis when 1-cm wedge was positioned under left foot at first evaluation of a scoliotic patient (right panels).

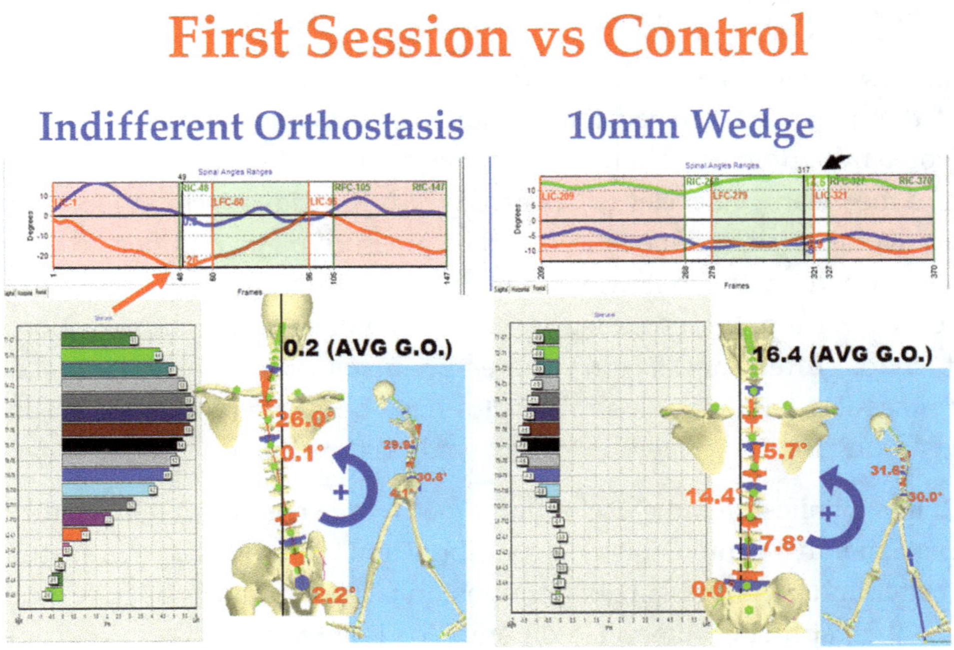

Figure 11. Composite figures representing a mean gait cycle comparison of the above-described scoliotic patient, during first evaluation (left panels) and at 6-month control (follow-up) (right panels). In each figure, the lower panels represent spine shape and computed spine torques at each inter-vertebral level taken at frames in which the spinal curves reach their maximum (at thoracic levels). The upper panels show spinal curves full ranges throughout the mean gait cycle, arrows pointing at reached maximum angular value. From these results, it can be noted that the inter-vertebral torque values, assessed at control session, fall below one-third with respect to the first-session values.

control (right panel). As can be seen, the spine shape remodelling and global posture rebalancing induce a complete transforming of the spinal inter-vertebral torques in the frontal plane, with a factor 4 reduction (i.e. the maximal values at follow-up are below 25% of the maximal values at first evaluation) at the upper thoracic level where the major deformity was present.

Theoretically, during neutral orthostasis, no inter-vertebral torques should be present in the frontal plane, if the spine was straight, aligned with gravity line and in the symmetry plane of the subject. Conversely, the occurrence of spinal deformities and postural unbalance determine an amount of not-negligible trunk torques loading each vertebra in an asymmetric way. Such behaviour could be dramatically worsened during a dynamic activity like walking. In fact, when static and dynamic values are compared (**Figures 10** vs. **11**), it is evident that during gait, spinal deformities increase and spine loads are higher. For instance, at thoracic level the Cobb angle value of the curve passes, from static to dynamic condition, from around 17° up to around 26°. Moreover, as it can be seen, also the values of assessed trunk torques, result during gait, of a magnitude of up to six times the values assessed during neutral erect standing. This phenomenon can be very important in the evolution of scoliosis inducing a spine deformities progression. In fact, taking into account the in vivo demonstration of the well-known Heuter-Volkmann principle, asymmetric loads on functional spinal unit (i.e. vertebrae plus inter-vertebral discs) determine a wedging process on both inter-vertebral disc and vertebrae during growth [39, 40]. In this way, any action inducing a reduction of such asymmetries results in beneficial effects. In the described case, in the comparison between the first session and follow-up at 6 months, the positive effect of customized foot orthoses complemented by wedge correction is greatly confirmed both in the static measurements and during gait.

Finally, to analyse the changes induced on the biomechanics of walking of a patient after 6 months of the use of customized foot orthoses, complemented by the wedge correction under left foot, baropodometric analysis outcomes have been compared. **Figure 12** shows the comparison of the mean gait cycles (as assessed from 10 strides each) at first evaluation (left panels) and at control (right panels) in terms of pressure maps and derived vertical forces measured by baropodometric foot insoles device during locomotion on the floor. This kind of baropodometric device provides measurements of the in-shoe direct interaction of the foot. So, to avoid obvious direct modification of pressure maps induced by customized foot orthoses at control session, the same neutral insoles have been used in patient's shoes for both sessions, but adding the 10-mm left underfoot wedge correction during the control session.

In **Figure 12**, it is manifest that the use of underfoot wedge correction (and of the customized insoles during 6 months) demonstrated to contribute in underfoot load asymmetries reduction as well as a better underfoot pressure distribution. In fact, by the analysis of vertical forces patterns it results that, at first evaluation, a different load between feet was occurring, being the left one more loaded along all the stance phase (upper-left panel). Moreover, a different heel to forefoot load transfer pattern is evident between the right and left foot showing that left foot stance phase was significantly longer than the contralateral, that is, the left foot pushes more and for longer time being more propulsive. In the pictures, to represent map pressures of stance phases, the so-called 'peak frames' are used. They are defined as the maps obtained by assigning to each pressure cell the peak pressure value reached during stance. Peak pressure maps enlighten (left-lower panel) the different loading patterns in each foot showing the pressure

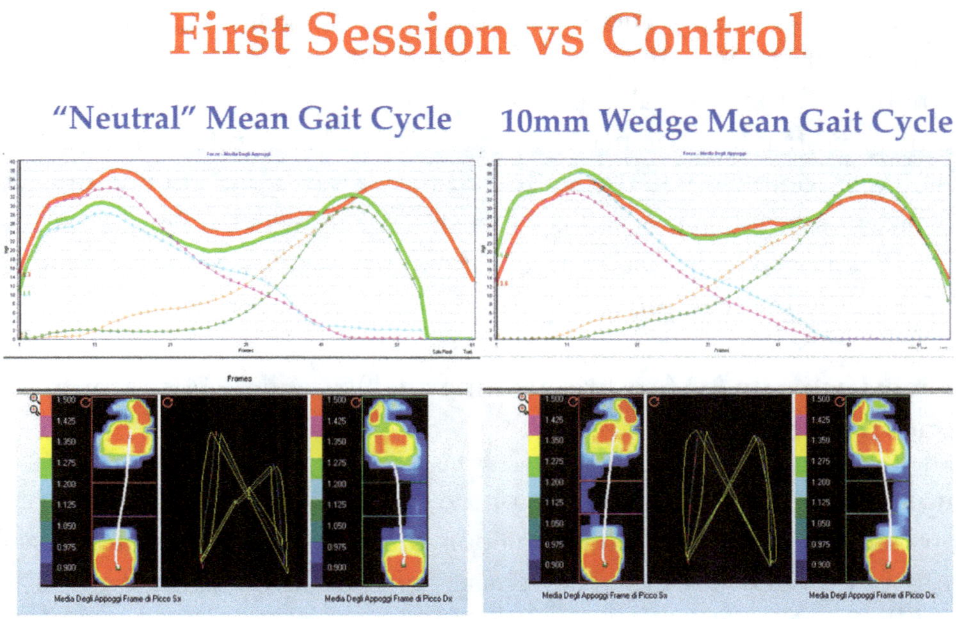

Figure 12. Baropodographic analysis of the mean gait cycle. The mean gait cycle characteristics obtained when the patient was walking wearing an underfoot wedge (right panel) and without underfoot wedge (left panel) are compared. Averaged force patterns, averaged peak pressure maps and COP patterns are represented pointing out the reduction of differences and asymmetries when underfoot wedge was worn.

values in different foot regions, with left foot presenting a cavo-valgus foot pattern due to ankle pronation during stance phase as it is evident by the absence of load on the lateral aspect of the foot between the heel and forefoot (isthmus). At control session, such asymmetries are really reduced. The stance phases of both feet present the same duration in time, vertical forces are almost superimposed and the lateral aspect of the left foot between the heel and forefoot (isthmus) started to be charged presenting a reduction of ankle pronation.

In this picture, a new introduced special graphical feature for gait analysis, the so-called 'butterfly' window, is displayed in the lower panels of the figure between the two peak pressure maps of the feet. This graphic is obtained by computing the frame-by-frame spatial weighted baricentre of both feet COPs actual positions (feet are considered as they were symmetrically positioned); such pattern allows an intuitive and immediate evaluation of the symmetry of subject's gait. In fact, at first evaluation, a strong asymmetry was evident between the left and right 'butterfly wings' of the diagram, pointing out different COP patterns for the left and right foot (both in their shape and in their time duration). Conversely, at control session, the two 'butterfly wings' resulted much more symmetrical, thus confirming the improvement obtained by underfoot wedge correction.

3.3. Case n.3 low back pain: 3D posture static and dynamic analysis first evaluation versus control

In this example, we want to show the fast-clinical intuitive use of the presented approach that provides quantitative support to the usual clinical observational analysis. To this aim, we superimposed the 3D reconstruction of the spine directly on the digital pictures of the patient. The subject was analysed at first examination during an acute phase of LBP and at follow-up after 1 month of treatment, when she recovered from acute phase (**Figure 13**). It is immediate to notice the improvement in both frontal and sagittal planes for orthostatic analysis as well as for spine mobility during lateral-bending test. At acute phase, the patient was presenting spine deformities and trunk unbalancing induced by pain. In sagittal plane, the physiological lordosis was almost completely flattened. In addition, a severe functional impairment in the range of movement as well as blocked compensation curves is evident. After the treatment programme that removed pain, the compensation curves disappeared sagittal spine shape and the spine mobility really improved.

3.4. Case n.4 low back pain 3D forward-bending analysis and SEMG recording: the flexion-relaxation phenomenon

In this example, we introduce the analysis of the so-called 'flexion-relaxation phenomenon' (FRP) to show that the 'stop' of such phenomenon, that is, usually related to muscular spasms due to pain in LBP patient during acute phase, can exist even when the pain disappears. Movements in the lumbar spine, including flexion and extension, are governed by a complex neuromuscular system involving both active (muscle) and passive components (vertebral bones, inter-vertebral disks, ligaments, tendons and fascia) [38]. There is evidence to suggest that EMG differences at paravertebral muscles exist between patients with back pain and healthy subjects during dynamic flexion tasks performed at peak flexion [38]. To this extent, several studies have examined the apparent myoelectric silencing of the low back extensor musculature during a standing to full trunk flexion manoeuvre named as FRP (**Figure 14**). The electrical signal reduction or silence that occurs in healthy subjects during lumbar spine flexion has been hypothesized to represent the extensor musculature being relieved of its moment-supporting role by the passive tissues, particularly the posterior spinal ligaments

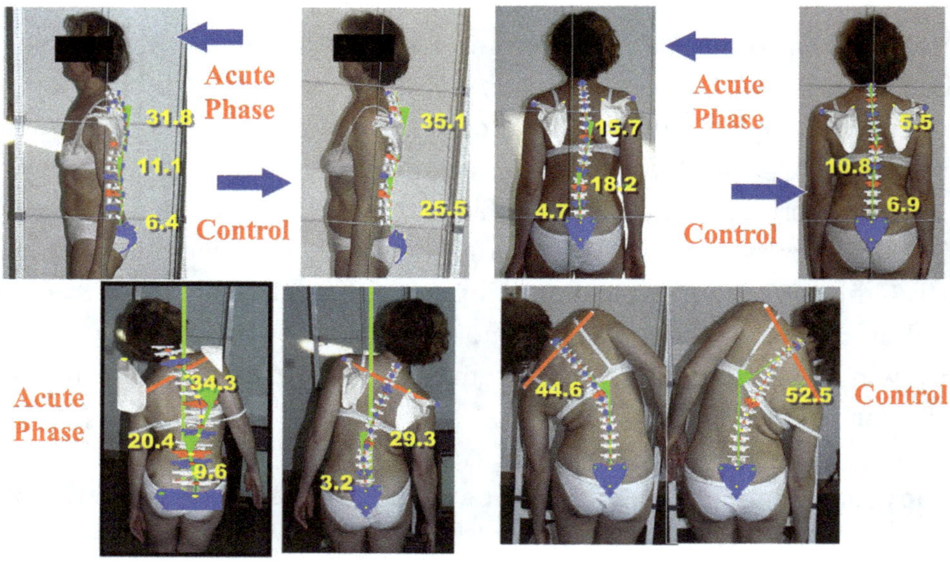

Figure 13. Upper panels: comparison between trunk unbalancing and spinal deformities induced by pain in LBP patient at acute phase and the postural improvement obtained after treatment (control evaluation). Lower panels: lateral bending tasks, revealing the patient's functional impairment of spinal mobility due to pain (left panels), compared with recovered range of movement after treatment (right panels).

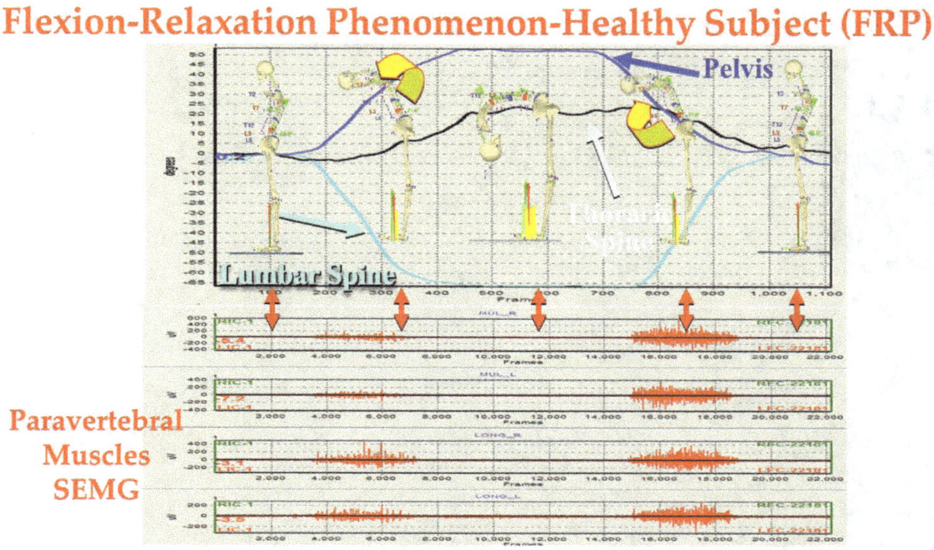

Figure 14. The FRP (a) in the upper panel, the ranges of variation of spinal sagittal angles and of pelvis tilt for a healthy subject performing a forward-bending manoeuvre are displayed. Full skeleton reconstructions (sagittal views) taken in the five most significant time events of the motor task are superimposed to graphs. (b) The lower panel represents paravertebral muscles activity recorded by SEMG, from which it can be emphasized that, in a healthy subject, a paravertebral muscles relaxation occurs when the maximum bending position is reached.

[41]. Likewise, a failure of the muscles to relax in patients with back problems is indicative of heightened erector spinae-resting potentials or underlying back muscle spasticity. Similar phenomena have been documented also in neck pain [42].

In this section, we present a case study to show and analyse some new aspects about the FRP connected to LBP and impaired functional behaviour at lumbar level. The upper panels of **Figure 15** describe the outcomes of the analysis of the execution of a forward-bending manoeuvre performed by a healthy subject and by LBP patient in acute phase and by the same patient at follow-up, after recovering from acute phase. The graphs represent the measurement of SEMG activities recorded in the left and right MF and ESLD paravertebral muscles as explained above in Section 2 (SENIAM recommendations [37]). The 3D skeleton reconstruction at maximum forward flexion and photos of the subjects are also shown. We remind here that the forward-bending test is defined by the following sequence: from erect standing to maximum forward flexion maintained for a few seconds and then a final extension movement back to erect standing. For this test, the most significant kinematic information comes from sagittal plane ROMs (see **Figure 14**) measured along the execution of the full movement of spine angles (thoracic kyphosis and lumbar lordosis) and pelvis tilt (measured as the inclination of the S1–S3 vertebral segment with respect to the vertical gravity line). By using the 3D skeleton model, the inter-vertebral trunk torques (in the sagittal plane) are assessed as well, during the performance of the test. While there are large obvious differences between healthy and LBP subject in acute phase (this latter being not able to perform a complete forward bending due to pain), more interesting is to focus the analysis on the differences that persist even after the LBP patient recovered from pain. **Figure 15** presents in the lower panels a comparison between a healthy subject versus LBP patient (at follow-up evaluation, when no more pain was present). As it can be noted, from the comparison of the time courses of both ROMs

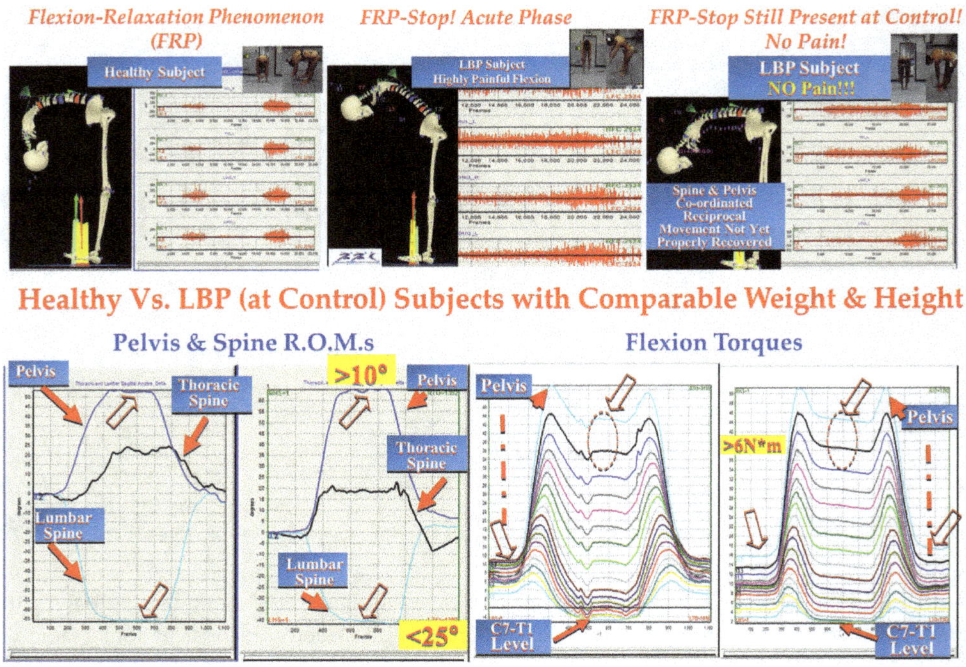

Figure 15. Forward bending results for healthy subject and LBP patient. 3D skeleton reconstruction at maximum forward trunk flexion and measured SEMG activity during the forward-bending test (upper-row panels). Comparison healthy subject versus LBP patient on spine and pelvis measured sagittal ROMs (lower-left panels) and flexion torques patterns (lower-right panels), respectively.

(of spine and pelvis sagittal angles) and flexion torques, the healthy subject presents with respect to the pathological one, both a noticeably lower trunk torques (especially at S1–L5 low lumbar levels) and a wider range of spinal angles, with a different pattern showing different strategies in task execution.

In particular, the LBP patient shows a lower mobility in the lumbar spine with a decrease of the ROM quantified in more than 25° lordosis angle value at maximum forward flexion, compensated by a higher mobility in the pelvis that presents an increase of the ROM quantified in more than 10°at maximum forward flexion. Conversely, thoracic spine mobility ranges are comparable in the two subjects. Such a condition reveals a stiffer behaviour in the lumbar spine of the LBP subject that could be connected to the still persistent FRP stop. In fact, SEMG recordings show, in the healthy subject, a clear presence of FRP as expected, while LBP subject still shows a full contraction activity in all the considered paravertebral muscles, that is, FRP stop. Further studies are currently in progress to determine, on a larger LBP population, if such described FRP stop could relate to modified stiffer pattern and reduced lumbar mobility as observed in this case.

4. Discussion and conclusion

The presented measurement system and approach contain three main sources of potential error: (1) the accuracy of the 3D stereo-photogrammetric capture, (2) operator-dependent skin marker positioning and (3) data processing.

The first instance is no more an issue because present-day high-resolution stereo-photogrammetric systems provide very high accuracy in 3D reconstruction of marker position (0.3–0.4-mm range on a 3-m wide by 3-m deep by 2-m high working volume in entry-level standard 6TVC 0.3 Mpix GOALS system) using well-established and easy-to-manage mature stereo-photogrammetric calibration procedure.

The second source of potential error was the cause for some initial scepticism that this methodology had to suffer from. In fact, notwithstanding characterized by a series of advantages, doubts about such an approach were mostly due to the improper belief of a certain inaccuracy of obtained results because of manual cutaneous positioning of the passive retro-reflective markers on the palpable bony landmarks. Additional concern was linked to supposed time-consuming nature of the marker-positioning process. However, studies [24, 43–45] showed that, obviously, operators need to be trained, as for each imaging-based technique but, when they reach the necessary skill, it has been demonstrated, via X-ray and MRI, that they are able to perform by palpation accurate marker positioning on pre-defined bony prominences. In particular on the spine, intra- and inter-examiner errors resulted relatively low with respect to subject postural adjustment variability. Furthermore, the same studies confirmed that, when the operators are trained, the marker placement takes only few minutes, in addition being a substantial first stage of examination that helps as guidance for the rest of the analysis.

Indeed, the third source of error, that is, data processing, could be a major source of data corruption if improper signal-processing techniques are used. Prior work by D'Amico et al. [7] originally introduced an efficient and specially devised numerical processing technique, showing maximal error of less than 1° (approximately) for the Cobb-computed angle on a curve of about 65°. A subsequent study on scoliotic patients [17] presented an in vivo comparison between frontal plane Cobb angles computed using stereo-photogrammetry and AP (anterior-posterior) X-ray images. Results showed that Cobb angles measured via X-ray matched those accessed via a stereo-photogrammetric system.

The advantages of the presented measurement system and approach are related to the ability to quantitatively capture both static and dynamic body postural expressions, including spinal shape, using 3D imaging of skeleton posture. It can achieve this for a static-erect posture and related oscillations, as well as additionally for the eventual behaviour of body segments during movement. This methodology has no harmful effects, so it provides a 'natural' approach for both capturing and monitoring the progression of pathology and/or the treatment outcomes. Moreover, researchers and clinicians can analyse the upright standing posture in real, neutral and unconstrained conditions, by obtaining, in a rapid and automatic way, a large number of useful 3D and 2D anatomical/biomechanical/clinical parameters. In addition, all possible postural characteristics are measured simultaneously and at a very fast frame rate. These features allow investigators to perform multiple different postural tests, within a same session, and to directly compare them in a statistically reliable way being the final assessment based always on averaged data either in static or in dynamic analysis. In addition, it allows a multi-factorial-multi-sensors approach that provides the capability to fully integrate all the measurement data into a unified view to correlate morphological-kinematic characteristics to full-functional evaluation and to use such results for clinical aims. When the analysis is focused only on 3D posture complemented by bending tests, multi-factorial clinical and biomechanical results (including the analysis and comparisons of standing-erect posture taken in different conditions) are immediately available, in the form of comprehensive report, both to the operator and to the subject at the end of acquisition session. In general, the mean duration of such analysis using the GOALS system lasts from 30 to 45 min. A longer duration is necessary when other more complex motor tasks (gait, run, FRP, etc.) are included in the acquisition session. The case studies presented in this chapter are only exemplary summarizing examples of a wider research activity that our group has carried on in more than 25 years. The obtained results demonstrated such methodology as being entirely suitable and effective for clinical application. This approach was not developed or intended to replace radiographs, from which much more information than spine morphology can be drawn. However, depending on the specific clinical purposes, this methodology could be used during screening and follow-up to reduce patient irradiation, evaluation time and cost.

This framework is extremely useful as a baseline reference at the diagnostic stage not only limited to orthopaedic field but its functional-biomechanical analysis capability can be naturally extended in neurological disorders. For this reason, it could be extremely useful at the stage of designing and developing treatment programmes in rehabilitation, in planning of orthopaedic surgical procedures and in monitoring the progression of pathology and/or treatment outcomes in any kind of postural disorders and pathologies. Additionally, it can be used beneficially for the study of postural characteristics connected to different sports activities as well as to evaluate postural change during growth and/or ageing processes. The GOALS system is under continuous development and improvement. Thousands of patients have been analysed and followed up with this methodology, identifying and precisely differentiating pathological patterns proving to be a type of analysis well accepted both by clinicians and by patients.

Author details

Moreno D'Amico[1,3]*, Edyta Kinel[2], Gabriele D'Amico[3] and Piero Roncoletta[3]

*Address all correspondence to: damicomoreno@gmail.com

1 G. D'Annunzio University, Chieti, Italy

2 Department of Rheumatology and Rehabilitation, Clinic of Rehabilitation, University of Medical Sciences, Poznan, Poland

3 Bioengineering and Biomedicine Company Srl, San Giovanni Teatino, Chieti, Italy

References

[1] Don R, Capodaglio P, Cimolin V, et al. Instrumental measures of spinal function: Is it worth? A state-of-the art from a clinical perspective. European Journal of Physical and Rehabilitation Medicine. 2012;**48**:255-273

[2] Roussouly P, Nnadi C. Sagittal plane deformity: An overview of interpretation and management. European Spine Journal. 2010;**19**:1824-1836

[3] Negrini S, Aulisa AG, Aulisa L, et al. 2011 SOSORT guidelines: Orthopaedic and rehabilitation treatment of idiopathic scoliosis during growth. Scoliosis. 2012;**7**:3

[4] Griegel-Morris P, Larson K, Mueller-Klaus K, et al. Incidence of common postural abnormalities in the cervical, shoulder, and thoracic regions and their association with pain in two age groups of healthy subjects. Physical Therapy. 1992;**72**:425-431

[5] Eric RK, James HS. Principles of Neural Science. 5th ed. New York, NY: McGraw-Hill Education/Medical; 2012

[6] D'Amico M, Roncoletta P. Joint segmental kinematic trunk motion and C.O.P. patterns for multifactorial posturographic analysis. Research into Spinal Deformities 3. 2002;**91**:149-152

[7] D'Amico M, D'Amico G, Roncoletta P. Algorithm for estimation, classification and graphical representation of clinical parameters in the measurement of scoliosis and spinal deformities by means of non-ionising device. Three Dimensional Analysis of Spinal Deformities. 1995;**15**:33-38

[8] D'Amico M, D'Amico G, et al. A 3-D biomechanical skeleton model and processing procedure. European Medical Physics. 2007;**43**:1-6

[9] Hay O, Dar G, Abbas J, et al. The lumbar lordosis in males and females, revisited. PLoS One. 24 August 2015;**10**. DOI: 10.1371/journal.pone.0133685. [Epub ahead of print]

[10] Takács M, Rudner E, Kovács A, et al. The assessment of the spinal curvatures in the sagittal plane of children using an ultrasound-based motion analysing system. Annals in Biomedical Engineering. 2014;**43**:348-362

[11] de Oliveira TS, Candotti CT, La Torre M, et al. Validity and reproducibility of the measurements obtained using the flexicurve instrument to evaluate the angles of thoracic and lumbar curvatures of the spine in the sagittal plane. Rehabilitation and Research Practice. 2012;**2012**:1-9

[12] Krawczky B, Pacheco AG, Mainenti MRM. A systematic review of the angular values obtained by computerized photogrammetry in sagittal plane: A proposal for reference values. Journal of Manipulative Physiological Therapy. 2014;**37**:269-275

[13] Ferreira EA, Duarte M, Maldonado EP, et al. Quantitative assessment of postural alignment in young adults based on photographs of anterior, posterior, and lateral views. Journal of Manipulative Physiological Therapy. 2011;**34**:371-380

[14] Saad KR, Colombo AS, Ribeiro AP, et al. Reliability of photogrammetry in the evaluation of the postural aspects of individuals with structural scoliosis. Journal of Bodywork and Movement Therapies. 2012;**16**:210-216

[15] Furlanetto TS, Sedrez JA, Candotti CT, et al. Photogrammetry as a tool for the postural evaluation of the spine: A systematic review. World Journal of Orthopaedics. 2016;**7**: 136-148

[16] Kotwicki T, Kinel E, Stryla W, et al. Discrepancy in clinical versus radiological parameters describing deformity due to brace treatment for moderate idiopathic scoliosis. Scoliosis. 2007;**2**:18

[17] D'Amico M, Vallasciani M. Non-ionising opto-electronic measurement and X-ray imaging. Two complementary techniques for spinal deformities evaluation and monitoring: Results of one year clinical activity. Research into Spinal Deformities 1. 1997;**37**:151-154

[18] Gracovetsky S, Newman N, Pawlowsky M, et al. A database for estimating normal spinal motion derived from noninvasive measurements. Spine. 1995;**20**:1036-1046

[19] Beaudoin L, Zabjek KF, Leroux MA, et al. Acute systematic and variable postural adaptations induced by an orthopaedic shoe lift in control subjects. European Spine Journal: Official Publication of the European Spine Society, the European Spinal Deformity Society, and the European Section of the Cervical Spine Research Society. 1999;**8**:40-45

[20] Zhao G, Ren L, Ren L, et al. Segmental kinematic coupling of the human spinal column during locomotion. Journal of Bionic Engineering. 2008;**5**:328-334

[21] Chong AK, Milburn P, Newsham-West R, et al. High-accuracy photogrammetric technique for human spine measurement. Photogrammetric Record. 2009;**24**:264-279

[22] Blondel B, Pomero V, Moal B, et al. Sagittal spine posture assessment: Feasibility of a protocol based on intersegmental moments. Orthopaedics & Traumatology: Surgery & Resection. 2012;**98**:109-113

[23] Ranavolo A, Don R, Draicchio F, et al. Modelling the spine as a deformable body: Feasibility of reconstruction using an optoelectronic system. Applied Ergonomics. 2013; **44**:192-199

[24] Schmid S, Studer D, Hasler CC, et al. Using skin markers for spinal curvature quantification in main thoracic adolescent idiopathic scoliosis: An explorative radiographic study. PLoS One. 2015;**10**:1-12

[25] Campos MH, de Paula MC, Deprá PP, et al. The geometric curvature of the spine of runners during maximal incremental effort test. Journal of Biomechanics. 2015;**48**:969-975

[26] Leroux MA, Zabjek K, Simard G, et al. A noninvasive anthropometric technique for measuring kyphosis and lordosis: An application for idiopathic scoliosis. Spine. 2000;**25**:1689-1694

[27] D'Amico M, D'Amico G, Paniccia M, et al. An integrated procedure for spine and full skeleton multi-sensor biomechanical analysis & averaging in posture gait and cyclic movement tasks. Research into Spinal Deformities 7. 2010;**158**:118-126

[28] D'Amico M, Bellomo RG, Saggini R, et al. A 3D spine & full skeleton model for multi-sensor biomechanical analysis in posture & gait. In: 2011 IEEE International Workshop on Medical Measurements and Applications Proceedings (MeMeA); 2011. pp. 605-608

[29] D'Amico M, Roncoletta P, Di Felice F, et al. LBP and lower limb discrepancy: 3D evaluation of postural rebalancing via underfoot wedge correction. Research into Spinal Deformities 8. 2012;**176**:108-112

[30] D'Amico M, Roncoletta P, Di Felice F, et al. Leg length discrepancy in scoliotic patients. Research into Spinal Deformities 8. 2012;**176**:146-150

[31] D'Amico M, Roncoletta P. Baropodographic measurements and averaging in locomotion and postural analysis. Research into Spinal Deformities 3. 2002;**91**:156-161

[32] Seidel GK, Marchinda DM, Dijkers M, et al. Hip joint center location from palpable bony landmarks—A cadaver study. Journal of Biomechanics. 1995;**28**:995-998

[33] de Leva P. Joint center longitudinal positions computed from a selected subset of Chandler's data. Journal of Biomechanics. 1996;**29**:1231-1233

[34] Zatsiorsky V, Seluyanov V, Chugunova L. In: Berme N, Capozzo A, editors. In Vivo Body Segment Inertial Parameters Determination using a Gamma-Scanner Method. OH, USA; Bertec Corporation-Worthington: 1990. pp. 186-202

[35] Liu YK, Wickstrom JK. Estimation of the inertial property distribution of the human torso from segmented cadaveric data. In: Kenedi RM, editor. Perspectives in Biomedical Engineering: Proceedings of a Symposium organised in association with the Biological Engineering Society and held in the University of Strathclyde, Glasgow. June 1972; London: Palgrave Macmillan UK. pp. 203-213

[36] Ferrigno G, Pedrocchi A, Baroni G, et al. ELITE-S2: The multifactorial movement analysis facility for the International Space Station. Acta Astronautica. 2004;**54**:723-735

[37] Hermens HJ, of the European Communities. Biomedical C, Programme HR. European recommendations for surface ElectroMyoGraphy: Results of the SENIAM project. Roessingh Research and Development. 1999. Available from: http://books.google.es/books?id=w7HgOwAACAAJ

[38] Colloca CJ, Hinrichs RN. The biomechanical and clinical significance of the lumbar erector spinae flexion-relaxation phenomenon: A review of literature. Journal of Manipulative Physiological Therapy. 2005;**28**:623-631

[39] Stokes IA, Burwell RG, Dangerfield PH. Biomechanical spinal growth modulation and progressive adolescent scoliosis—A test of the 'vicious cycle' pathogenetic hypothesis: Summary of an electronic focus group debate of the IBSE. Scoliosis and Spinal Disorders. 2006;**1**:16

[40] Meir AR, Fairbank JCT, Jones DA, et al. High pressures and asymmetrical stresses in the scoliotic disc in the absence of muscle loading. Scoliosis. 2007;**2**:4

[41] McGill SM, Kippers V. Transfer of loads between lumbar tissues during the flexion-relaxation phenomenon. Spine. 1994;**19**:2190-2196

[42] Nederhand MJ, Hermens HJ, IJzerman MJ, et al. Chronic neck pain disability due to an acute whiplash injury. Pain. 2003;**102**:63-71

[43] Negrini A, Negrini S, Santambrogio GC. Data variability in the analysis of spinal deformity: A study performed by means of the AUSCAN System. Three Dimensional Analysis of Spinal Deformities. 1995;**15**:101-106

[44] Negrini S, Negrini A, Atanasio S, et al. Postural variability of clinical parameters evaluated in orthostatic position in idiopathic scoliosis. European Medicophysics. 2001;**37**:135-142

[45] Zemp R, List R, Gulay T, et al. Soft tissue artefacts of the human back: Comparison of the sagittal curvature of the spine measured using skin markers and an open upright MRI. PLoS One. 2014;**9**:1-8

10

Sagittal Alignment in Spinal Deformity: Implications for the Non-Operative Care Practitioner

Prachi Bakarania, Hagit Berdishevsky, Kelly Grimes and John Tunney

Abstract

Sagittal alignment has become a hot topic in the world of orthopedics, particularly as it pertains to adults with spine deformities and coexisting pain, activity limitations, and health-related quality of life. It is reported that the prevalence of spinal deformity in the older adult will continue to increase. Clinicians across disciplines recognize the myriad of variation that exists in sagittal alignment, and that there is not one ideal norm to ascribe to. Relatively new to the spine deformity community has been the discovery of the relationship between the pelvis and the femur (pelvic incidence) in dictating lumbar lordosis and overall spinal alignment. While it is acknowledged that variation exists, there is now evidence that there is a limited range within which we can compensate for loss of sagittal alignment and still function well. When compensations run out, the quality of life becomes affected. These alignment variations, compensations, and in some cases, loss of alignment all together have clinical implications for the physiotherapist working with the older adult population. The purpose of this chapter is to describe the current state of evidence-informed knowledge around spinopelvic parameters as they relate to the adult with spine deformity and offer clinical implications for the conservative care practitioner.

Keywords: adult spinal deformity, scoliosis, sagittal alignment, pelvic incidence, lumbar lordosis, sagittal vertical axis

Learning objectives

1. Explain why the sagittal profile is important from an evolutionary and biomechanical perspective.
2. Appreciate the historical evolution of our understanding of sagittal alignment.

3. Define key sagittal parameters.
4. Explain the correlations between the various parameters that are key in understanding the sagittal relationships.
5. Describe how spinal deformity may lead to compensatory changes in sagittal alignment.
6. State implications in terms of assessment strategies for the conservative care practitioner (physiotherapists/orthotists).

1. Introduction

Spinal Deformity may be defined as an abnormality in alignment, formation, or curvature of one or more portions of the spine [1]. Spine deformities can occur in one or a combination of the axial, coronal, and sagittal planes. Scoliosis is a spinal deformity defined by the Scoliosis Research Society (SRS) as a lateral curve measuring 10° or more on an anterior-posterior radiograph with the presence of vertebral rotation [2].

In recent years, attention to the role of sagittal plane alignment in the overall health and function of adults with spine deformity has increased [3]. The purpose of this chapter is to shed light on the body of literature surrounding sagittal alignment variations and hypothesize about clinical implications for the conservative care practitioner managing spinal deformity in clinical practice.

2. Main body

2.1. Definition of posture

Alignment and postural control have long been fundamental to the clinical decision-making process of the physiotherapist. The Guide to Physical Therapy Practice lists "Posture" as a key test and measure to be included in a physiotherapist's objective examination [4]. Indeed, there exists no universal definition of posture and within postural control, alignment [5]. However, health-care practitioners from various backgrounds make similar statements when describing posture. Basmajian in 1965 understood posture to be the "upright, well-balanced stance of the human subject in a 'normal' position" [6]. The Posture Committee of the American Academy of Orthopedic Surgeons (AAOS) defines posture as "the state of muscular and skeletal balance which protects the supporting structures of the body against injury or progressive deformity, irrespective of the attitude in which the structures are working or resting. Under such conditions, the muscles will function most efficiently and the optimum positions are afforded for the thoracic and abdominal organs" [7].

2.2. Evolutionary perspective on upright posture

In evolutionary terms, it is upright stance and the ability of humans to achieve bipedalism that differentiates humans from the majority of the animal world. This ability was made possible by the evolution of the structure of the pelvis and lumbar spine as well as their muscular attachments.

Several changes have been critical to this evaluation. First, the human lumbar spine is exceedingly longer and more mobile, which has allowed for lumbar lordosis (LL)/extension to align the trunk over the pelvis from a lateral view [8].

Second, the sacrum in humans is broader/wider. It contributes to the mobility of the lower lumbar segments to form lordosis, where the narrowness of the sacrum and length of the ilia in other primates "lock" the lower lumbar segments [9]. In addition to the sacrum being shorter in length and broader in width, the ilia are also broader in width and more flared anteriorly [9]. This adaptation brings the anterior gluteal muscles (gluteus medius and minimus) from their former roles as hip extensors and migrates them laterally and anteriorly to perform their current roles as hip abductors and stabilizers of the pelvis during the single limb stance phase of gait. In partnership with a longer femoral neck, the gluteals create a longer lever arm, allowing the hip abductors to function more effectively in stabilizing the pelvis during the stance phase of gait.

Other muscular changes include hypertrophy of the gluteus maximus in humans, particularly during running, where it serves to keep the trunk from falling forward during heel strike [9]. Additionally, the hamstrings, while they played a "power" function in quadrupedal locomotion, play more of a stabilizing/control role in human bipedal locomotion. Furthermore, humans have smaller erector spinae muscles most likely owing to the center of mass being at the second sacral vertebrae, which creates a shorter lever arm in which the erector spinae have to work [9]. Therefore, the muscles do not need to be under such constant activation.

A general understanding of the evolution of spinopelvic alignment and upright stance helps us understand how the loss of this congruent relationship is potentially problematic in individuals with spinal deformity.

2.3. Historical perspective on understanding of sagittal alignment

The evolution of our understanding of sagittal alignment has been developing for over 150 years. It is von Meyer who is credited with the discovery of the weight center of the human body at the level of the second sacral vertebra [6]. Although highly variable, most clinicians and researchers reporting on alignment agree that the line of gravity should pass near the mastoid process of the temporal bone, just anterior to the second sacral vertebrae, just posterior to the hip joint, and just anterior to the knee and ankle joint [6, 7, 9, 10]. Thus, balanced about this line of gravity, man is able to remain upright with mild anterior/posterior sway and minimal energy expenditure.

The German orthopedist, Franz Staffell, in 1889, is credited with further sub-classification of ideal posture into categories (i.e., round, flat, lordotic) [11].

Statements such as that made by Schulthess in 1905 are indicative of the openness of clinicians to the variation in the sagittal plane versus the assumption of one ideal posture and all else faulty [12].

Kendall, Kendall, and Boynton in 1952 described an ideal postural type and three faulty postural types (kyphotic-lordotic, flat back, and swayback) [7]. Rex McMorris in 1961 described what he termed faulty postural types in children [13]. Roussouly in 2005 identified lordotic types, which will be discussed in further detail later in this chapter [14]. Mac-Thiong in 2010 described six postural types [15].

Our evolution in understanding the relationship of the pelvis to the spine can be traced to the early 1960s. Joanne Bullock-Saxton, in her narrative review in 1988, citied work by Hollinshead in 1962 observing a relationship between the position of the pelvis and the amount of lumbar lordosis [16]. Indeed, others also discussed the interaction between pelvic obliquity or pelvic inclination and its role in determining the degree of lumbar lordosis. Additionally, the obliquity of the sacrum was determined to be related to the degree of lumbar lordosis [16]. During et al. explained the relationship between the position of the sacrum and the depth of lumbar lordosis as functional. The steeper the slope of the upper portion of the sacrum, the deeper the lumbar lordosis needs to be in order to maintain optimal position of the upper part of the body over the lower along the line of gravity [17].

The advent of instrumentation with spinal fusion in the surgical management of scoliosis and spinal deformity has led to a greater push to understand sagittal alignment. Although early surgical instrumentation was effective in addressing the frontal plane aspect of the scoliotic alignment, follow-up revealed often deleterious effects on the sagittal plane [18]. Doherty, in 1973, described what was later coined by Moe and Denis as "flatback syndrome," characterized by a fixed forward inclination of the trunk due to the loss of normal lumbar lordosis [18]. The early instrumentation combined the use of a straight rod with distractive forces and, when intervention extended to lower lumbar levels, the combination of these forces led to a loss of lumbar lordosis [18]. Recognition of this postoperative outcome led to advancements in surgical technique, which is beyond the scope of this text, as well as the understanding of the need to not only preserve but also enhance lumbar lordosis in order to minimize the risk of postoperative flatback syndrome. The identification of pelvic incidence, a morphological parameter that describes the relationship of the sacrum to the femur, represented a turning point in the movement to better address the sagittal plane from an operative perspective [19]. These parameters and their clinical implications may also be useful, as we will see, for the physiotherapist working with the older adult with spine deformity, as it gives us parameters within which we can better prognosticate the type of client we may be able to work with successfully.

2.4. Measuring spinopelvic alignment

Assess a patient's sagittal alignment allows the practitioner to objectively understand its potential role in contributing to a patient's pain and dysfunction. In 2006, the Scoliosis Research Society published the first classification system to develop a common language around adult spinal deformity (ASD). This classification grew out of an understanding that the existing adolescent scoliosis classifications were not entirely applicable to the adult population when making clinical decisions around operative management. The most recent update on this classification emphasizes the importance the sagittal plane plays in maintaining healthy upright spinal postures. Their work is valuable for the conservative care practitioner to help make clinical predictions as to the contribution of alignment to pain in our patients with spinal deformity [20].

The first step of the classification is to identify the coronal curve type, depending on the location of the curve apices and convexities. The categories are thoracic, thoracolumbar/lumbar, or double curve. The second step is to assess for the presence of sagittal modifiers. These modifiers include pelvic incidence (PI), global alignment via sagittal vertical axis (SVA), pelvic tilt (PT), degree of lumbar lordosis (LL), as well as subluxation or listhesis in the frontal or sagittal plane [20].

2.4.1. Pelvic incidence

Pelvic incidence is an anatomical or morphological measurement that is unique to each individual and is independent to the spatial orientation of the pelvis (**Figure 1**). It is specific to each individual and remains constant throughout the life span. The steps in measuring PI are as follows: (1) Draw a line across S1 superior end plate. (2) Find the midpoint from #1 and draw a downward perpendicular line. (3) Draw a line from the center of the femoral head line to the center of the center sacrum line. Often in the presence of pelvic obliquity you will need to find the midpoint of both femoral heads. (4) The angle between these lines is the pelvic incidence.

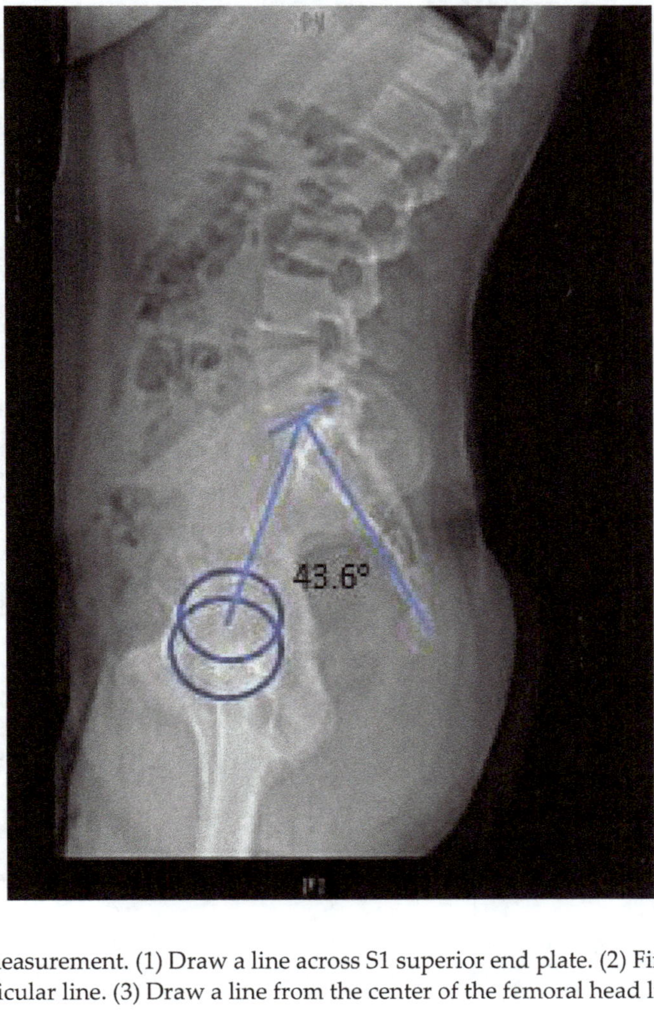

Figure 1. Pelvic incidence measurement. (1) Draw a line across S1 superior end plate. (2) Find the midpoint from #1 and draw a downward perpendicular line. (3) Draw a line from the center of the femoral head line to the center of the center sacrum line.

2.4.2. Lumbar lordosis

Lumbar lordosis is measured by the angulation from the inferior angle of T12 and the superior end plate of S1 (**Figure 2**).

2.4.3. SVA

Sagittal vertical axis is used to measure the degree of forward or backward angulation of a patient's posture. SVA is one of the easiest radiological parameters to measure, since the

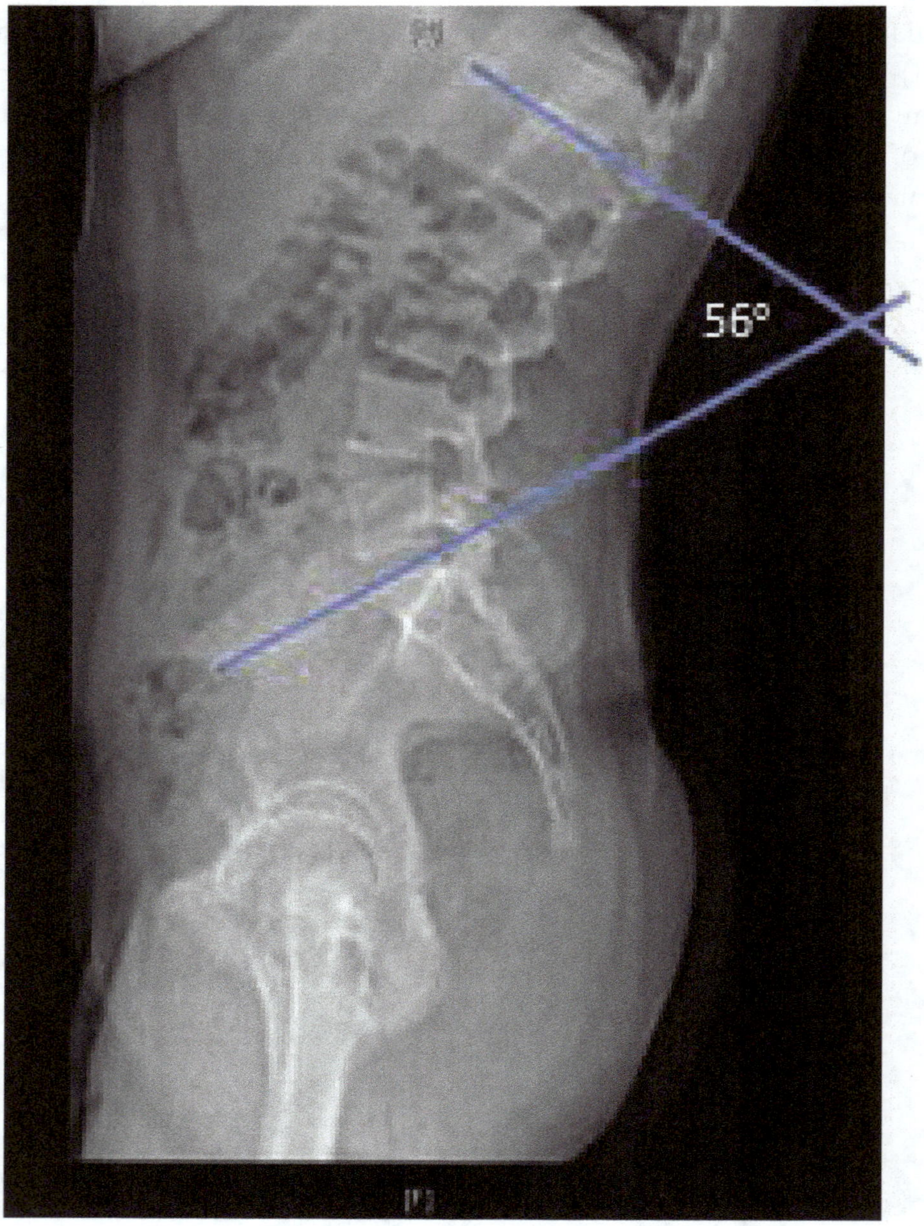

Figure 2. Lumbar lordosis measurement: From inferior end plate of T12 and superior end place of sacral. This patient has a lumbar lordosis of 56.2°.

femoral heads do not have to be visualized. For this reason, the authors have found it to be a clinically relevant and useful measure to incorporate into clinical practice. The steps to measure SVA on a standard lateral view radiograph are as follows: (1) Identify the center of C7—inferior end plate, and draw a line straight down perpendicular to the bottom of the film. (2) Draw a vertical line from the posterior-superior corner of the sacrum. (3) Measure the distance between lines 1 and 2 [21]. A positive number indicates that C7 is in front of sacrum. On a clinical examination, the patient's head is likely to be in front of the torso as well as his trunk in a more forward flexed position. A negative number indicates that a C7 is behind the sacrum. This type of posture is often called swayback. Clinically, the patient likely stands with their pelvis more in front than their head (**Figure 3A** and **B**).

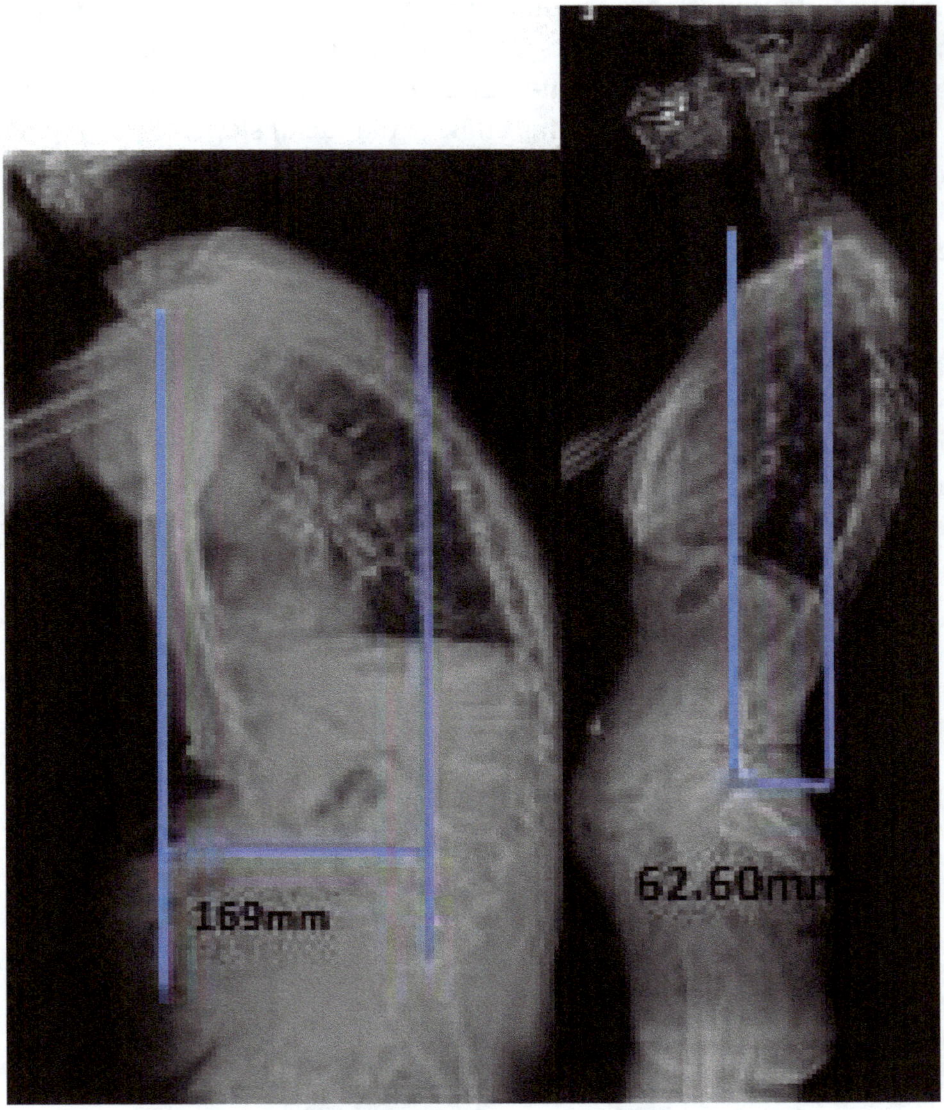

Figure 3. SVA—Sagittal vertical axis: The steps to measure SVA are as follows: (1) Identify the center of C7—inferior end plate, and draw a line straight down perpendicular to the bottom of the film. (2) Draw a vertical line from the posterior-superior corner of the sacrum. (3) Measure the distance between lines 1 and 2. (A) This individual has a (+) SVA of 169.98 mm. (B) This indivdual has a (-) SVA of 62.6mm.

2.4.4. Pelvic tilt

Radiological pelvic tilt is a sagittal measurement that can be assessed on a lateral radiograph. Refer to **Figure 4** for specifics. The following are the measurement steps: (1) Draw a line from the midpoint of the sacral end plate running perpendicular down to the bottom of the X-ray. (2) Draw a line from the center of the femoral heads to the center of the sacrum. (3) The angle between these two lines is the pelvic tilt. Also, pelvic tilt + sacral slope (SS) = pelvic incidence (**Figure 4**) [21].

2.4.5. Sacral slope

The last radiological measure discussed here is the least discussed as it is often difficult to measure. However, its importance is vital to understanding the relationship of the other parameters. Refer to **Figure 5** for specifics. The steps to measurement are as follows: (1) Draw a line along the superior sacral end plate. (2) Draw a line from the anterior superior edge parallel to the bottom of the X-ray. (3) This angle is the sacral slope. Pelvic incidence = sacral slope + pelvic tilt [22].

2.5. Inter-relationships between spinopelvic parameters

A significant chain of interdependence exists between pelvic and spinal parameters. Pelvic incidence, as previously stated, is an independent and anatomic parameter that determines pelvic orientation and the optimal size of lumbar lordosis [19]. In practice, the PI of an individual is correlated together with his or her sacral slope. In this section, both SS and PI will be described in relation to LL and sagittal balance as well as the consequences of mismatch between the pelvic parameters and LL for the adult individual with spinal deformity.

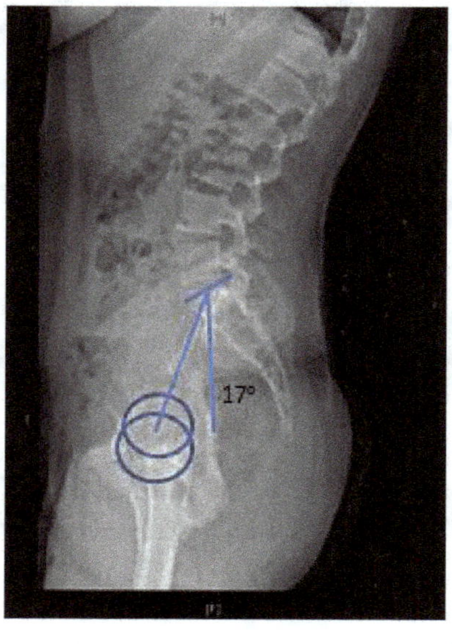

Figure 4. Pelvic tilt. (1) Draw a line from the midpoint of the sacral end plate running perpendicular down to the bottom of the X-ray. (2) Draw a line from the center of the femoral heads to the center of the sacrum. (3) The angle between these two lines is the pelvic tilt. This individual's pelvic tilt measures 17°.

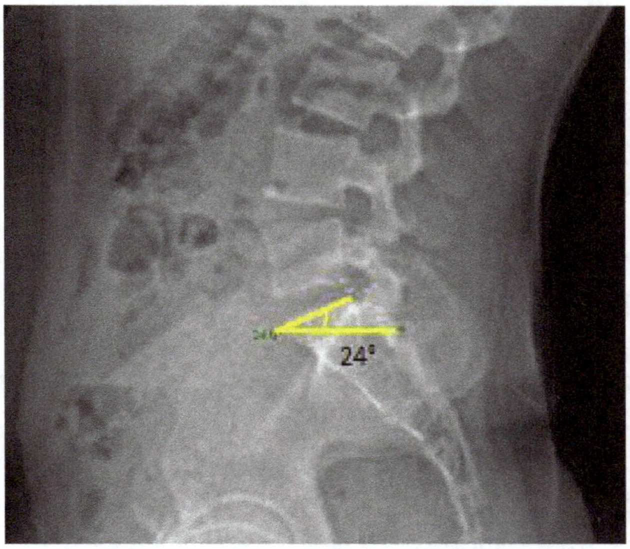

Figure 5. Sacral slope: (1) Draw a line along the superior sacral end plate. (2) Draw a line from the anterior superior edge parallel to the bottom of the X-ray. (3) This angle is the sacral slope. This individual's sacral slope measures 24°.

2.5.1. *Influence of sacral slope on global sagittal alignment*

In a well-balanced spine, the SS is between 35 and 45° and the LL has an apex at L3–L4 [23] (**Figure 6**). In an individual with a low SS angle (<35°), a regional hypolordotic lumbar deformity with a compensatory hypo-kyphosis or normal thoracic and lumbar apex at L5 may be observed [23]. *Regional deformity* is defined as sagittal kyphotic misalignment that affects a limited number of segments of the spine (i.e., the lumbar spine, the thoracic spine, the thoracolumbar junction (TLJ), or the lower lumbar spine). *Compensatory mechanisms* are changes in the sagittal alignment of spinal or non-spinal segments, different from those involved in regional deformity, to restore the

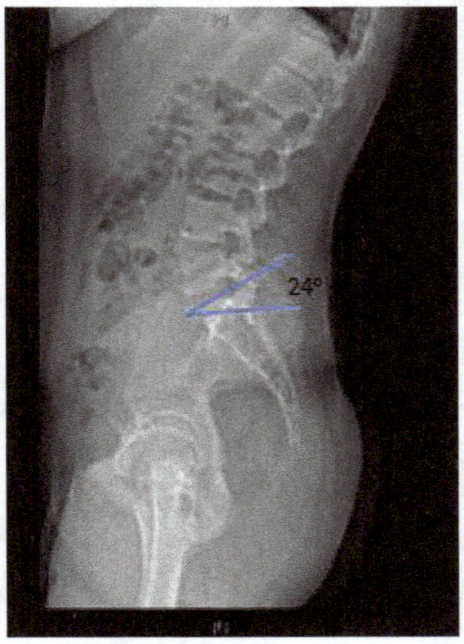

Figure 6. Drawings of sacral slope and sagittal spinal alignments. Left: Sacral slope (SS) < 35°, apex of lumbar lordosis (LL) at middle L5, the spine is hypolordotic and relatively normal kyphotic; middle: 35° < SS < 45°, apex of LL at middle L3–L4, the spine is well balanced; right: SS > 45°, apex of LL at base L3, the spine is hyperlordotic and hyper-kyphotic.

alignment of the gravity line or the horizontal gaze. Compensatory mechanisms need active muscle contraction by the subject [24, 25]. When the SS is high (>45°), a regional hyper-lordosis lumbar deformity along with compensatory thoracic hyper-kyphosis may commonly be observed [23].

2.5.2. *Pelvic incidence and its relationship to LL and sagittal balance*

A mean value PI was documented in 2011 to be 55 ± 10° [24], and a mean value of LL and thoracic kyphosis (TK) was documented in 1989 to be 44 and 36° [26]. These mean values do not imply ideal but simply a fixed angle providing anatomical characteristics of the pelvis and lumbar spine. Ranges of value are more appropriate for describing normal, but in this section, the mean values give an easier way of understanding the concept of match versus mismatch between the two. A ±10° difference between PI and LL was documented as an ideal match for optimal maintenance of sagittal balance [27]. A *match* occurs when both PI and LL are within the margin of 10° difference (known as PI-LL = 10 or PI − LL = 10). PI and LL can be high or low in degrees and still be considered a match. For example, a PI of 70° and an LL of 65° would be considered a high degree. A PI of 30° and an LL of 35° would be considered a low degree. In both cases, the difference between them is 5° and thus considered a match and a harmonious sagittal plane alignment (**Figure 7**).

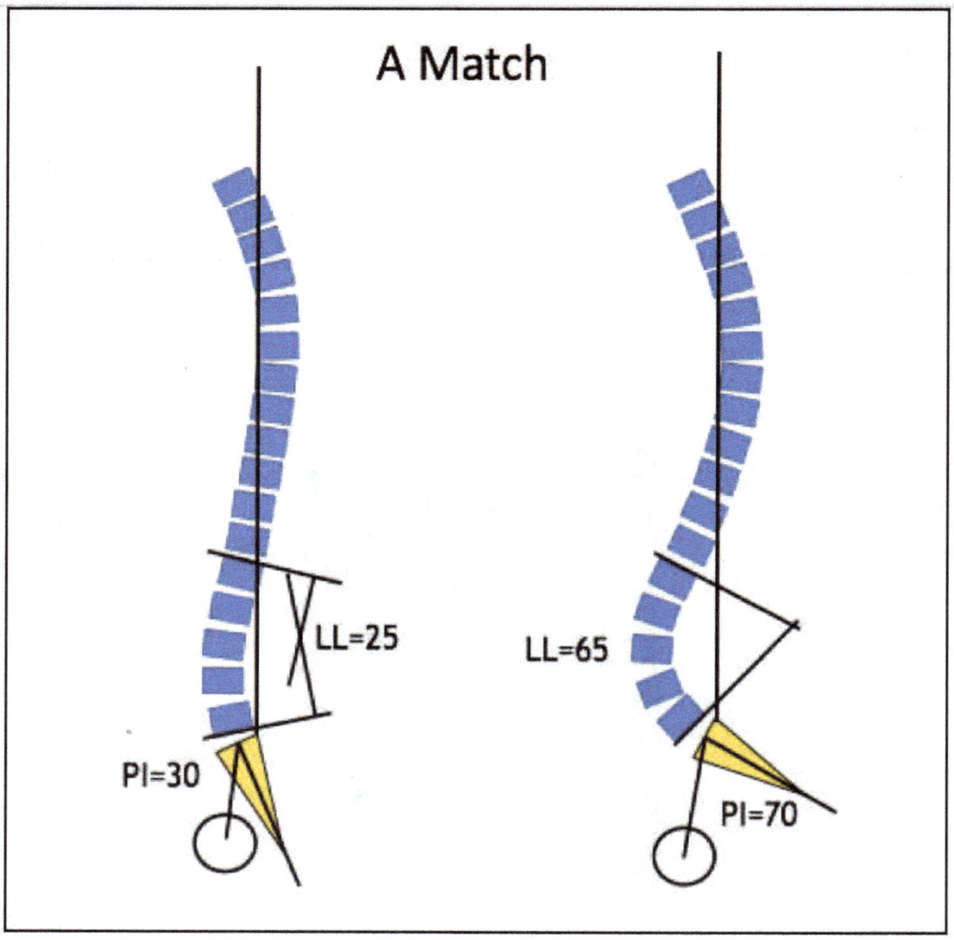

Figure 7. Representative drawing of harmonious spine in the sagittal plane: high PI and LL (left) and low PI and LL (right). Both are a match between PI and LL of two possible separate individuals.

A *mismatch* occurs when there is a greater than 10° difference between PI and LL and can lead to a disharmonious sagittal plane alignment. A mismatch can be presented by high PI and low LL (PI-LL >10) or the opposite (**Figure 8**).

The most documented [24–26] types of mismatches in adolescent idiopathic scoliosis (AIS) and ASD include those with PI-LL >10° where the PI is high and the LL is low (**Figure 9**).

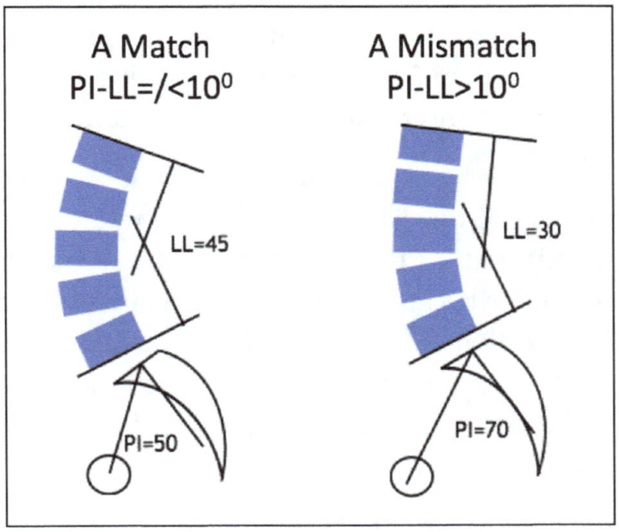

Figure 8. Representative drawing of match (left) and mismatch (right) PI and LL.

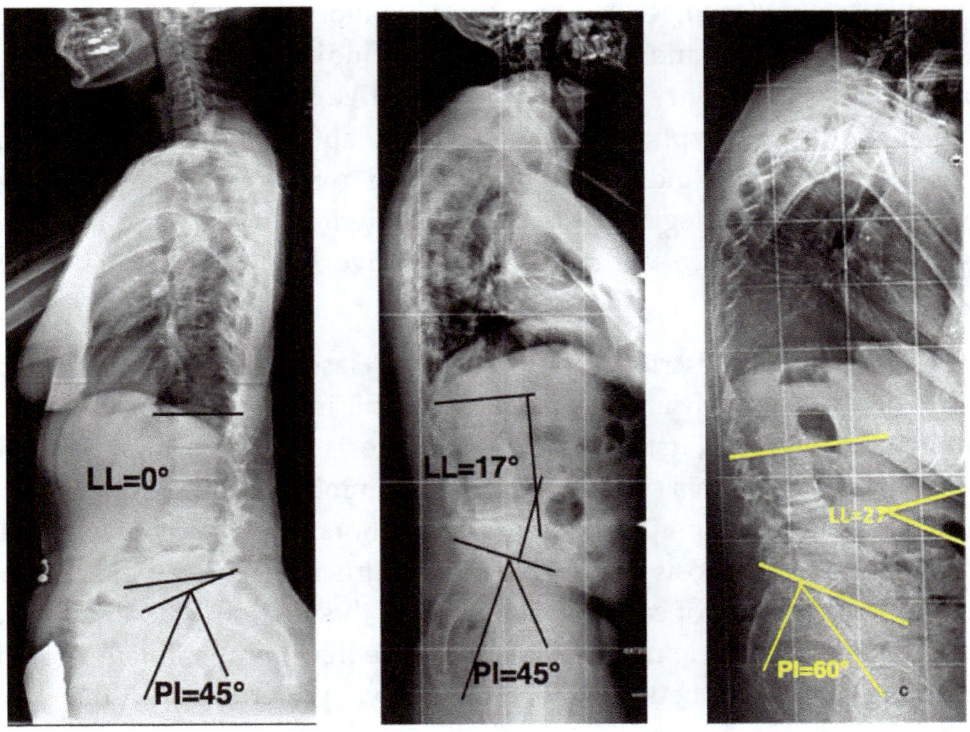

Figure 9. Mismatch PI-LL in adolescent (left) and older adults (middle and right).

2.5.3. Clinical implications

Radiological parameters that most highly correlate with pain, disability, and low quality of life are sagittal vertical axis, pelvic tilt, and the PI-LL relationship and are thus key components of the SRS-Schwab ASD classification [20, 27–29].

In a multi-center, prospective cohort trial in 2013 related radiological parameter thresholds to clinical findings as being predictive of worse clinical symptoms and poorer quality of life [28]. They proposed and concluded that a PI-LL of 10° or less, global alignment (positive SVA) of less than 4 cm, and PT of less than 20° were the ideal spinopelvic alignment for reducing operative intervention procedures and postoperative pain and disability [28].

Overall, literature demonstrates increased surgical complexity with increased severity of sagittal deformity modifiers. A significantly higher osteotomy rate was reported with increasing positive sagittal malalignment and a PI-LL mismatch [29–31]. Iliac fixation was more commonly used as global alignment became increasingly positive. Berjano and Aebi reported the value of the pedicle subtraction osteotomy (PSO), a procedure to restore lumbar lordosis in patients with lumbar/thoracolumbar scoliosis, concurrent loss of lumbar lordosis, and PI-LL mismatch [32]. This procedure has been demonstrated to restore sagittal alignment and improve patient self-reported pain and function.

The incorporation of spinopelvic parameters into surgical decision making has provided greater insight into the relationship between spine deformity and compensatory strategies to attempt to maintain upright alignment. It is theorized, for example, that a person with a low PI may adapt well to a situation if their lumbar lordosis is reduced (due to degenerative changes or scoliosis) because their sagittal alignment, based on the existence of low PI, may more readily "accept" changes that will cause hypolordosis in the lumbar spine and still maintain a match between PI and LL. Conversely, an individual with a high PI and low or loss of lumbar lordosis (secondary to lumbar degenerative changes or scoliosis or to compensate for a decreased thoracic kyphosis) will likely not adapt as well as the one described first. The high PI may not allow the individual to adapt well to the low lumbar lordosis, and after exhausting compensatory strategies at the pelvis (through pelvic tilt) and lower extremities, they may tend toward a positive sagittal balance (positive SVA) and potential compensations in the thoracic spine as well.

Lamartina and Berjano [24] describe a comprehensive classification of sagittal imbalance. In their classification, two compensatory mechanisms occur in response to reduced lumbar lordosis (i.e., lumbar kyphosis). First, local lumbar kyphosis may be compensated for by thoracic lordosis (**Figure 10**). In this situation, the thoracolumbar junction is normal or lordotic. Second, lumbar kyphosis may not be compensated by thoracic lordosis but by thoracic hyperkyphosis causing global kyphosis. In this case, the TLJ is in kyphosis, and the whole spine demonstrates an anterior loss of sagittal balance. In both situations, there will be additional compensations, including pelvic retroversion and knee flexion to maintain upright posture. The reason for the differences between the two is not yet understood but the most accepted theory is that the differences in compensation in the thoracic region are based on the preexisting alignment of the thoracic (being originally hypo-kyphotic vs. normal or hyper-kyphotic)

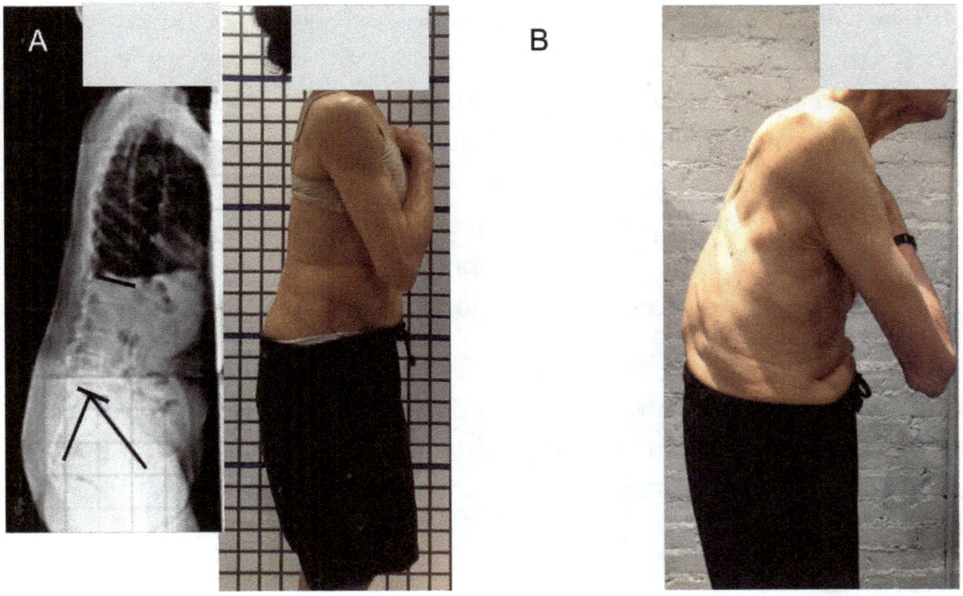

Figure 10. (A) Lumbar kyphosis with a compensatory thoracic lordosis, pelvic retroversion (increased pelvic tilt), and knee flexion. (B) global kyphosis—lumbar kyphosis is not compensated by thoracic lordosis. The TLJ is kyphotic. Compensatory pelvic tilt and flexed knees are present.

and the TLJ. Lumbar kyphosis differs from global kyphosis in that in *lumbar kyphosis*, there is a local kyphosis (at the lumbar region) with compensatory thoracic hypo-kyphosis (**Figure 10A**). In this alignment strategy, thoracic extensor muscles are active, and patients may benefit from remodeling of the lumbar lordosis conservatively or by selective lumbar osteotomy and fusion where the patient may regain a balance with reversal of the compensatory mechanism of the thoracic spine. In *global kyphosis*, the thoracic spine fails to compensate to the lumbar kyphosis and the whole trunk becomes kyphotic (**Figure 10B**).

2.5.4. Summary

The literature review of this section demonstrates that the sagittal plane is vital to understanding pain and disability in patients with ASD, and that SVA, PT, and PI-LL mismatch are the main drivers that affect disability and decreased function [27–32]. Becoming proficient in defining radiographically the above parameters, values and limits, can help guide a better therapeutic decision-making process conservatively and operatively with the aim and focus on maintaining or creating the best sagittal alignment for the individual that will improve function, as well as decrease pain and disability.

2.6. Assessment of the patient with ASD

The objective examination should begin with the assessment of alignment using a posture grid. In this section, we only discuss the evaluation of the sagittal alignment. With the patient standing sideways to the posture grid, the examiner can obtain sagittal alignment in a variety of ways, utilizing tools such as an inclinometer, a flexi-ruler, or a plumbline. The amount of cervical lordosis, thoracic kyphosis, lumbar lordosis, thoracolumbar junction transitional area, pelvic tilt, as well as description of hip and knee position can be measured. An increase in thoracic kyphosis (hyper-kyphosis), and loss of lordosis either in the cervical or in the lumbar/thoracolumbar region, may lead to alignment faults accompanied by muscle length/strength/activation changes that will need to be tested and addressed. See **Table 1** for a description of predicted implications of various alignment faults on mobility, muscle length, strength, and muscle performance. This is not an all-inclusive list and does not substitute for a careful evaluation of alignment and contributing factors to the clinical presentation of the client. See **Table 2** for take-home messages regarding radiological parameters as were discussed in this chapter.

Specific intervention strategies are beyond the scope of this chapter. The authors recommend that clinicians interested in working with this patient population pursue additional training in scoliosis education as most experts view it as a sub-specialty in physiotherapy practice [34].

Thoracic hyper-kyphosis	Loss of LL with TLJ in kyphosis	Loss of LL with TLJ normal or lordotic	PI and hip pathology
Compensatory alignment faults • excess cervical lordosis with forward head • excess lumbar lordosis **Mobility deficits** • shoulder range of motion (ROM): flexion and external rotation • thoracic mobility • ribcage mobility **Muscle length deficits** • short/stiff pectorals • short/stiff latissimus dorsi • short/stiff rectus abdominus **Muscle performance deficits** • abdominals (imbalance of coordination/recruitment of abdominal musculature) • scapular adductors • thoracic extensors	**Compensatory alignment faults** • increased thoracic and global kyphosis • increased pelvic tilt • increased hip/knee flexion **Mobility deficits** • shoulder range of motion (ROM): flexion and external rotation • thoracic mobility • ribcage mobility **Muscle length deficits** • short/stiff pectorals • short/stiff latissimus dorsi • short/stiff rectus abdominus **Muscle performance deficits** • abdominals (imbalance of coordination/recruitment of abdominal musculature) • scapular adductors • global trunk extensors and hip extensors, knee extensors	**Compensatory alignment faults** • increased thoracic hypo-kyphosis (usually preexisting) **Mobility deficits** • thoracic mobility • ribcage mobility **Muscle length deficits** • short/stiff or overactive thoracic extensors • short/stiff rectus **Muscle performance deficits** • abdominals (imbalance of coordination/recruitment of abdominal musculature) • scapular adductors • global trunk extensors and hip extensors, knee extensors	Novel theory hypothesizing relationship between low PI and femoral acetabular impingement (FAI) [33] Low PI → anterior pelvic tilt with gait → artificial anterior acetabular over coverage and recurrent FAI that increases risk for CAM morphology

Table 1. Common sagittal alignment faults and predicted impairments.

Take-home messages on radiological measurements: [20–22, 27, 28]
1. Pelvic incidence = sacral slope + pelvic tilt—This is a radiological measurement
2. Lumbar lordosis should be within ±10° of pelvic incidence (PI)
3. Pelvic tilt should be <25°
4. SVA (sagittal vertical axis)- should be within 46mm
5. Frontal or sagittal plane listhesis, 0 cm

Table 2. Take-home messages on radiological measurements.

2.7. Implications of sagittal alignment and spinopelvic parameters for the orthotist managing adolescents with spine deformity

2.7.1. The evolution of orthoses for patients with spinal deformity

Spinal bracing has evolved significantly since the days of Dr. Sayre's tripod device and Dr. Taylors "spinal assistant," both notable historical reference points [35]. The ideas that they employed are still found in orthoses designed today. The concepts of spinal elongation, application of pressure to the prominence of the deformity, and "windows" to create areas of relief are still basic concepts of almost all bracing types still used today. This demonstrates to us that we are not starting a new form of treatment but merely using research to advance ideas started long ago. For further reference, please refer to the SRS bracing manual [36].

The pivotal *Bracing in Adolescent Idiopathic Scoliosis trial* (BrAIST) has altered the medical community's recommendation on bracing in the AIS population. The study was originally designed as a randomized controlled study, but when enrollment goals were not being met, a preference arm was added. This meant that families who opted against randomization were able to choose which group they would like to enter [37]. The study used 44% of patients assigned to the randomized cohort to calculate their intention to treat analysis. They found that the Number Needed to Treat (NNT) in order to prevent one case of curve progression was 3.0 and reduction in relative risk with bracing was 56% [37]. This is no small matter as scoliosis fusion surgery was second only to appendicitis in terms of the total cost in children aged 10–17 years [37, 38]. The BrAIST study linked the success of the brace with more hours of wear time, an average of 17.7 h per day [37].

2.7.2. Role of the sagittal profile in scoliosis orthoses—our theory

It has long been known that scoliosis is a three-dimensional deformity, and even in the presence of spinal deformity, the body will try to regain balance. Historically, the focus of intervention has been on the control of the frontal and transverse plane. However, the sagittal plane may play a larger role in spinal deformity than previously suspected. The pelvic incidence parameter, described earlier in this chapter, may be a key factor in driving sagittal alignment and an important factor in brace design [19]. It is known that spinal loading occurs mainly via axial compression. However, vertebral bodies are also subjected to shear forces in an anterior or posterior direction. The more posterior the shear force, the less stable the spine is in rotation [39]. It may be theorized that increased posteriorly directed shear forces increase the risk of scoliotic deformity. A study by Schlosser in 2015 noted that the spines of girls during the peak growth spurt are more posteriorly inclined [40]. If accounting for sagittal forces during the peak growth phase can reduce this rotational instability, it may lead to further efforts both clinically and research-wise to address scoliosis based on parameters in addition to the Cobb angle. It may be, according to the hypothesis of the authors, that an increase in Cobb angle is a reaction to the above-described imbalance and instability. Is it possible to predict at-risk patients based on parameters other than the Cobb angle and treat these patients proactively? These questions warrant more clinical research.

2.7.3. Brace construction

Up to now, the goal in orthoses fabrication has been to maintain "normal" lumbar lordosis and kyphosis values. However, there is a wide range of "normal" ranges in pediatrics. The original scoliosis TLSO used 0° of lordosis as its default value. It was noted that orthoses may achieve the same coronal correction with a lumbar lordosis of 15°, which led to increased patient comfort level. This point is referenced in the SRS bracing manual and in an editorial response in which research has proven the original Boston brace set at 0° of lordosis "produced significant curve correction of the spinal deformity in the frontal plane at the expense of a significant reduction of thoracic kyphosis in the sagittal plane" [36, 41] (**Figure 11**). With respect to the sagittal profile, the authors feel it is imperative to match a patient's individual pelvic incidence to their ideal lumbar lordosis when constructing a brace. In a study using biomechanical modeling, we have the first opportunity to trial several braces on the same patient to observe outcomes based on 15 different design factors [42] (**Figure 12**). This study had some interesting conclusions which may help guide the future of brace treatment.

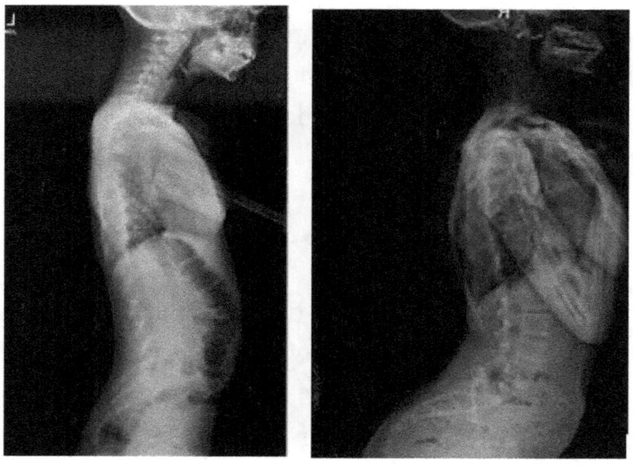

Figure 11. It would be difficult to treat both of these patients when using a "standard" amount of lumbar lordosis. Both of these patients require individualized parameters for treatment success.

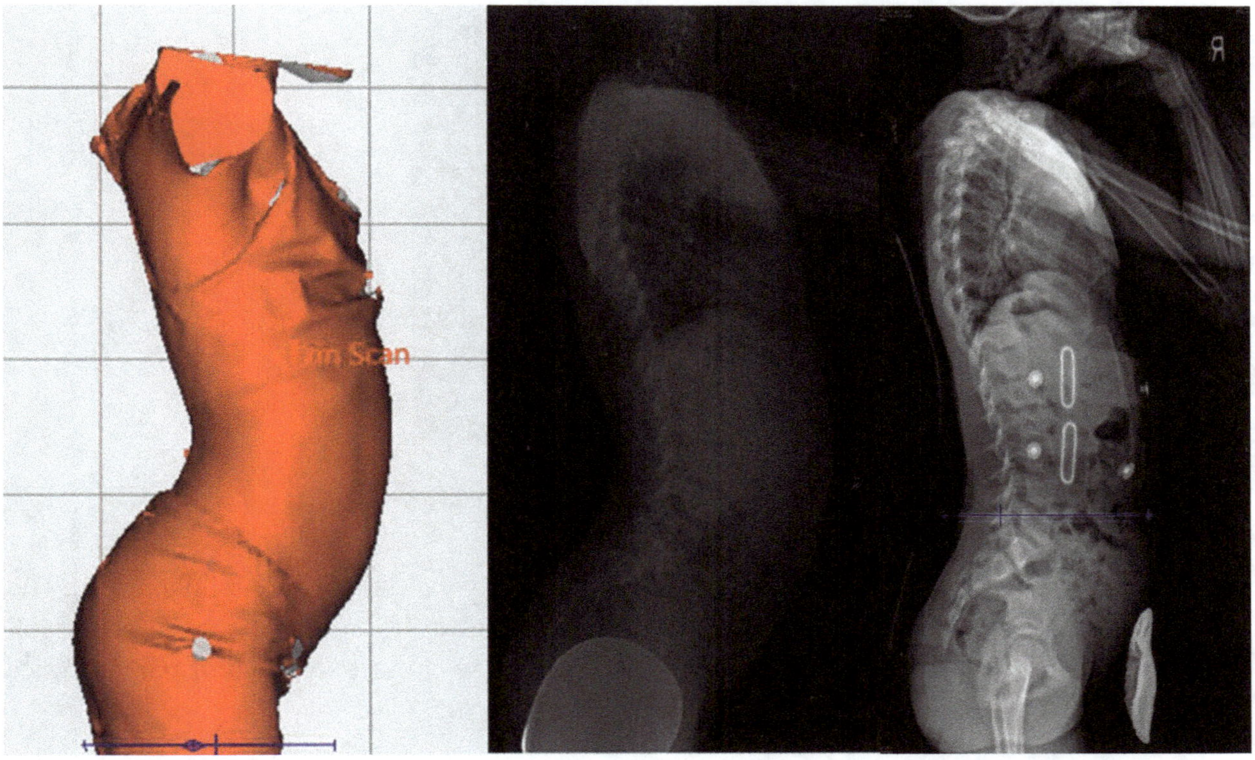

Figure 12. Example of a brace correcting sagittal balance while maintaining thoracic kyphosis.

1. When a thoracic pad was placed in a more posterior position, it controlled axial rotation better but caused decreased kyphosis.
2. Placing pads below the curve apex was not optimal. In a questionnaire of the Society on Scoliosis Orthopaedic and Rehabilitation Treatment (SOSORT) members, 11 of the 21 surveyed said the pad should be at the level of the apex. Ten indicated pad placement below the apex [43].
3. No correlation was found between the reduction of the lordosis and the correction of the coronal curves (**Figure 13**).
4. The reduction of the lordotic profile of the brace only had a negative effect on sagittal curves (hypo-kyphosing and hypo-lordosing). This is actually the way that Schuermans kyphosis is treated with the brace to have the effect of reducing hyper-kyphosis.
5. An asymmetric rigid shell was more efficient in correcting the coronal curves than a symmetric one.
6. Strap position has a great effect on rotational control of the brace. Anterior opening seems to control rotation better.

All of these concepts need to be tested in the real world and on a much larger scale but they are great starting points for developments of new treatments. A global method to assess bracing

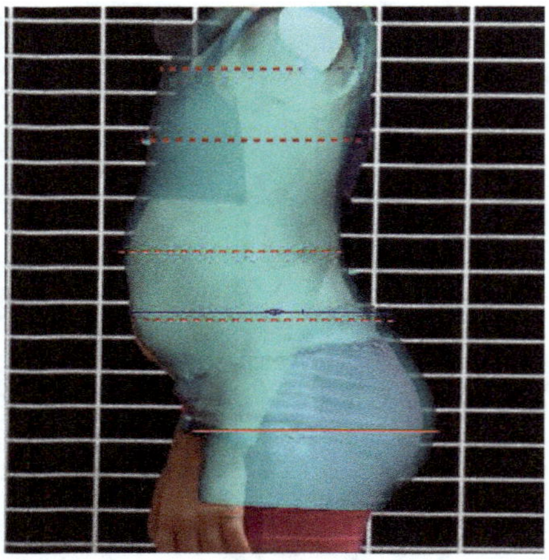

Figure 13. New digital imaging can be used to match clinical photos and digital X-rays to patient-specific morphology.

is the concept of overall balance summation, but this is only valid in the frontal plane [44]. The implications for sagittal plane malalignment that continues into adulthood have been well documented and discussed in this chapter; therefore, they should also play a part in brace design [27].

In conclusion, further work is needed with regard to the role of the orthotist in treating sagittal deformity in scoliosis patients, and clear protocols need to be developed. This field is ripe for an infusion of new ideas. The paper that found the number to treat to be three patients also reported that this number was only for patients who were considered compliant. It also reads "routine bracing without efforts to maximize brace compliance are likely to be less effective than the brace trial indicates" [45]. It has been suggested that all conservative care centers should make a strong effort to maximize brace compliance and this should be the new routine, or standard of care as Karol has shown in a recent article. Karol's study demonstrated that if patients engage in compliance counseling, then patients will wear their brace an extra 3 h per day. This increase in bracing compliance also correlated with a decreased surgical rate of 11% [45]. This topic requires further consideration of factors involved in setting up clinics that can handle this portion of treatment.

3. Conclusion

This chapter has introduced current concepts and evidence-informed practice patterns around knowledge of sagittal alignment and its implications for the conservative care practitioner managing adults with spinal deformity and for the orthoptist managing adolescents with idiopathic scoliosis. Much research and clinical practice lie ahead for practitioners in this field, and it has been the intention of the authors to begin to start a deeper conversation around the role of sagittal alignment in the clinical decision-making process with this unique patient population.

Acknowledgements

The authors wish to thank the orthopedics department of Columbia University Medical Center, especially Dr. Charla Fischer, and East Coast Prosthetics/Orthotics for their support and expertise in our professional and personal learning journeys, and for the opportunity to work collaboratively for the optimal health of our patients. Additionally, the authors wish to thank Patricia Orthwein, Nicholas Feinberg, and Anas Minkara for their contributions to editing this chapter. Many thanks!

Author details

Prachi Bakarania[1], Hagit Berdishevsky[1], Kelly Grimes[1*] and John Tunney[2]

*Address all correspondence to: kg2648@cumc.columbia.edu

1 Columbia University Medical Center, New York, NY, USA

2 East Coast Orthotics & Prosthetics, New York, NY, USA

References

[1] Ailon T, Smith JS, Shaffrey CI, et al. Degenerative spinal deformity. Neurosurgery. 2015;**77**(Suppl 4):S75–S91

[2] Schwab F, el-Fegoun AB, Gamez L, Goodman H, Farcy JP. A lumbar classification of scoliosis in the adult patient: Preliminary approach. Spine. 2005;**30**(14):1670-1673

[3] Schwab FJ, Blondel B, Bess S, Hostin R, Shaffrey CI, Smith JS, et al. Radiographical spino-pelvic parameters and disability in the setting of adult spinal deformity: A prospective multicenter analysis. Spine. 2013;**38**(13):E803–E812

[4] American Physical Therapy Association. Guide to physical therapist practice 3.0. Alexandria: American Physical Therapy Association; 2014. Available from: http://guidetoptpractice.apta.org/ [Accessed: February 1, 2017]

[5] Shumway-Cook A, Woollacott MH. Normal postural control. In: Shumway-Cook A, Woollacott MH, editors. Motor control: Translating research into clinical practice. 4th ed. Philadelphia: Lippincott Williams and Williams; 2012. pp. 161-194

[6] Basmajian JV. Man's posture. Archives of Physical Medicine and Rehabilitation. 1965;**46**:26-36

[7] Kendall FP. Muscles, Testing and Function with Posture and Pain. 5th ed. Philadelphia: Lippincott Williams & Wilkins; 2005

[8] Schultz AH. Vertebral column and thorax. Primatologia. 1961;**5**:1-66

[9] Lovejoy CO. The natural history of human gait and posture. Part 1. Spine and pelvis. Gait Posture. 2005;**21**(1):95-112

[10] Neumann DA, Kinesiology of the Musculoskeletal System: Foundations for Rehabilitation. 3rd ed. St Louis: Elsevier; 2017

[11] Staffell F. Die menschlichen Haltungstypen und ihre Beziehungen zu den Buckgratsverkrummungen. Wiesbaden: J. F. Bergmann; 1889

[12] Bonne AJ. On the shape of the human vertebral column. Acta Orthopaedica Belgica. 1969;**35**(3):567-583

[13] McMorris RO. Faulty posture. Pediatric Clinics of North America. 1961;**8**:213-224

[14] Roussouly P, Gollogly S, Berthonnaud E, Dimnet J. Classification of the normal variation in the sagittal alignment of the human lumbar spine and pelvis in the standing position. Spine. 2005;**30**(3):346-353

[15] Mac-Thiong JM, Roussouly P, Berthonnaud E, Guigui P. Sagittal parameters of global spinal balance: normative values from a prospective cohort of seven hundred nine Caucasian asymptomatic adults. Spine. 2010;**35**(22):E1193-E1198

[16] Bullock-Saxton JE. Normal and abnormal postures in the sagittal plane and their relationship to low back pain. Physiotherapy Practice. 1988;**4**:94-104

[17] During J, Goudfrooij H, Keessen W, Beeker TW, Crowe A. Toward standards for posture. Postural characteristics of the lower back system in normal and pathologic conditions. Spine. 1985;**10**(1):83-87

[18] Potter BK, Lenke LG, Kuklo TR. Prevention and management of iatrogenic flatback deformity. Journal of Bone and Joint Surgery-American Volume. 2004;**86-A**(8):1793-1808

[19] Legaye J, Duval-Beaupere G, Hecquet J, et al. Pelvic incidence: A fundamental pelvic parameter for three-dimensional regulation of spinal sagittal curves. The European Spine Journal. 1998;**7**:99-103

[20] Schwab F, Ungar B, Blondel B, et al. Scoliosis Research Society—Schwab adult spinal deformity classification: A validation study. Spine. 2012;**37**(12):1077-1082

[21] Lafage V, Schwab F, Patel A, et al. Pelvic tilt and truncal inclination two key radiographic parameters in the setting of adults with spinal deformity. Spine. 2009;**34**(17):E599-E606

[22] Joseph SA, Jr, Moreno A, Brandoff J. Sagittal plane deformity in the adult patient. The Journal of the American Academy of Orthopaedic Surgeons. 2009;**17**:378-388

[23] Hu P, Yu M, Sun Z, Li W, Jiang L, Wei F, Li, X, Chen Z, Liu Z. Analysis of global sagittal postural patterns in asymptomatic Chinese adults. Asian Spine Journal. 2016;**10**(2):282-288

[24] Lamartina C, Berjano P. Classification of sagittal imbalance based on spinal alignment and compensatory mechanisms. European Spine Journal. 2014;**23**:1177-1189

[25] Senteler M, Weisse B, Snedeker JG, Rothenfluh DA. Pelvic incidence-lumbar lordosis mismatch results in increased segmental joint loads in the unfused and fused lumbar spine. European Spine Journal. 2014;**23**(7):1384-1393

[26] Bernhardt M, Bridwell KH. Segmental analysis of the sagittal plane alignment of the normal thoracic and lumbar spines and thoracolumbar junction. Spine (Phila Pa 1976). 1989;**14**(7):717-721

[27] Glassman SD, Bridwell K, Dimar JR, et al. The impact of positive sagittal balance in adult spinal deformity. Spine. 2005;**30**(18):2024-2029

[28] Terran J, Schwab F, Shaffrey CI, Smith JS, Devos P, Ames CP, Fu KM, Burton D, Hostin R, Klineberg E, Gupta M, Deviren V, Mundis G, Hart R, Bess S, Lafage V. The SRS-Schwab adult spinal deformity classification: Assessment and clinical correlations based on a prospective operative and nonoperative cohort. Neurosurgery. 2013;**73**(4):559-568

[29] Schwab F, Farcy JP, Bridwell K, et al. A clinical impact classification of scoliosis in the adult. Spine (Phila Pa 1976). 2006;**31**(18):2109-2114

[30] Schwab F, Lafage V, Farcy JP, et al. Surgical rates and operative outcome analysis in thoracolumbar and lumbar major adult scoliosis: Application of the new adult deformity classification. Spine (Phila Pa 1976). 2007;**32**(24):2723-2730

[31] Berjano P, Aebi M. Pedicle subtraction osteotomies (PSO) in the lumbar spine for sagittal deformities. European Spine Journal. 2015;**24**(Suppl 1):S49-S57

[32] Morris WZ, Fowers AC, Yuh RT, Gebhart JJ, Salata MJ, Liu RW. Decreasing pelvic incidence is associated with greater risk of cam morphology. Bone and Joint Research. 2016;**5**:387-392

[33] Berdishevsky H, Lebel VA, Bettany-Saltikov J, Rigo M, Lebel A, Hennes A, Romano M, Białek M, M'hango A, Betts T, de Mauroy JC, Durmala J. Physiotherapy scoliosis-specific exercises—A comprehensive review of seven major schools. Scoliosis and Spinal Disorders. 2016;**11**:20

[34] Zampini JM, Sherk HH. Lewis A Sayre: The first professor of orthopedic surgery in America. 2007;**466**:2263-2267

[35] Scoliosis Research Society. SRS Bracing Manual [Internet]. Photovoltaic Modules [Internet]. 2014. Available from: http://www.srs.org/professionals/online-education-and-resources/srs-bracing-manual [Accessed: March 30, 2017]

[36] Weinstein SL, Dolan LA, Wright JG, Dobbs MB. Effects of bracing in adolescents with idiopathic scoliosis. New England Journal of Medicine. 2013;**369**:1512-1521

[37] HCUP Kids' Inpatient Database (KID). Healthcare Cost and Utilization Project (HCUP). Rockville: Agency for Healthcare Research and Quality; 2009. Available from: http://www.hcup-us.ahrq.gov/kidoverview.jsp

[38] Kouwenhoven JW, Smit TH, van der Veen AJ, Kingma I, van Dieën JH, Castelein RM. Effects of dorsal versus ventral shear loads on the rotational stability of the thoracic

spine: A biomechanical porcine and human cadaveric study. Spine (Phila Pa 1976). 2007;**32**:2545-2550

[39] Schlösser TP, Vincken KL, Rogers K, Castelein RM, Shah SA. Natural sagittal spino-pelvic alignment in boys and girls before, at and after the adolescent growth spurt. European Spine Journal. 2015;**24**(6):158-167

[40] Labelle H, Dansereau J, Bellefleur C, Poitras B. Three-dimensional effect of the Boston brace on the thoracic spine and rib cage. Spine (Phila Pa 1976). 1996;**21**(1):59-64

[41] Clin J, Aubin CE, Parent S, Sangole A, Labelle H. Comparison of the biomechanical 3D efficiency of different brace designs for the treatment of scoliosis using a finite element model. European Spine Journal. 2010;**19**(7):1169-1178

[42] Rigo M, Negrini S, Weiss HR, Grivas TB, Maruyama T, Kotwicki T. SOSORT consensus paper on brace action: TLSO biomechanics of correction (investigating the rationale for force vector selection). Scoliosis. 2006;**1**:11

[43] Carlson M, Smith M. Description for new overall balance: Summation for the conservative treatment of idiopathic scoliosis in determining orthosis design. Academy Today. 2007;**3**:A-13-A-15

[44] Sanders JO, Newton PO, Browne RH, Katz DE, Birch JG, et al. Bracing for idiopathic scoliosis: how many patients require treatment to prevent one surgery? Journal of Bone and Joint Surgery-American Volume. 2014;**96**:649-653

[45] Karol L, et al. Effect of compliance counseling on brace use and success in patients with adolescent idiopathic scoliosis. Journal of Bone and Joint Surgery-American Volume. 2016;**98**(1):9-14

11

Fusionless Correction of Moderate Adolescent Idiopathic Scoliosis with a New Minimally Invasive Dynamic Implant (ApiFix®) and Postoperative Schroth Scoliosis Specific Exercises-Case Series

Yizhar Floman and Michael A. Millgram

Abstract

The standard surgical management of AIS is spinal fusion. Nonfusion solutions for addressing moderate AIS curves are desirable. ApiFix® is a new posterior dynamic device consisting of an expandable ratcheting rod anchored by two pedicle screws to the concave side of the scoliotic spine. It was designed to address single, moderate Lenke type 1 or 5 curves. Surgery is performed without the addition of spine fusion of the instrumented segments. The surgical procedure is short with negligible blood loss and rapid recovery. Deformity correction is achieved by distraction leading to rod elongation. Curve correction is achieved not only during surgery but also after the surgical procedure by performing scoliosis specific exercises. These exercises activate the ratchet with further rod expansion and curve reduction. The reported cases demonstrate the efficacy of the combined approach of surgery and exercises in controlling moderate AIS. This clinical experience with the ratchet device shows consistent curve improvement and stabilization. It lends support to the concept that surgery with this new posterior dynamic device may be a viable alternative to fusion and or as an internal brace in non-compliant brace users for managing moderate AIS curves.

Keywords: moderate AIS, Lenke 1 and Lenke 5 curves, non-fusion surgery combined with Schroth SSE

1. Introduction

Adolescent idiopathic scoliosis (AIS) is a condition that affects 1–3% of children aged 10–16 years [1]. A structural lateral curvature of the spine with a rotational component develops in otherwise healthy teenagers during puberty. Mild or moderate curves pose no health threats but may be associated with cosmetic concerns. Teenagers with mild deformities are placed under clinical surveillance and are encouraged to exercise, those with larger curves (more than 25°) are braced, while skeletally immature patients with thoracic curves exceeding 45° are candidates for surgical intervention [2]. Patients with thoracolumbar or lumbar curves usually undergo surgery with a lower than the traditional 45°Cobb angle threshold [3]. The standard surgical procedure for AIS is a spinal fusion of 8–10 vertebrae. Although surgical fusion is a successful solution for progressive spinal deformity, fusion leads to loss of spine mobility and may cause painful disc degeneration at the junctions of the mobile spine with the fused segments.

Non-fusion surgical solutions addressing moderate AIS curves may, therefore, be desirable alternatives to the traditional standard care of fusion. To this end, growth-modulating nonfusion procedures have been developed such as convex vertebral body stapling and/or convex vertebral body tethering as a surgical alternative for idiopathic scoliosis [4–6]. Stapling or tethering necessitate an anterior surgical approach to the spine and are both relatively extensive procedures. An intermediate posterior fusionless and less complex surgical approach for moderate AIS may be helpful. The ApiFix® system was developed to fill this missing gap [7].

ApiFix® is a new posterior dynamic device consisting of an expandable ratcheting rod anchored by two pedicle screws to the concave side of the scoliotic spine. Surgery is performed without the addition of spine fusion of the instrumented segments. Deformity correction is achieved by distraction leading to rod elongation. Curve correction is achieved not only during surgery but also after the surgical procedure by performing scoliosis specific exercises. These exercises activate the ratchet with further rod expansion and curve reduction.Early experience with the ApiFix® device showed it to be a viable alternative to fusion in reducing and maintaining correction of moderate AIS curves [7].

2. Indications, implant design, surgical technique, postoperative exercises

2.1. Indications

The implant is designed to be used in patients with AIS, aged 10–17 years, with a single major curve, either Lenke type 1 or Lenke type 5 curves, with a Risser sign between 0 and 4. The magnitude of the major curve should be between 30° and 60° and adequate flexibility on supine side bending views showing curve diminution to 35° or less. The device may be also used in individuals with smaller curves as an internal brace, especially in non-compliant external brace users.

2.2. Implant design

The device has a mini-ratchet mechanism that allows unidirectional elongation of an expandable rod. It is made out of titanium alloy with an Amorphous Diamond-Like Ceramic coating

(**Figure 1**). The expandable rod with polyaxial rings (eye joint) at its' extremities is anchored to the spine with two pedicle screws that are implanted around the apex of the main curve (**Figure 1**). The rod screw connection has a 50° freedom of motion. The rod can expand by 40 mm, depending on the pre-distraction rod length. Rod expansion is incremental and gradual, making the deformity correction safer. The implant has a control pin that can abort the ratchet mechanism and put the device in a neutral mode or in a locked position to create a fusion-like rod (**Figure 1**).

The implant has a CE mark.

2.3. Surgical technique

The concave side of the spine is exposed through a 10–12 cm incision usually from end to end vertebrae. The convex side of the spine is left undisturbed. Two pedicle screws are inserted into the end vertebrae and connected by the eye joints to the expandable ApiFix® device. The construct usually spans five to six disc spaces around the curve apex.

The distraction of the ratchet mechanism during surgery allows immediate correction of the deformity. No fusion is performed. The surgical procedure takes about 1 h, and blood loss is negligible. Intra-operative neuro-monitoring is utilized during surgery. Hospitalization is very short, i.e., 1–2 days. Patients are immediately mobilized without external support.

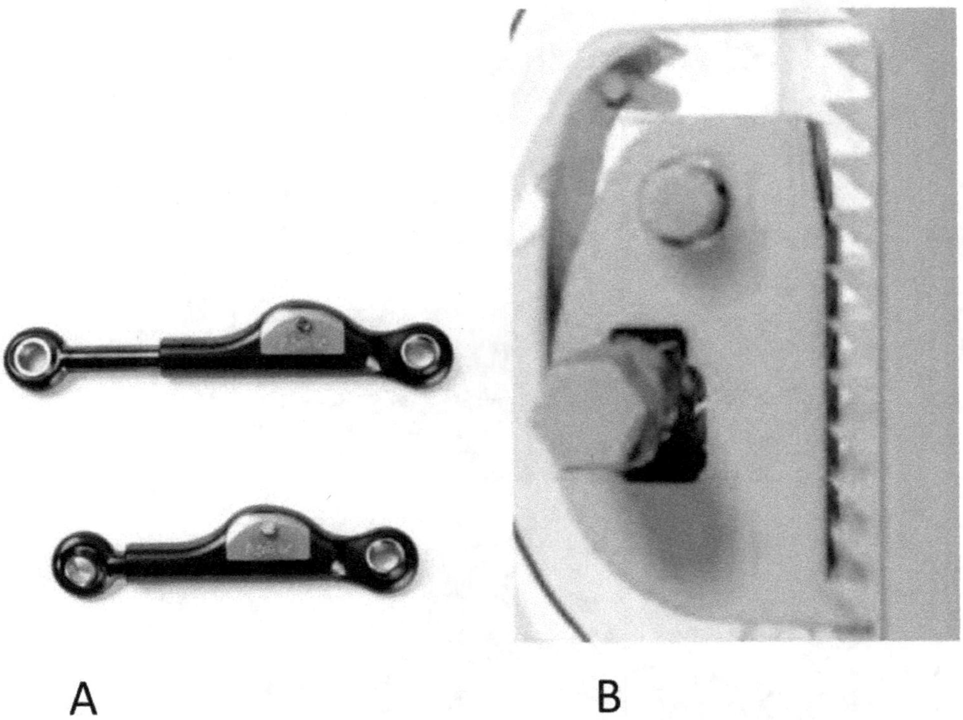

A B

Figure 1. (A) The ApiFix® device, the expandable rod, and the control pin and (B) close-up of the ratchet and the control pin.

2.4. Postoperative exercises

Postoperative exercises were designed to activate the ratchet mechanism and to further elongate the distance between the pedicle screws. Two to three weeks after surgery, patients are directed to perform five basic Schroth-like exercises that enabled gradual elongation of the ratchet mechanism, leading to further curve reduction (**Figure 2**). The patients bend towards the corrective direction, and the device maintains the designated correction after the patients' return to the neutral position. There are five basic exercises:

(1) Hanging from an open door or bar; the exercise begins with both hands holding the door top with the hips and knees bent at 90°, while the knees and toes lean on the door. By extending the

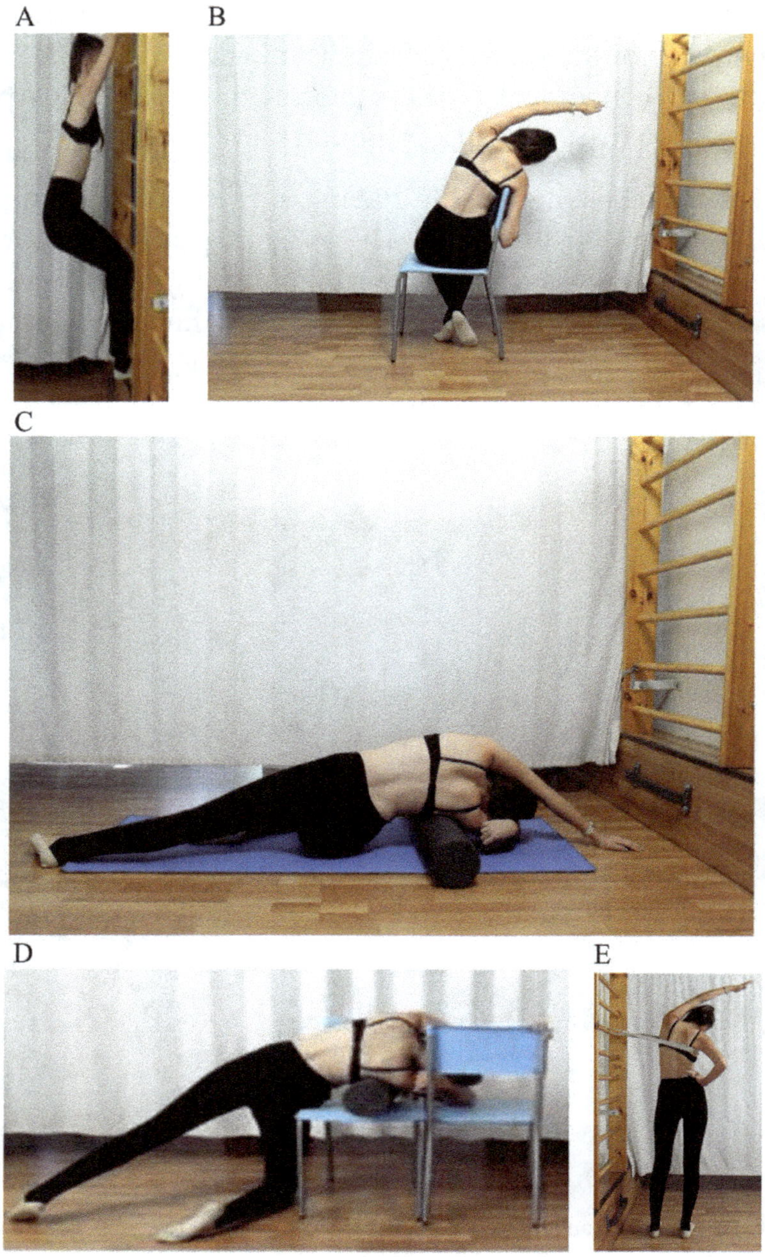

Figure 2. (A) Hanging from a door or bar, (B) chair bends, (C) bending on a roll, (D) lying on two chairs, and (E) bending over the band.

hips and knees, a traction force along the instrumented spine is exerted elongating the device. The maneuver is repeated five times. (2) Sitting on a chair with the backrest against the right rib cage (in Lenke type 1 curves). The right-hand leans on the backrest and the left one is placed over the head. The torso is leaned toward the backrest and right hand. The exercise is repeated 10–15 times. (3) Side bending on a rigid cylinder or roll placing the roll under the right rib cage. The right hand is bent under the head and the left one is placed over the head. The left arm is stretched above the head. (4) Lying on two chairs and a roll. A bolster is placed on the chair closer to the exercising individual. The patient lies on the bolster over the right side. The left hand is stretched over the head toward the second chair. (5) Standing tilts with a band. The band is placed on the right rib cage creating a fulcrum over which the torso is bent to the corrective side.

For Lenke type 5 curves, exercises are slightly modified by applying the band or bolster to the lower ribs or even to the waist usually on the left side of the body.

The patients are instructed to perform the exercises for 30 min daily, for 3–6 months after surgery. No braces are used and no restrictions on physical activity are imposed on the adolescents.

3. Illustrative case reports

Case 1: 15-year-old male presented with a Lenke type 1 curve of 48°, Risser sign was 3 (**Figure 3A**). The curve was considered too big to be controlled by bracing. He was subjected to surgery with ApiFix®. The procedure lasted about an hour, and blood loss was negligible. Hospitalization was 2 days. Initially, the curve was reduced to 26° (**Figure 3B**). After 3 months of performing the designated exercises, the curve was reduced to 18° (**Figure 3C**).

The patient is pain-free and satisfied with his cosmetic appearance.

Case 2: An 11-year-old female presented with a Lenke type 5 curve T8–L2 of 20° Risser 0. Family history revealed that her elder sister who also had AIS underwent posterior spine fusion from T4–L1. A TLSO was prescribed but the curve progressed to 43° during a period of 2 years (**Figure 4A**). At age 13, she underwent surgery with ApiFix® between T8–L1 (**Figure 4B**). The surgery lasted 50 min, and blood loss was insignificant. The immediate postoperative Cobb angle was 24°. She began exercises and the rod had elongated considerably with the exercises. At 9 months, the curve measured 20° (**Figure 4C**). Angle trunk rotation as measured by the Scoliometer was reduced from 7° preoperatively to 2° after surgery (**Figure 4D1** and**D2**).

4. Discussion

The current communication describes a unique approach to moderate AIS curve correction. The new approach combines operative curve correction followed by additional correction with exercises performed after the surgery. The designated scoliosis specific exercises become an integral part of the treatment protocol with the ratchet device. This differs dramatically from scoliosis correction by spinal fusion. By avoiding spinal fusion, natural spinal motion

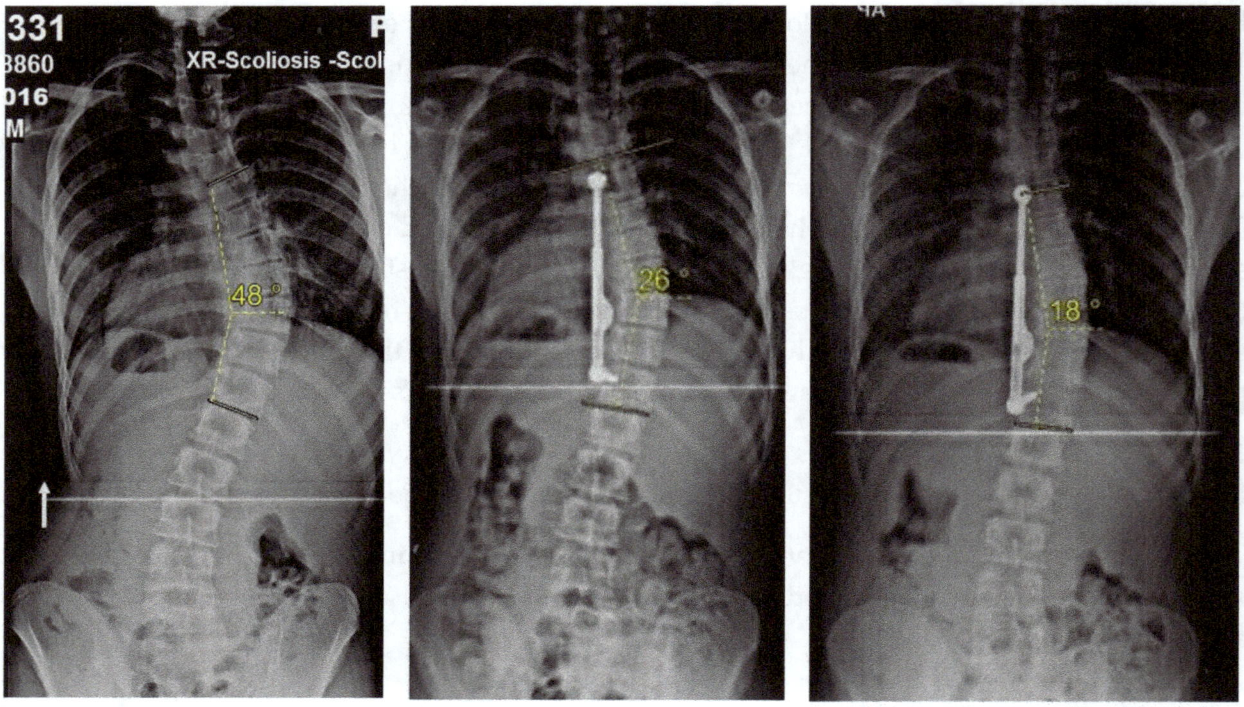

A B C

Figure 3. Case 1: (A) Preoperative standing AP X-ray, (B) postoperative standing AP X-ray, and (C) after 3 months of exercises. The expandable rod has elongated with further curve reduction.

is preserved by in large and allows further curve correction by exercising. The novel ratchet spinal implant may be looked upon as an internal brace. It is, therefore, logical to combine the internal brace with scoliosis specific exercises. Schreiber et al. in a randomized controlled study on nonoperative management of AIS reported that a combination of standard of care of AIS including bracing with Schroth scoliosis specific exercises gave a better curve correction than care without exercises [8]. Our novel concept and method also combine a brace, although internal, and exercises in the management protocol. The postoperative quasi Schroth corrective exercises help in reducing the final Cobb angle. Schreiber suggested that Schroth exercises should be considered as an add-on to the standard of care of AIS. Likewise, the correcting exercises after ApiFix® implantation should also be viewed as an add-on to surgical treatment. Theoretically, the combination of exercises with ApiFix® surgery may be more efficient than external bracing and Schroth maneuvers as the ratchet mechanism captures the correction gained during exercises.

The biomechanical properties of the ApiFix® ratchet device were investigated by Holewijn et al. [9]. They performed a biomechanical study on cadaveric thoracic spines in which they compared spinal motion with the ApiFix® device or with rigid pedicle screw fixation. The ratchet device caused a 40% decrease in range of motion in flexion/extension and about 18% in lateral bending, while the range of motion in axial rotation remained unaffected. In comparison, rigid instrumentation caused a significantly ($p < 0.05$) larger decrease in range of motion in flexion/extension (−80.9%), lateral bending (−75.0%), and axial rotation (−71.3%). The study of Holewijn et al. [9] showed that spinal range of motion was significantly less constrained by the ratcheted device as compared to rigid pedicle screw-rod instrumentation. Therefore, it can

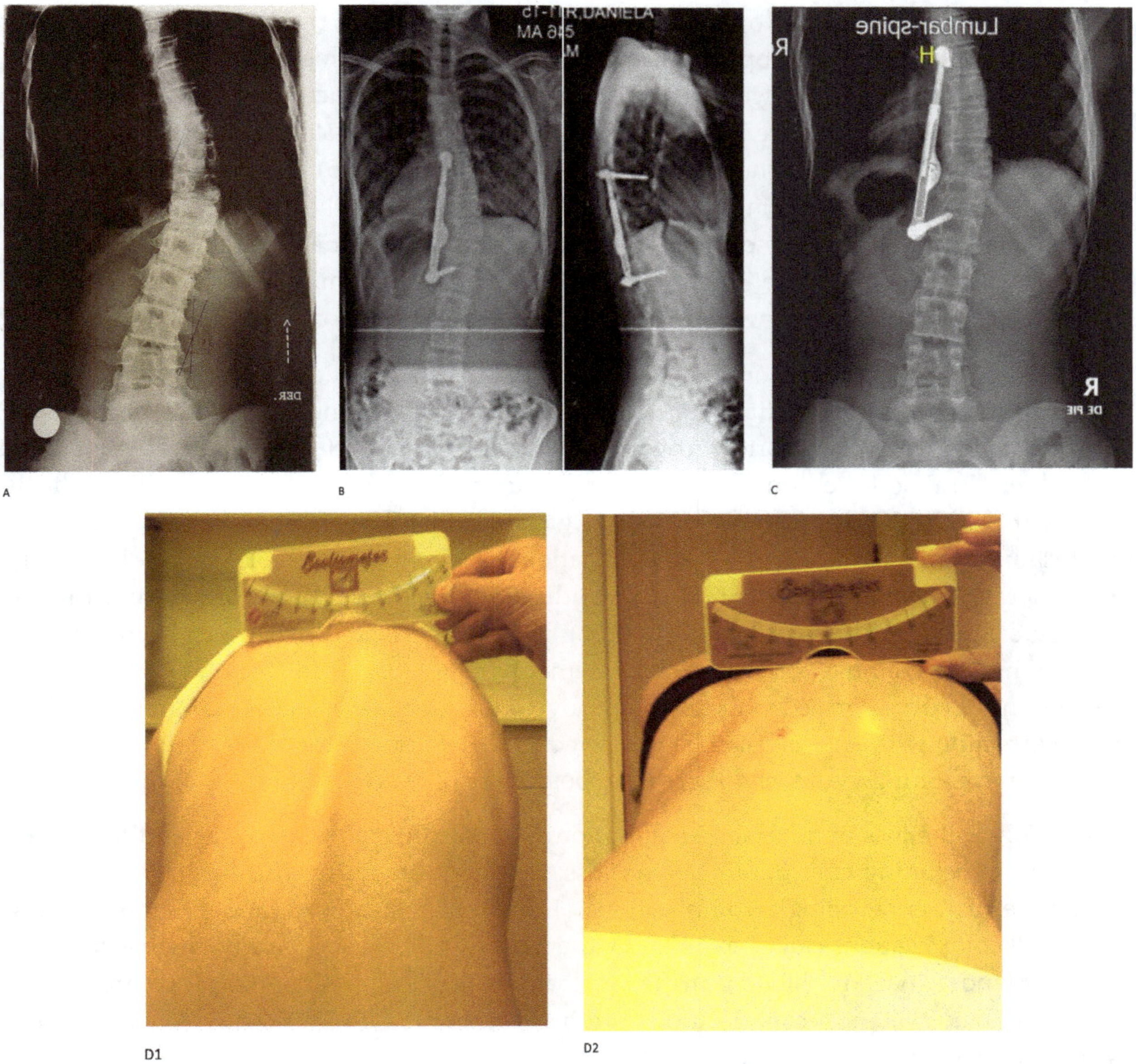

Figure 4. Case 2: (A) Preoperative standing AP X-ray and (B) postoperative standing AP & lateral X rays, and (C) after 9 months of exercises. The expandable rod has elongated with further curve reduction. D1: Scoliometer measurement before surgery 7. D2: Scoliometer measurement after surgery 2.

be assumed that the concave ratchet device enables scoliosis correction with preservation of a more physiological spinal motion. Holewijn et al. [9] also found that adjacent segment biomechanics were not significantly altered. These beneficial biomechanical characteristics can be attributed to the polyaxial connectors between the implant and screws. Therefore the risk of implant failure is deemed low as implant loads in the absence of spinal fusion are expected to be minimal.

At the time of writing, the new dynamic device was utilized in over 100 cases in Europe and Israel. The clinical outcome observed in those cases documented that curve correction and stabilization of moderate AIS without concomitant fusion were both efficient and durable (unpublished results). Although there were few failures, analysis of the failed cases revealed that each failure was related to operation on curves bigger than 60°, rigid curves or to improper pedicle screw placement. In properly selected candidates for instrumentation with ApiFix®, no implant failures or loosening were observed. The clinical experience gained lends support to the view that the ratchet device is a valid alternative to traditional standard surgery with long instrumentation and fusion. The main curves (Lenke 1 or Lenke 5) were reduced, and curve reduction was maintained during the follow-up period. Although the ApiFix® device operates in a distraction mode that may produce kyphosis, there was no clinically significant change in the sagittal curves of the spine in the operated patients. Long term, 2–4 years follow-up, of a cohort of operated patients showed no curve progression, adding on, or implant failure.

Curve correction without fusion in the management of AIS is not a new concept. Fusionless scoliosis surgery has the benefit of curve correction without limiting spinal motion. Betz et al. [5] and Samdani et al. [6] reported growth-modulating convex vertebral body stapling and/or convex vertebral body tethering as a nonfusion surgical alternative for idiopathic scoliosis that occurs before the onset of the adolescent growth spurt. The published clinical results of that technique are promising [4–6]. The indications chosen for the use of ApiFix® in managing moderate AIS are almost identical to the indications of vertebral body tethering, although the surgical approach (posterior vs. anterior) and the age of the patients are different [6]. Some of the shortcomings of vertebral body tethering/stapling include the inability to predict the amount of curve correction and whether overcorrection will occur. In contrast, the final curve correction with ApiFix® can be predicted to closely match the magnitude seen on the preoperative bending views, and there is no possibility of overcorrection.

In addition to the loss of natural spinal motion, standard fusion surgery has additional disadvantages, including considerable blood loss, requiring blood transfusions [10, 11], a 12% prevalence of non-neurologic complications [11, 12], late infections, and pseudoarthrosis. Almost all complications can be avoided by the use of ApiFix®: specifically, there is minimal blood loss and no need for blood transfusion, the prevalence of non-neurologic complications is negligible, neurological complications can be expected to be significantly reduced by the use of only two pedicle screws and the gradual nature of the deformity correction, and there is no risk of pseudoarthrosis since fusion is not attempted. The ultra-short operative time and hospital stay are also significant advantages.

In conclusion, our experience with this novel dynamic device demonstrated consistent curve improvement and stabilization. It lends support to the concept that surgery with this new posterior dynamic device combined with postoperative scoliosis specific exercises may be a viable alternative to fusion and and non-compliant brace users for managing moderate AIS curves.

Author details

Yizhar Floman* and Michael A. Millgram

*Address all correspondence to: yizharfloman@gmail.com

Israel Spine Center, Assuta Hospital Tel Aviv, Israel

References

[1] Weinstein SL, Dolan LA, Cheng JCY, Danielson A, Morcuende JA. Adolescent idiopathic scoliosis. Lancet 2008;**371**:1527-1537

[2] de Kleuver M, Lewis SJ, Germscheid NM. et al. Optimal surgical care for adolescent idiopathic scoliosis: An international consensus. European Spine Journal. 2014;**23**:2603-2618

[3] Souder C, Newton PO, Shah SA, Lonner BS, Bastrom TP, Yaszay B. Factors in surgical decision making for thoracolumbar/lumbar AIS: It's about more than just the curve magnitude. Journal of Pediatric Orthopaedics. 2016; 3 Mar. DOI: 10.1097/BPO.000000 0000000746. [Epub ahead of print]

[4] Betz RR, Kim J, D'Andrea LP. et al. An innovative technique of vertebral body stapling for the treatment of patients with adolescent idiopathic scoliosis: A feasibility, safety, and utility study. Spine. 2003;**28**:S255-S265

[5] Betz RR, Ranade A, Samdani AF. et al. Vertebral body stapling: A fusionless treatment option for a growing child with moderate idiopathic scoliosis. Spine. 2010;**35**:169-176

[6] Samdani AF, Ames RJ, Kimball JS. et al. Anterior vertebral body tethering for idiopathic scoliosis: Two-year results. Spine. 2014;**39**:1688-1693

[7] Floman Y, Burnei G, Gavriliu S. et al. Surgical management of moderate adolescent idio pathic scoliosis with ApiFix®: A short peri-apical fixation followed by post-operative curve reduction with exercises. Scoliosis. 2015;**10**:4

[8] Schreiber S, Parent EC, Moez EK. et al. Schroth physiotherapeutic scoliosis-specific exer cises added to the standard of care lead to better Cobb angle outcomes in adolescents with idiopathic scoliosis-an assessor and statistician blinded randomized controlled trial. PLoS One. DOI: 10.1371/journal.pone.0168746. 29 December 2016

[9] Holewijn RM, de Kleuver M, van der Veen AJ. et al. A novel spinal implant for fusionless scoliosis correction: A biomechanical analysis of the motion preserving properties of a posterior peri-apical concave distraction device. Global Spine Journal; First Published April 7, 2017. DOI: 10.1177/2192568217699377. In press

[10] Shapiro F, Sethna N. Blood loss in pediatric spine surgery. European Spine Journal. 2004;**13**(Suppl 1):S6-S17

[11] Newton PO, Marks MC, Bastrom TP. et al. Surgical treatment of Lenke 1 main thoracic idiopathic scoliosis. Spine. 2013;**38**:328-338

[12] Reames DL, Smith JS, Fu KM. et al. Complications in the surgical treatment of 19360 cases of pediatric scoliosis. A review of the scoliosis research society morbidity and mor tality data base. Spine. 2011;**36**:1484-1489

12

Computational Simulation as an Innovative Approach in Personalized Medicine

Bauer Sabine and Paulus Dietrich

Abstract

Background: Statistical analyses show that both the spine curvature and the morphological properties of the vertebral bodies can differ considerably. Therefore, the best outcome of a surgery for the individual patient could be achieved by developing patient specific implants to prevent inadequate anchorage of implants that don't optimally fit to the anatomy and can cause damages of spinal structures.

Objective: The aim of our work is to develop patient-specific biomechanical simulation models of the spine to determine the patient-specific load situation and to open up the possibility of developing implant designs that are adapted to the morphological contours of the patients' endplates, which ensures an optimal fit and a balanced load distribution.

Methods: Our approach is the scientific fusion of the fields "medical imaging" and "biomechanical computer modeling." The individual characteristics of patients will be visualized and analyzed through medical imaging. The surface models together with the estimated biomechanical properties can be transferred into biomechanical multibody simulation models.

Results: Taking the patient-specific characteristics and the material properties of the implant into account, simulation models are created to simulate preoperatively the biomechanical effects of new implant designs. In this way, the load situation of the modeled spinal structures can be determined.

Keywords: personalized medicine, computational simulation, medical imaging, surgical planning, patient-specific implants

1. Introduction

Each human has individual physical characteristics and differs not only in his individual anthropometry and morphology but also in the biomechanical properties of his various biological structures. In order to take these individual factors into account, medicine is going to great lengths to offer tailor-made intervention to individual patients. In the last few years, "individualized medicine" has been addressed as a significant development in medicine. In individualized medicine, products are only suitable for the target patient, but not in a comparable way for others. Overall, individualized medicine can be divided into five different typologies [1]:

1. Biomarker-based stratification
2. Genome-based information about health-related characteristics
3. Determination of risk of disease
4. Differential offers for intervention
5. Therapeutic unique devices.

Therapeutic uniqueness is understood as an individual patient's tailor-made therapeutic device. The idea of individualized devices is not restricted to a specific medical area, but is used in different medical applications. Examples of such individual medical devices are as follows:

- Artificial pancreas device system, as a device under clinical investigation that automatically monitors patient's glucose levels and delivers patient-tailored insulin doses in people with diabetes.
- Software-based quantitative electrocardiogram (EEG) analysis to predict an individual's response to various psychotropic drugs.
- Tinnitus masker, which is personalized by the manufacturer to patient tinnitus.
- Zenith Fenestrated AAA Endovascular Graft as an indicator for the endovascular treatment of patients with abdominal aortic or aortoiliac aneurysms having morphology suitable for endovascular repair [2].

In spinal surgery, it is common practice to use magnetic resonance imaging (MRI) or computed tomography (CT) imaging to assemble, for example, pedicle screw spinal systems consisting of a rod, screw, hook-connector kit to take the patient's individual physiology into account. Currently, the pedicle screw spinal systems are available in different standardized sizes, which fulfill different requirements. In some of these standard implants, for example, there is also the possibility of adjusting the inclination angles of the contact surfaces of the implant to the vertebral body. Despite these adjustment possibilities, due to the very different anatomical conditions of the patents, in some cases only an insufficient anchoring of the implant can be achieved. Further reasons for the need of more precise individualized implants are disease-specific requirements. The aim is to improve the surgical outcome through an exact individual adaptation and adequate fitting to individual anatomical needs [3]. A modern manufacturing process for such therapeutic uniqueness is a patient-specific production by means of "rapid prototyping," in which the individualization is based on the manufacturing process of the single-unit production [1].

A further step in individualized manufacturing process could be the integration of a preoperative simulation of the spinal stress situation taking the biomechanical conditions of the respective patient into account. This will allow a prediction of the effects of the surgical procedure and an identification of the best possible surgical option. How this would be implemented in a clinical workflow practice is discussed in the subsequent section by means of an extended process chain of rapid prototyping.

2. Process chain for the production of therapeutic unique products

The existing process chain without considering the biomechanical simulation includes the image acquisition, the image post-processing and the rapid prototyping [4, 5]. The image raw data acquired using CT or MRI are segmented, visualized and transferred in a suitable data format by image post-processing. In the next step, a computer-aided design (CAD) model of the segmented objects is generated. Finally, these CAD data can be used to create a customized implant design [6]. This process chain can be expanded by biomechanical simulations to determine the patient-specific stress situation in spinal structures preoperatively. Based on this simulation, a patient-specific implant with an optimal fitting can be designed to reduce the risk of complications, incorrect loading conditions due to insufficient adapted implant design and adjacent segment degeneration. A possible expanded process chain could look like **Figure 1**, based on Hüsing et al. [1] and Rengier et al. [3].

The expanded process chain starts with the medical imaging or technical construction as the basis for the following three-dimensional (3D) reconstruction. After the three-dimensional reconstruction of the data, a biomechanical simulation model can be created. In a simulation model, morphological information and biomechanical properties of the patent-specific spine as well as of the corresponding implant are obtained. The aim of this biomechanical simulation is to ensure a "natural" stress distribution on the various spinal structures by the modeling of a patient-specific implant. Thus, overloading, which can lead to degenerative damage to the

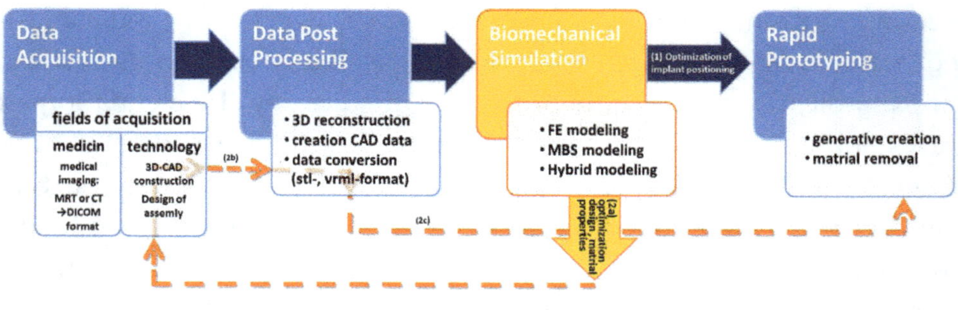

Figure 1. Expanded process chain with implemented biomechanical modeling.

head, should be avoided. This aim can be achieved by optimized positioning of the implant, an optimization of the implant design as well as of the implant material properties.

The goal of finding an optimal positioning (1) of an implant is in focus, which ensures, for example, a "natural" stress distribution, can be determined by the patient-specific simulation model. If desired, the exact coordinates of the positioned implant can be exported. These can then be taken into account in the operation planning. The rapid prototyping can be realized sequentially or in parallel.

If the baseplate design of a "standardized" implant is not suited to the morphological conditions of the contact surface of a patient-specific vertebral body, alternative baseplate designs can be demonstrated by means of a biomechanical simulation. In addition, corresponding modifications in implant material properties can also be analyzed and its effect on the spinal structures can be evaluated (see **Figure 1** process chain, loop (2a)). Thus, the risk of complications is minimized through, for example, an insufficient anchoring and the concomitant loosening of the implant or the occurrence of load peaks by point contact. On the basis of the simulation results, the implant can be re-designed specifically for a patient (see **Figure 1** process chain, loop (2b)), and corresponding input data (see **Figure 1** process chain, loop (2c)) can be generated for the further processing of rapid prototyping.

In the field of rapid prototyping, generative creations and processes with material removal can be different. Generative creation is the production of 3D physical models by applying material in thin layers and solidifying them. Established techniques are stereolithography, selective laser sintering, fused deposition modeling, laminated object manufacturing, and inkjet-printing techniques. A more detailed explanation can be taken from [3].

With such an expanded process chain, patient-specific implants can be produced not only with optimally shaped contact surfaces, which ensure a permanent fit of the implant without sinking and slipping, but also preoperative predictions can be made about the biomechanical effects of the implant and an optimized positioning can be proposed.

3. Medical imaging

Medical imaging is used as a basis for biomechanical modeling of the spine. Depending on the scientific question, these may be obtained from MRI cone beam computer tomography (CBCT), positron emission tomography (PET), single photon emission computed tomography (SPECT), and ultrasonography (US) [3]. From appropriate image data, using a specific image post-processing algorithm, 3D visualizations can be generated as well as an analysis of the biomechanical behavior of the tissue.

3.1. Segmentation and visualization

Since decades, the fully automatic segmentation of images—not only in the medical domain—is a challenge that is still unsolved in general [23, 35]. Not only the algorithms are the topic of research but also the question, how to evaluate the result of an image segmentation [33, 34].

Many modern segmentation algorithms in medical image processing use level sets; a review of these techniques can be found in [32]. State-of-the-art systems use the input of an expert to initialize segmentation and also allow for manual correction of the segmentation results.

To provide the input for modeling, the shape of the bones of a patient is required in three dimensions, which requires accurate segmentation. The key to success is to provide a computer assistance to speed up segmentation and to provide an interface that allows for fast and simple computer tools.

Bone structures are segmented in CT data. In those cases, where an MR image is also available, CT data and MR data are registered [36, 37] and fused. Most modern medical workstations provide such tools.

3.2. Defining biomechanical parameters

One possible way to determine the mechanical behavior of the spinal bony structures is to determine them from CT data. The radiation emitted during the scanning process penetrates the object and is weakened to varying degrees by the tissue. On the basis of the measured intensity reduction, an attenuation coefficient is calculated for each beam direction, to which a CT number is assigned. The unit of the CT number is given in Hounsfield [Hu] [6]. The Hounsfield unit is defined by the following equation:

$$H = 1000 * \frac{CT - CT_w}{CT_w - CT_a} \tag{1}$$

where CT_w and CT_a are the CT values of water and air [7]. According to Sun et al. [8], the CT number can be correlated to the density, for example, of the bone by a linear interpolation using relations available in published literature. The determined density can then be related to the so-called Young's modulus E. The heterogeneous elasticity, for example, of the cancellous and cortical bone, can in turn be defined by the following relationships [5]:

For cancellous bone, $CT < 816$:

$$\rho = 1.9 * 10E - 3 * CT + 0.105 \tag{2}$$

$$E = 0.06 + 0.9 * \rho * 2 \tag{3}$$

For cortical bone $CT > 816$:

$$\rho = 7.69{*}10 - E * 4 * CT + 1.028 \tag{4}$$

$$E = 0.09 + 0.9\rho 7.4 \tag{5}$$

In addition to determining biomechanical parameters by means of the CT number, it is also possible to obtain biomechanical information of, for example, the degree of intervertebral disc degeneration by a radiographic grading system. To determine more objective assessment of lumbar and cervical intervertebral disc degeneration, a new radiographic grading system [9, 10] is developed. The classification of this radiographic grading system is based on the three variables "height loss," "steophyte formation," and "diffuse sclerosis." According to Wilke et al. [9], each of these three variables first has to be graded individually on lateral and postero-anterior radiographs. Finally, the so-called overall degree of degeneration is assigned on a four-point scale from 0 (no degeneration) to 3 (severe degeneration).

Recent approaches try to estimate biomechanical properties of humans by tracking motions both in color image sequences as in distance measurements. Such data are available from devices that were designed for consumer games, but have also been used experimentally in medical applications, for example, in Ref. [38].

4. Biomechanical modeling and simulation

Biomechanical modeling is an established method to simulate physics and physiology of a human body. Depending on the scientific question, it is possible to create whole body models for humans [11, 12] or parts of the body like the human heart [13, 14] or the spine [15, 16]. A distinction can be made between the multibody simulation (MBS) modeling and the finite element (FE) modeling. Depending on the scientific question, either the MBS or the FE simulation method can be used. For analyzing highly sophisticated problems, the FE modeling is the appropriate modeling method. The system is divided into a finite number of small geometric elements, called the finite elements. At the connection point, the so-called nodes, boundary and transition conditions are defined in accordance to specific material laws [17]. If the biomechanical behavior of high dynamic movements or larger parts or the entire of the human body is the focus, the MB simulation is the suitable method. A further possibility is to combine MBS and FE to ensure a higher degree of fine specific structure modeling. Due to such hybrid models (e.g. MBS-coupled with FE models), short computing times are guaranteed. The rapid availability of results enables a future usability in medical routine for spinal operation planning. Further detailed explanations of the basics of simulations can be taken out of [18].

4.1. Application examples implant design

The possibility of using the biomechanical simulation in the area of spinal surgery is diverse. Preoperatively, the effects of mono- or multisegmental spinal fusion on adjacent segments can be analyzed. In addition, an optimized positioning of the inserted implant can be demonstrated by taking into account the reconstruction of the sagittal balance or an adequate stress distribution. One can also compare the effects of minimally invasive surgical methods to surgical procedures with high degree of resections of spinal structures.

Although most manufacturers of implants offer different sizes of implants, a full-area contact of the implant with the vertebral body is not always ensured. An insufficient anchorage can lead to local stress peaks at the contact points. With the help of computer-assisted simulations, such stress peaks can be analyzed. To ensure the best possible anchoring, the effects of different contact surface designs of the implant can be determined. Thus, the simulation can contribute to a development of patient-specific shaped implant surfaces, which ensure a permanent fit of the implant without sinking and slipping. Preoperatively, the effects of different implant lengths can also be analyzed.

The following simulations are intended as examples for a patient-specific problem and do not include the entire "expanded process chain," but only the subsection of the "biomechanical simulation." Thus, the following examples serve to illustrate the added value by the biomechanical modeling with regard to operation planning.

4.1.1. Effects of different standardized cage sizes

This example is intended to show the effects of the cage size on the biomechanics of the lumbar spine. For this, a biomechanical simulation a model of a person was created, which considers gender (male), age (35 years), weight (75 kg, body mass index (BMI) 22), and body height (1.85 m), including detailed lumbar spine structures (**Figure 2**). The lumbar spine model includes the biomechanical properties of the intervertebral discs, the facet joints, the ligamentous structures and the muscle groups left, right m. erector spinae, left and right m. rectus abdominus according to [21]. The exact model configuration as well as the validation can be found in Refs. [18–20].

To investigate the effects of fusing implants with five different sizes, the size of this optimally fitted implant is varied about ±2.5 and ±5%. In this context, an optimal fit is the planar resting of the cage on the endplates of the corresponding vertebral body. It should be noted that the entire cage base area is not in contact with the vertebral endplate, because it is a standardized implant without considering the patient-specific vertebral endplate morphology. The load situation, which is simulated, is the upright position under load of the body weight and a fused functional spinal unit (FSU) L4-L3. The weight force solves the kinematics of the MBS model and the motion equations, which form a system of coupled differential equations, are integrated for each simulation time step. This means that this weight force causes small movements in the spinal structures, and they are brought out of their equilibrium state. The reaction forces of the individual spinal structures build up until a new equilibrium state is reached. The following results refer to this new equilibrium state.

The basic implant size is chosen so that the implant fills the entire space between the corresponding vertebral bodies, and thus has contact with the endplates of the vertebral bodies. This basis cage is named in the **Figures 3–5** as "optimal fit." The cage is increased or reduced by a certain percentage and is shown in **Figures 3–5** as follows: "plus 2.5%" and "plus 5%" for the cages, which are enlarged 2.5 and 5%, respectively, and "minus 2.5%" and "minus 5%" for the size reduction of 2.5 and 5%, respectively (**Figure 3**).

When the basic cage is implemented in the FSU L3-L4, the other FSUs will undergo the least load compared to a smaller or larger cage size.

In the simulation cage "optimal fit," the lowest FSU sac-L5 is loaded the highest of all the FSU (**Figure 4**). The smallest stress is recorded in the FSU L5-L4. When a larger or smaller implant is selected, the load in all FSUs increases sharply. The load of the different FSUs hardly differ in height, whether the choice of a larger (plus 2.5% or plus 5%) or smaller (minus 2.5% or minus 5%) cage. The difference is marginal when comparing the simulations of the simulation cases "plus 2.5%," "plus 5%," "minus 2.5%," and "minus 5%" within the FSUs. The results show how

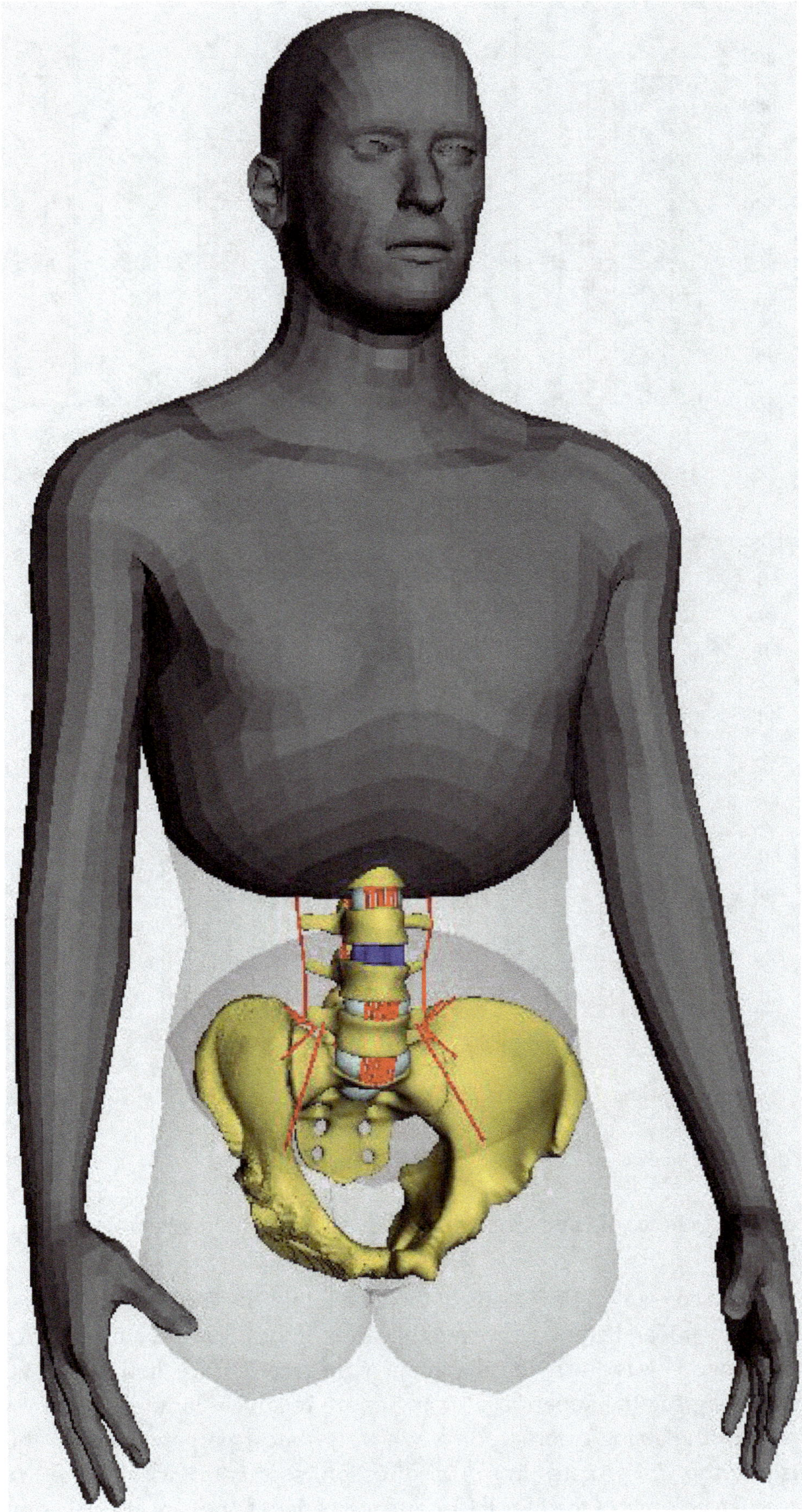

Figure 2. Simulation model of a person.

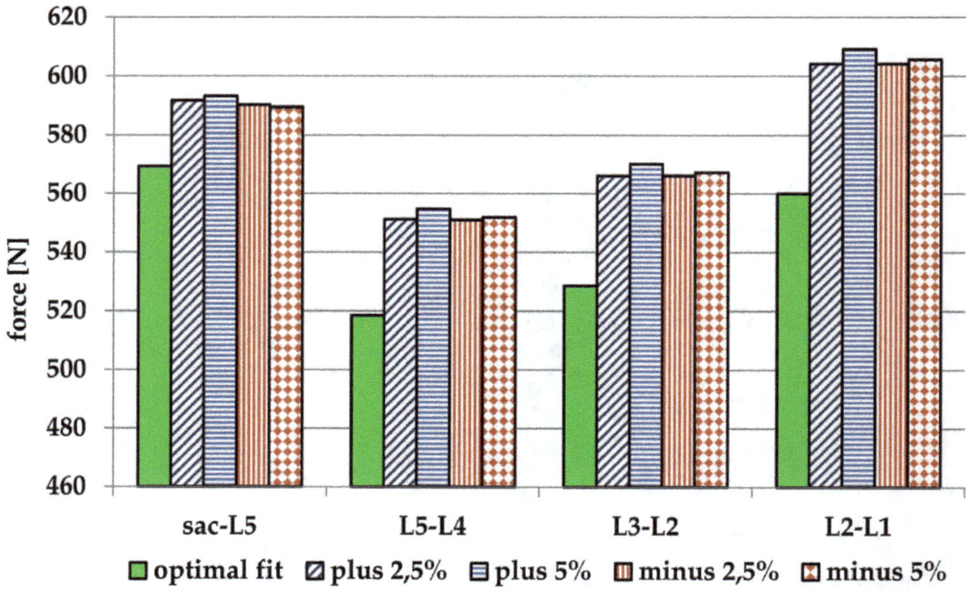

Figure 3. Vertical force intervertebral discs.

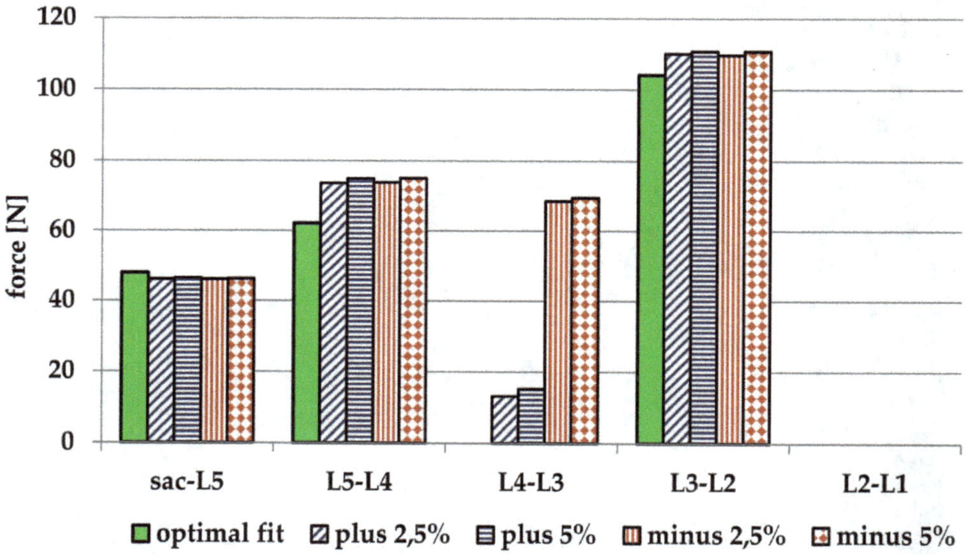

Figure 4. Loads of the facet joints.

important the correct choice of cage size could be, so that the intervertebral discs are not loaded more heavily.

On the other hand, if considering the loads of the facet joints, the choice of the implant size has a small influence on their load height. However, the facets of the FSU L3-L2 are much more heavily loaded than any other. This is due to the alignment of the facet surface. In the case of the FSUs L3-L2, the corresponding sagittal superior facet angles are relatively large so that the value of the force component of the acting external force, which is almost perpendicular to this surface, is high. Furthermore this FSU rotates in dorsal direction, so this boosts also the load situation. What's more, the facets joints of the FSU L4-L3 are not loaded in the cage when choosing the cage size "optimal fit." The reason is that the spinal alignment is modified by the body weight, so that the vertebral bodies above the implemented cage FSU situated move in such a position that the lower endplate of FSU is in contact with the cage. As a result, the cranial facet joint surfaces of L4 and the caudal facet joint surfaces of L3 come directly and strongly into contact, and are therefore correspondingly highly loaded. The uppers facet joint L2-L1 are loaded in none of the simulation cases. The reason could be that the alignment of the facet joints is nearly parallel to the direction of movement, and so the facet surfaces "slide" through each other.

In general, the direction of rotation of the FSU is determined by the acting torque resulting from the lever arm and the acting weight force. Thereby, a force whose line of action runs vertically in front of the axis of rotation produces a positive torque, and a force whose line of action runs dorsally behind the axis of rotation produces a negative torque. A positive torque results in flexion movement, and a negative torque results in an extension movement of the affected vertebral body segments. From this model configuration or rather specific spinal alignment, the rotations seen in **Figure 5** are obtained. It should be noted, however, that these results are only valid for this model configuration and cannot be transferred to other patients. Already in the case of a changed spinal alignment, completely different results can occur [22]. But this example shows the effects of choosing a non-optimal fitting cage and the significance of the appropriate choice of the right cage size.

4.1.2. *Cervical vertebral replacement*

The superior surface of a cervical vertebral body is shaped like a tub. On its sides, it has small branches which are called uncinate processes. These margins build the uncovertebral joints (**Figure 6**) [23]. Thereby, the angle of the uncovered joints of the different vertebral bodies is not of the same magnitude, but increases significantly from C5 to C7 [24].

Due to the special anatomical conditions, the implantation of a vertebral body replacement implant or its baseplates cannot be optimally brought into contact with the corresponding superior or inferior anchor vertebra (**Figure 7**).

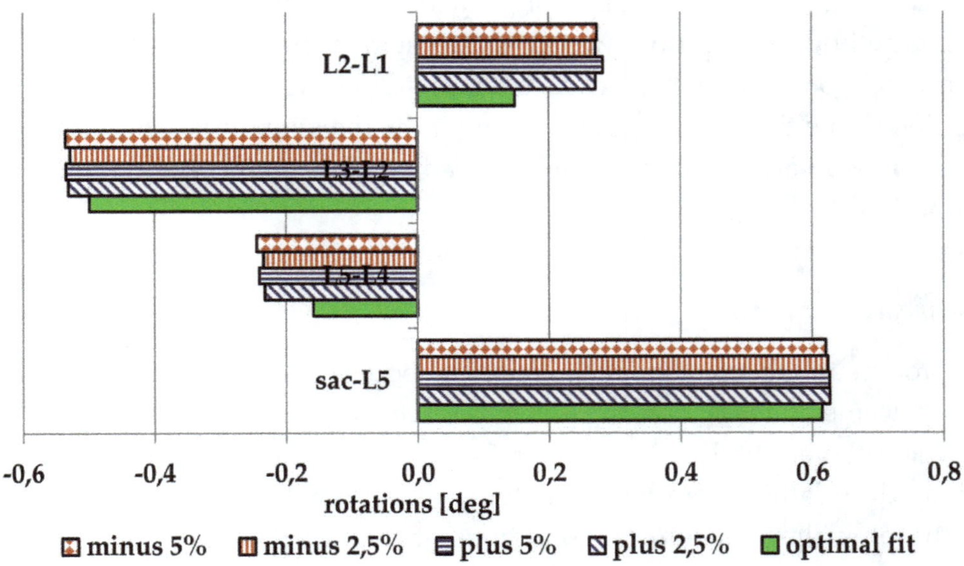

Figure 5. Rotation of the intervertebral discs.

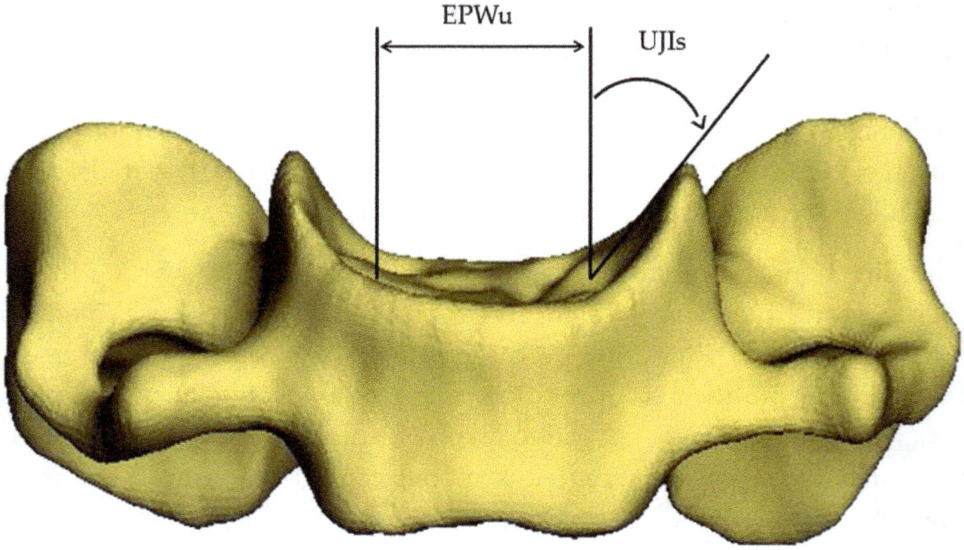

Figure 6. Illustration of the uncovertebral joint inclination.

In order to guarantee planar rest of the implant, the implant base should either be relatively narrow, so that it preferably rests only on the endplate surface of the corresponding vertebral body or be a "negative replica" of the patient-specific vertebral body surface, including consideration of the uncovered joint angle. A small implant baseplate has the disadvantage that the stress on the vertebral body is thereby increased by the reduced contact surface. A baseplate adapted to the superior vertebral surface could result in a much larger area of contact, and therefore a more balanced load distribution is achieved. Because this is a recently launched research project, the following examples are not intended to be final versions, but merely should represent the possibilities of a future implementation of biomechanical simulation in a process chain. The main focus will be to demonstrate the model creation and not to present validated results. The multibody simulation model is therefore a prototype. It should also be noted that we focus on the MBS modeling because this type of simulation is a much faster calculation method than the finite element method. In addition, we aim to implement fine-structured parts, such as the spine, into a whole-body model in order to simulate the dynamic situation of everyday life and thus to determine the stresses. Depending on the question, it is also possible to create a hybrid model of MBS and FE parts. A more detailed explanation can be found in Ref. [18] and in Section 5.

4.1.2.1. Basic model description

The MBS prototype model consists of the vertebral bodies C3-C6, where an extractable vertebral body replacement implant is implemented between the anchor vertebrae C3 and C6 (**Figure 8**). The intervertebral body surfaces C4 and C5 are adapted accordingly to the real operative procedure laminectomy. The anatomy of vertebral bodies C6 and C3 is retained. Because of the prevailing anatomical conditions of the uncovertebral joint and the relating lateral margins, a complete contact of the implant baseplates with the vertebral endplate of the anchor vertebra cannot be realized. As a result of the typically slightly corrugated form of the

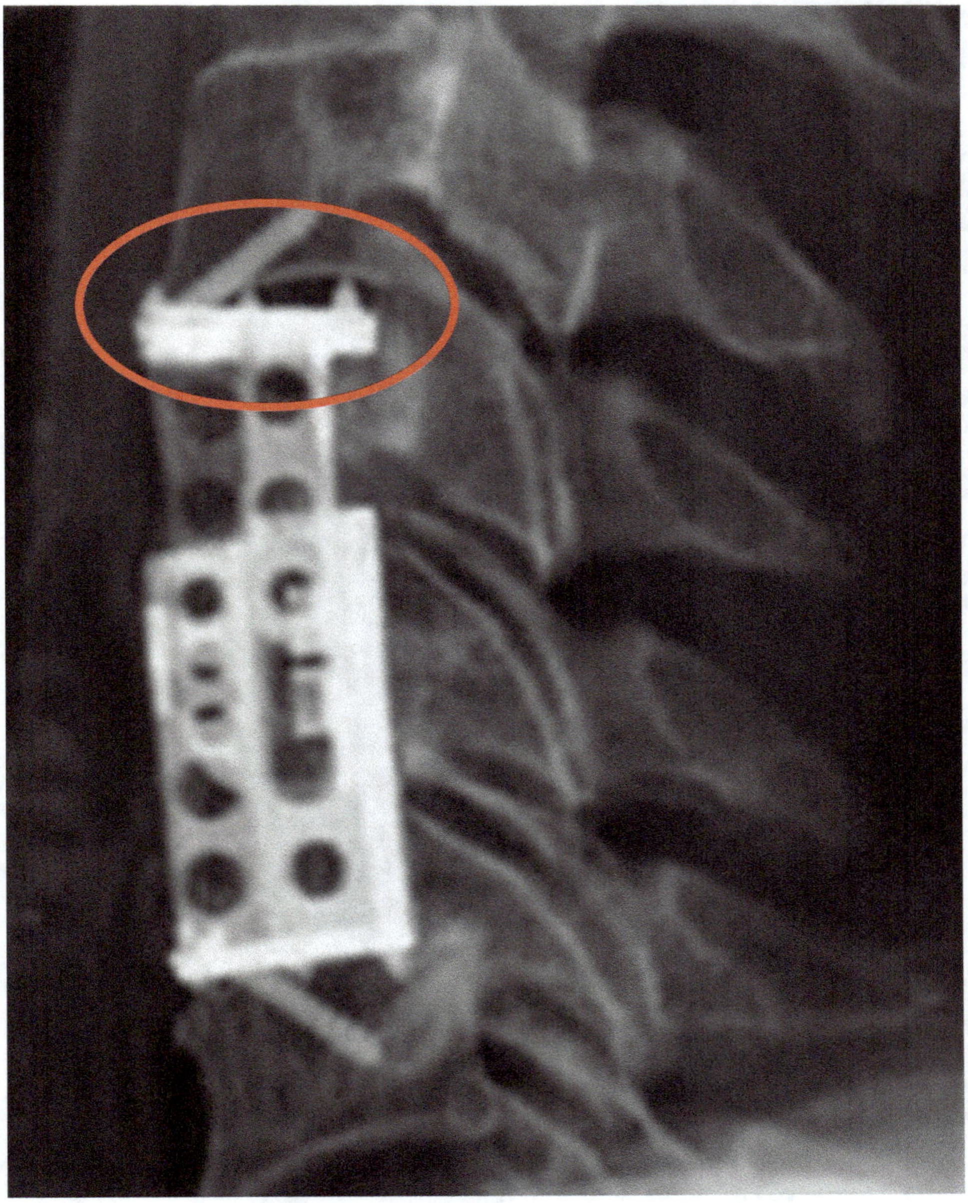

Figure 7. X-ray image of an implemented vertebral body replacement implant.

anchor vertebra, the parts of the implant base located medial have no direct contact with the anchor vertebra in the unload state. The cervical vertebral curvature corresponds to an average spine curvature and is 28 degrees [25]. The biomechanical properties of the ligaments and facet joints are taken from literature [26, 27].

4.1.2.2. Realization of the surface contact

The modeling of the contact between the vertebral body and the implant is realized by means of a special three-dimensional contact force element. The contacting surfaces, the baseplate of the implant, and the superior or inferior vertebral surface of the C3 and C6 are tessellated in such a way that the surfaces of the objects are composed of equally large polygons. In addition,

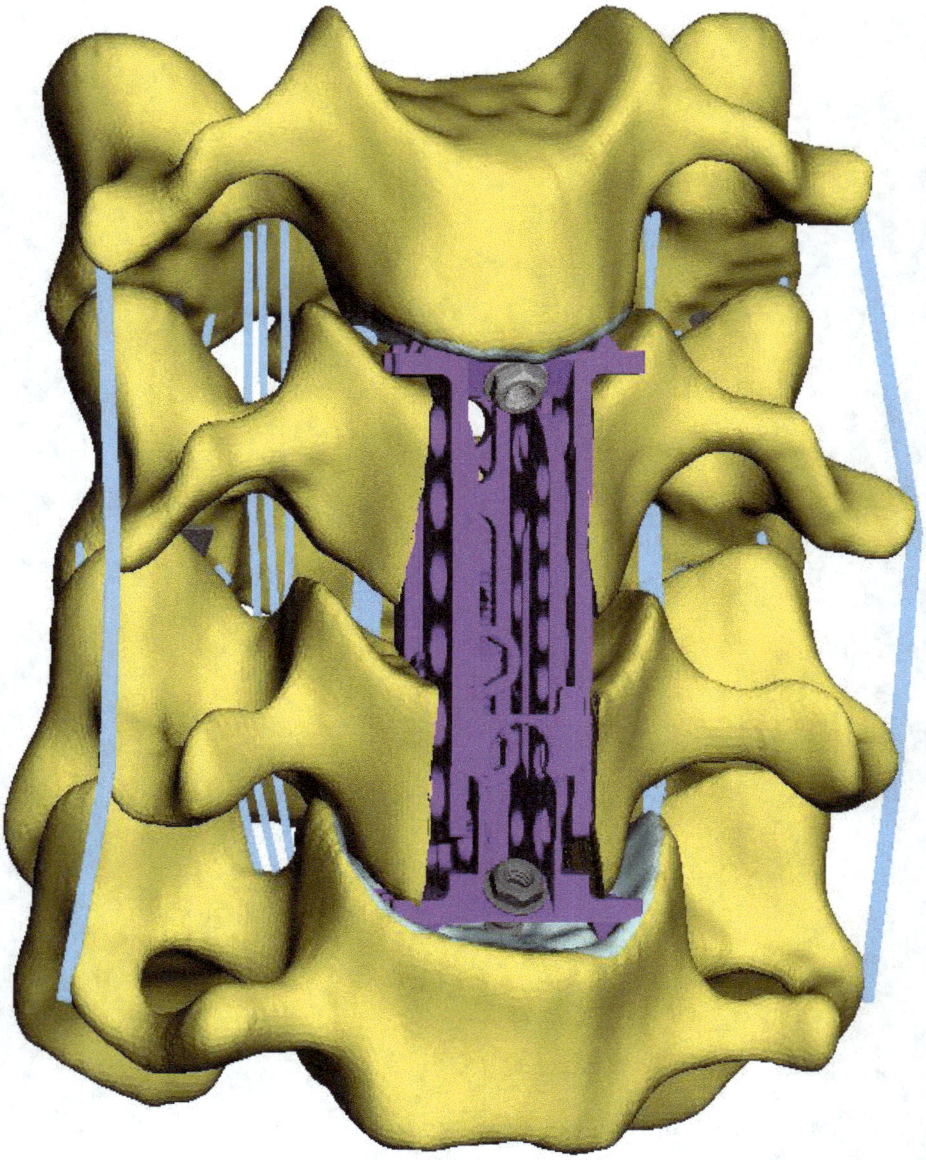

Figure 8. MBS model C6-C3 including vertebral body replacement implant.

the baseplate was dissected into smaller subunits to allow a more detailed analysis of the contact behavior (**Figure 9**).

For each of these polygons, a contact force is determined which is essentially oriented according to Hippmann [28] on the boundary layer model, and combined with a half-space approximation and contact force elements. So the contact force F_k is composed of a normal force F_{nk} and a tangential force F_{tk}. The normal force F_{nk} is composed as follows:

$$F_{nk} = \begin{cases} F_{ck} + F_{dk} : F_{ck} + F_{dk} > 0 \\ 0 : F_{ck} + F_{dk} \leq 0 \end{cases} \quad (6)$$

Annotation: in the following the subscript E and F stand for the corresponding bodies E and F. For the case $F_{ck} + F_{dk} > 0$, the equation is composed of a stiffness term,

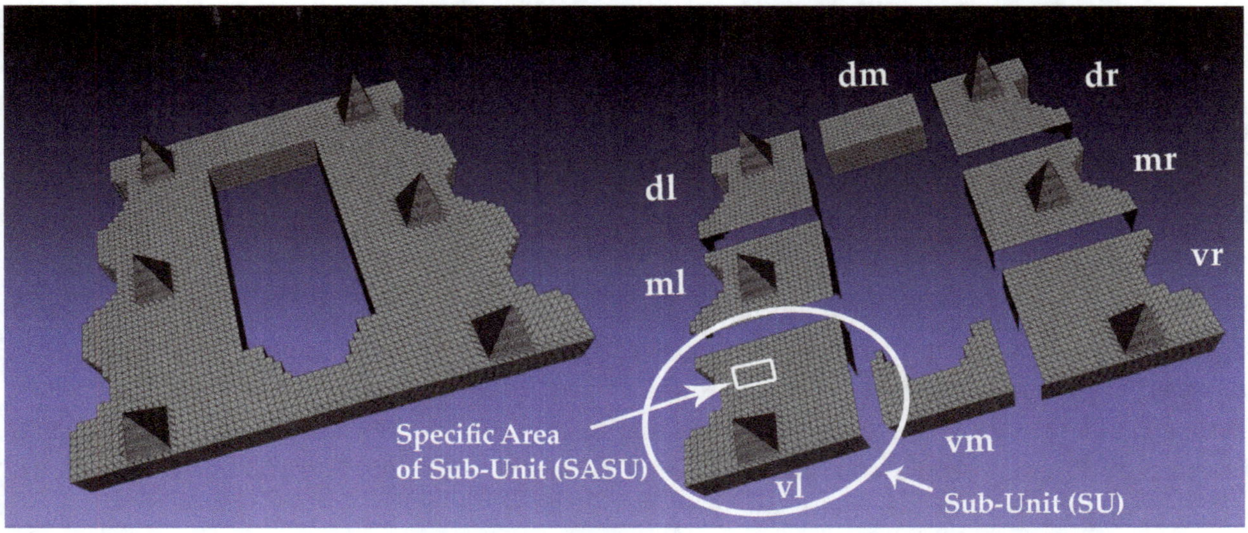

Figure 9. Illustration of the tessellated polygon meshes of the caudal implant base and explanation of terms.

$$F_{ck} = c_l * A_k * u_{nk} \tag{7}$$

c_l : stiffness of the contact element; A_k : total area of the contact element; u_{nk} : penetration of the contact element.

which results from

$$c_l = \frac{c_{lE} * c_{lF}}{c_{lE} + c_{lF}} \tag{8}$$

with

$$c_{lE} = \frac{K_E}{b_E} = \frac{1 - \nu_E}{(1 + \nu_E) + (1 - 2\nu_E)} * \frac{E_E}{b_E} \tag{9}$$

for c_{lF} analog and a damping term

$$F_{dk} = \begin{cases} d_l * A_k * v_{nk} : u_{nk} \geq u_d \\ d_l * A_k * v_{nk} * \dfrac{u_{nk}}{u_d} : u_{nk} < u_d \end{cases} \tag{10}$$

where

$$v_{nk} = n_k * v_k \tag{11}$$

stands for the relative speed projected in the normal direction

$$v_k = v_{M_e M_f} + \omega_{M_e M_f} \times r_{M_f C_k} \tag{12}$$

of both contact bodies at the position c_k of the contact element.

According to Hippmann [28], the parameter u_d can be used to define a penetration depth up to which the damping force acts linear. This makes it possible to avoid unrealistic forces during rapid contact processes. Further input parameters are the layer depth b, the E-modulus, and Poisson's ratio v of each surface and the damping constant d. Because the vertebral body replacement implant consists of a titanium alloy, the corresponding material property for E and v has been entered into the model. The E-modulus and Poisson's ratio v for the superior and inferior vertebral body surfaces are taken from [29, 30]. The damping is 10% of the E-modulus of the vertebral body replacement implant. The resulting total force of the contact surface is determined by summing the acting forces of all contact elements. Because the vertebral body replacement implant is actually fastened to the vertebral body by means of a screw, this fixation has been realized by a force element that realizes spring and damper forces and moments between bodies in multiple axis direction. These parameters (c = 108 N/m, $d = c$ * 0.1 Ns/m) are determined by means of sensitivity analysis.

The tangential force F_{tk} is calculated as follows [28] and is determined in dependence of the tangential relative velocity

$$v_{tk} = v_k - v_{nk} * n_k \tag{13}$$

$$v_{tk} = |v_{tk}| \tag{14}$$

and the normal force F_{nk} of the contact element

$$F_{tk} = \begin{cases} \mu * F_{nk} : \ v_{tk} \geq v_\varepsilon \\ \mu * F_{nk} * \dfrac{v_{tk}}{v_\varepsilon} * \left(2 - \dfrac{v_{tk}}{v_\varepsilon}\right) : \ v_{tk} < v_\varepsilon \end{cases} \tag{15}$$

To avoid a set-valued static friction, the frictional force is disabled when the sliding speed falls below a given small value v_ε.

The total force F_k and the torque M_k of the single contact element are now:

$$F_k = F_{nk} * n_k + F_{tk} * \frac{\mathrm{v}_{tk}}{v_{tk}} \tag{16}$$

$$M_k = r_{M_f C_k} \times F_k \tag{17}$$

Finally, the forces and torques of all contact elements are summed to the resulting total force screw:

$$F_E^{M_f} = \sum\nolimits_k F_k \tag{18}$$

$$M_E = \sum\nolimits_k M_k \tag{19}$$

A detailed description of the determination of the contact force and further information can be found in [28].

4.1.2.3. Simulation results

The external force that causes the kinematics of the model is 50 N, which corresponds to the average weight force of the corresponding upper body segments and is taken from [31]. In general, it is possible to analyze both the kinematic and kinetic parameters of the modeled spinal structures in this model configuration, such as the ligaments or facet joints, as well as the contact behavior "vertebral body surface-implant plate." In the following, the contact behavior is analyzed and the parameters "total contact patch area," "weighted penetration," "maximum penetration," "maximum contact pressure," and "weighted contact pressure" are discussed.

The surfaces of the subunits of the caudal implant base surface, which comes into contact with the superior anchor vertebral surface, are of different size (**Table 1**). The sinister regions are more in contact than the dexter regions.

Both the dorsally central (dm) and dorsally dexterous region (dr) of the implant baseplate have no contact with the vertebral body C6. The percentage total contact surface is 52%.

The average penetrations and the maximum penetrations of the subunits are shown in **Figure 10**. The right front (vr) and central front (vm) subunits penetrate the superior vertebral body surfaces on average most strongly. The weighted penetration of the left middle (ml) and right middle (mr) subunits is half as high. Due to the missing contact in the subunits "dm"and "dr," there is no penetration.

The maximum penetration behaves in an analogous manner. The difference between the "weighted penetration" and the "maximum penetration" of the ventral right "vr" and the left dorsal "ld" subunit stands out. The maximum penetration is 2.5 times and 2 times higher than the weighted penetration. In the remaining subunits, the maximum penetration is more than 1.5 times higher than the weighted penetration. We concluded that within the different subunits (SU) the penetration depth of the specific areas of this subunit (SASU) can be very different in some cases.

	Percentage contact patch area (%)
vr	15.0
vm	9.8
vl	1.3
ml	15.7
dl	1.2
dm	0.0
dr	0.0
mr	8.9

Table 1. Percentage contact of the subunits of the implant base with the vertebral endplate.

Looking at the contact pressure in **Figure 11**, the right ventral (rv) subunit of the implant baseplate is much more heavily loaded than the other subunits. The maximum contact pressure in this subunit of the implant base is 6 times stronger and the weighted contact pressure is 5 times stronger. Comparing the maximum and the weighted contact pressure of the right ventral (rv) subunit, the subunit "rv" certain specific areas of subunit are loaded up to 2.5 times more than others.

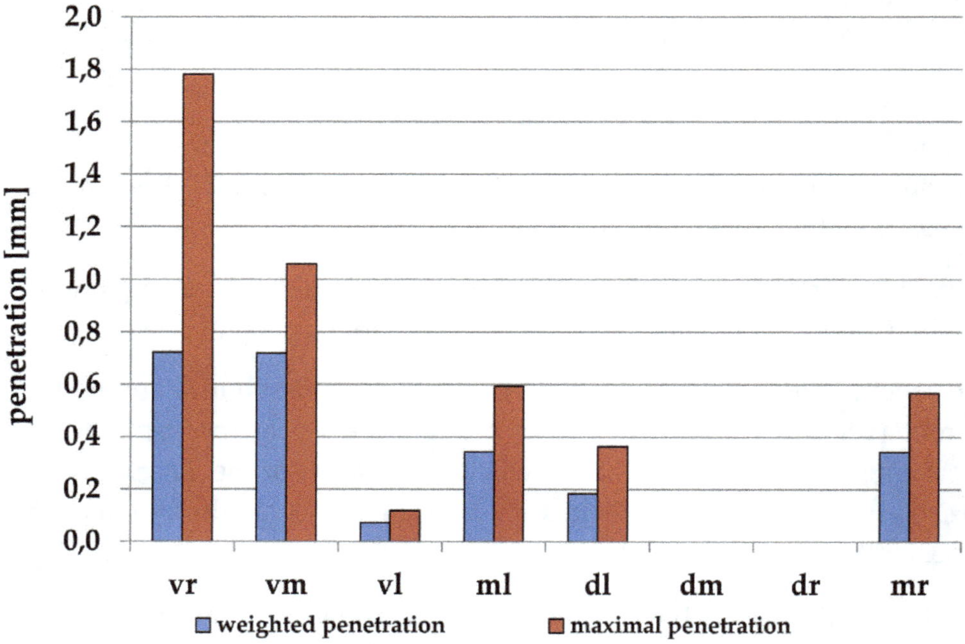

Figure 10. Penetration of the contact surfaces.

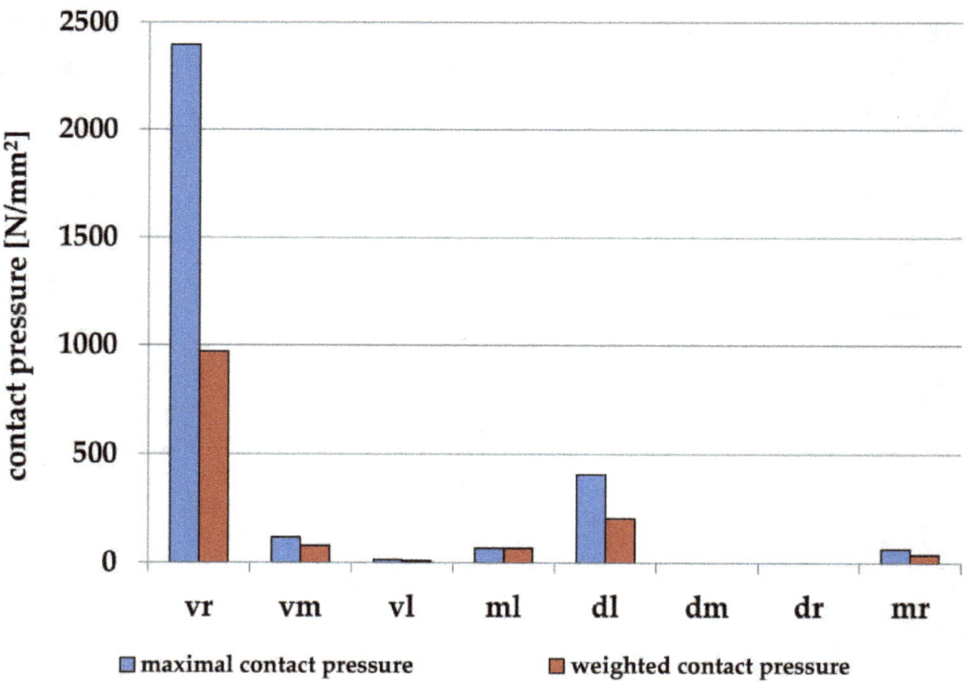

Figure 11. Contact pressure of the different subunits.

5. Summary and discussion

In many fields, personalized medicine has already been successfully introduced. In spinal implant surgery, patient-specific implants with an optimized fit shape could minimize severe complications. Depending on the question of cause, it is also possible to disassemble the basis plate of the implant into even smaller subunits in order to be able to make more detailed statements. If necessary, a hybrid model consisting of MBS and FE parts can also be created. However, it is always important to consider how exact the model must be. The desired precision determines how many more parameters, whose biomechanical properties must be known, flow into the model. However, some of these biomechanical parameters can only be inadequately determined. Furthermore, the calculation time increases with the increase in the fine structure of the model.

The presented modeling should not be seen as a competition to the FE modeling because our aim is to pursue a holistic way of looking at patients. Therefore, detailed models should be implemented in a whole-body model to simulate dynamic everyday situations and to obtain patient-specific knowledge about the stress situation in the fine-structured area. A valid modeling is indispensable, which can be ensured by selecting suitable input parameters. Because personalized input parameters of the model are often difficult to determine, we try to develop a procedure for the determination of patient-specific biomechanical properties of the human structures, which also guarantees rapid availability of these data as input parameters for the modeling.

Author details

Bauer Sabine[1*] and Paulus Dietrich[2]

*Address all correspondence to: bauer@uni-koblenz.de

1 Institute for Medical Engineering and Information Processing, University Koblenz-Landau, Koblenz, Germany

2 Institute for Computer Science, University Koblenz-Landau, Koblenz, Germany

References

[1] Hüsing B, Hartig J, Bührlen B, Reiß T, Gaisser S. Individualisierte Medizin und Gesundheitssystem. Future Report. 2008;126:1–348 Available from: http://www.tab-beim-bundestag.de/de/pdf/publikationen/tab-brief/TAB-Brief-034.pdf

[2] FDA USA Food and Drug Administration. Paving the Way for Personalized Medicine: FDA's Role in a New Era of Medical Product Development. 1st ed. U.S. Department of Health and Human Services; 2013; Silver Spring, USA. p. 62. DOI: http://www.fda.gov/downloads/.../PersonalizedMedicine/UCM372421....

[3] Rengier E, Mehndiratta A, von Tengg-Kobligk H, Zechmann C, Unterhinninghofen R, Kauczor H.-U, Giesel F. 3D printing based on imaging data: Review of medical applications. International Journal of Computer Assisted Radiology and Surgery. 2010;**5**(3):335-341. DOI: 10.1007/s11548-010-0476-x 2010

[4] Sauer A, Beneke F, Bergers D, Witt G. Modelle und Prototypen für die Medizin. RTejournal. 2005;**2**(2):1-10. Available from: http://. www.rtejournal.de/ausgabe2/69

[5] Ay M, Kubat T, Delilbasi C, Ekici B, Yuzbasioglue H, Hartomacioglub S. 3D Bio-Cad modeling of human mandible and fabrication by rapid-prototyping technology. Usak University Journal of Material Sciences. 2013;**2**:135-145. DOI: 10.12748/uujms.201324255

[6] Kauffmann G, Sauer R, Weber W. Radiologie: Bildgebende Verfahren, Strahlentherapie, Nuklearmedizin und Strahlenschutz. 4th ed. München, Jena: Urban & Fischer Verlag/Elsevier GmbH; 2011. p. 320

[7] Rho J, Hobantho M, Ashman R. Relations of mechanical properties to density and CT numbers in humanbone. Medical Engineering and Physics. 1995;**17**(5):347

[8] Sun W, Starly B, Nam J, Darling A. Bio-CAD modeling and its applications in computer-aided tissue engineering. Computer-Aided Design. 2005;**37**:1097-1114

[9] Wilke H-J, Rohlmann F, Neidlinger-Wilke C, Werner K, Claes L, Kettler A. Validity and interobserver agreement of a new radiographic grading system for intervertebral disc degeneration: Part I. Lumbar spine. European Spine Journal. 2006;**15**(6):720-730. DOI: 10.1007/s00586-005-1029-9

[10] Kettler A, Rohlmann F, Neidlinger-Wilke C, Werner K, Claes L, Wilke, H-J. Validity and interobserver agreement of a new radiographic grading system for intervertebral disc degeneration: Part II. Cervical spine. European Spine Journal. 2006;**15**(6):732-741. DOI: 10.1007/s00586-005-1037-9

[11] Rajagopal A, Dembia C, DeMersm M, Delp D, Hicks J, Delp S. Full-body musculoskeletal model for muscle-driven simulation of human gait. IEEE Transactions on Biomedical Engineering. 2016;**63**(10):2068-2079 DOI: 10.1109/TBME.2016.2586891

[12] Östh J, Brolin K, Bråse D. A human body model with active muscles for simulation of pretensioned restraints in autonomous braking interventions. Traffic Injury Prevention. 2014;**16**:304-313. DOI: 10.1080/15389588.2014.931949

[13] Stapleton S, Moreira R, Jockenhoevel S, Mela P, Reese S. Effect of reinforcement volume fraction and orientation on a hybrid tissue engineered aortic heart valve with a tubular leaflet design. Advanced Modeling and Simulation in Engineering Sciences. 2015;**2**(21):1-17. DOI: 10.1186/s40323-015-0039-3

[14] Baillargeon B, Rebelo N, Fox D, Taylor R, Kuhl E. The living heart project: A robust and integrative simulator for human heart function. European Journal of Mechanics A/Solids. 2014;**48**:38-47. DOI: 10.1016/j.euromechsol.2014.04.001

[15] Ignasiak D, Sperr R, Ferguson S. The effect of age-related changes in spinal kinematics on vertebral loading during daily living activities. In: 22nd Congress of the European Society

of Biomechanics; July 10-13, 2016; Lyon, France. 2016. DOI: https://esbiomech.org/conference/index.php/congress/lyon2016/paper/view/188

[16] Schmidt H, Heuer F, Wilke H-J. Interaction between finite helical axes and facet joint forces under combined loading. Spine. 2008;**33**(25):2741-2748. DOI: 10.1097/BRS.0b013e31817c4319

[17] Schwertassek R, Wallrapp O. Dynamics of flexible multibody systems. Methods of mechanics for computer-aided design and analysis of mechatronic systems. Wiesbaden: Vieweg+Teubner Verlag; 1999. p. 476 DOI: 10.1007/978-3-322-93975-3

[18] Bauer S. Basics of multibody systems: Presented by practical simulation examples of spine models. In: Lopez-Ruiz R, editor. Numerical Simulation—From Brain Imaging to Turbulent Flows. Rijeka, Croatia: Intech; 2016. pp. 29-49. DOI: 10.5772/62864

[19] Bauer S, Paulus D. Analysis of the biomechanical effects of spinal fusion to adjacent vertebral. International Journal of Simulation-Systems, Science and Technology—IJSSST. 2015;**15**(2):1-7. DOI: 10.1109/EMS.2013.28

[20] Bauer S, Keller E, Paulus D. Rückenschmerz durch Übergewicht? Biomechanische MKS-Modellierung der Belastungssituation der Lendenwirbelsäule bei unterschiedlichem Körpergewicht. In: Handels Heinz, Thomas Martin D, Hans-Peter M, Thomas T, editors. Bildverarbeitung für die Medizin 2015; 15. bis 17. März 2015 ; Lübeck. Berlin, Heidelberg: Springer; 2015. pp. 323-328. DOI: 10.1007/978-3-662-46224-9

[21] Rohlmann A, Bauer L, Zander T, Bergmann G, Wilke H-J. Determination of trunk muscle forces for flexion and extension by using a validated finite element model of the lumbar spine and measured in vivo data. Journal of Biomechanics. 2006;**39**(6):981-989

[22] Juchem S, Hausen U, Gruber K. Effects on individual spine curvatures—A comparative study with the help of computer modelling. In: Olaf D, editor. Biomedical Engineering; 16.09.2016–19.09.2016; Jena, Germany. De Gruyter; 2012. pp. 132-135. DOI: https://doi.org/10.1515/bmt-2012-4052

[23] Tubbs R, Rompala O, Verma K, Mortazavi M, Benninger, B, Loukas, M, Chambers R: Analysis of the uncinate processes of the cervical spine: An anatomical study. Journal of Neurosurgery: Spine. 2012;**16**:401-407. DOI: 10.3171/2011.12.SPINE11541

[24] Panjabi M, Duranceau J, Goel V, Oxland T, Takata K. Cervical human vertebrae—quantitative three-dimensional anatomy of the middle and lower regions. Spine. 1991;**16**(8):861-869. DOI: 10.1007/s00586-003-0586-z

[25] Grob D, Frauenfelder H, Mannion H. The association between cervical spine curvature and neck pain. European Spine Journal. 2007;**16**:669-678. DOI: 10.1007/s00586-006-0254-1

[26] Yoganandan N, Kumaresan S, Pintar FA. Biomechanics of the cervical spine Part 2. Cervical spine soft tissue responses and biomechanical modeling. Clinical Biomechanics. 2001;**16**:1-27. DOI: http://dx.doi.org/10.1016/S0268-0033(00)00074-7

[27] White A, Panjabi M. Clinical Biomechanics of the Spine. University of Michigan: Lippincott; 1978. p. 534

[28] Hippmann G. Modellierung von Kontakten komplex geformter Körper in der Mehrkörperdynamik [dissertation]. Wien: TU Wien; 2004. p. 175. Available from: http://elib.dlr.de/12219/

[29] Kurutz M. Finite element modeling of the human lumbar spine. In: Moratal D, editor. Finite Element Analysis. Rijeka, Croatia: InTech; 2010. pp. 209-236. DOI: http://www.intechopen.com/books/finiteelement-

[30] Kumaresan S, Yoganandan N, Pintar F, Maiman D. Finite element modeling of the cervical spine: Role of intervertebral disc under axial and eccentric loads. Medical Engineering & Physics. 1999;**21**:689-700

[31] Panjabi M, Summers D, Pelker R, Videman T, Friedlaender G, Southwick W. Three-dimensional load-displacement curves due to forces on the cervical spine. Journal of Orthopaedic Research. 1986;**4**:152-161. DOI: 10.1002/jor.1100040203

[32] Cremers D, Rousson M, Deriche R. A review of statistical approaches to level set segmentation: Integrating color, texture, motion and shape. International Journal of Computer Vision. 2007;**72**:195-215. doi:10.1007/s11263-006-8711-1

[33] Zhang YJ. A survey on evaluation methods for image segmentation. Pattern Recognition. 1996;**29**(8):1335-1346. DOI: 10.1016/0031-3203(95)00169-7

[34] Fenster A, Chiu B. Evaluation of segmentation algorithms for medical imaging. In: Proceedings of Annual International Conference of the IEEE Engineering in Medicine and Biology Society. IEEE Engineering in Medicine and Biology Society Conference; 2005. DOI: 10.1109/IEMBS.2005.1616166

[35] Zhu H, Meng F, Cai J, Lu S. Beyond pixels. A comprehensive survey from bottom-up to semantic image segmentation and cosegmentation. Journal of Visual Communication and Image Representation. 2016;**34**:12-27

[36] Fitzpatrick J, Hill D, Maurer C. Image Registration. Handbook of Medical Imaging. Medical Image Processing and Analysis. 2000;**2**:447-514

[37] Wyawahare MV, Patil PM, Abhyankar HK. Image registration techniques: An overview. International Journal of Signal Processing, Image Processing and Pattern Recognition. 2009;**2**(3):11-28

[38] Junyi X, Alfredo S. A real-time respiratory motion monitoring system using KINECT: Proof of concept. Journal of Medical Physics. 2012;**39**(5):2682-2685. doi:10.1118/1.4704644

13

Surgical Treatment of Spinal Meningiomas

Antonino Raco, Alessandro Pesce and
Massimo Miscusi

Abstract

Spinal meningiomas are common spinal tumors; in most cases they are benign and with a good surgical prognosis. However, specific location, infiltration of spinal cord, vascular encasement, or spinal root involvement can bring to a less favorable prognosis. We reviewed a series of 173 consecutive patients with spinal meningiomas treated from 1976 to 2011 in our institution, and data were stratified according to sex, age, symptoms, axial location, Simpson resection grade, and functional pre-/postoperative status. Particular attention was paid to description of those factors leading to a poor outcome. Functional improvement at follow-up was observed in 86.7% of cases, 6.4% of patients resulted stable, and 6.9% worsened; a low functional grade before surgery was connected to a lesser improvement after. Anterolateral meningiomas were the most represented (42.2%); a gross total resection (Simpson grade I and II) was conducted in 98.8% and a macroscopically complete removal without dural resection or coagulation (Simpson grade III) was performed in 1.2%. According to data from our series, negative prognostic factors seem to be: anterior or anterolateral axial implant, long-lasting symptoms before diagnosis, WHO grade > I, Simpson grade II and III resection, sphincter involvement, and worse functional grade at onset.

Keywords: spinal meningiomas, surgery, spinal tumors, recurrence, surgical outcome

1. Introduction

Spinal meningiomas (SM) account for 1.2–12% of CNS meningiomas, being relatively uncommon [1–3]. The typical clinical presentation consists of pain [4], followed by gait, sensory, and sphincter disturbances. The constant improvement of neuroimaging techniques, the use of intraoperative neuromonitoring, and the increasing reliability of the contemporary surgical tools have further improved the prognosis of SM, already recognized as excellent by Cushing and Eisenhardt [5], more than 80 years ago, in their historical monograph. Since this cornerstone in SM literature, many series confirmed this finding [1, 6–9]. However, cases of anteriorly located or calcified lesions, cases of recurrences, and cases in which there is violation of the arachnoidal layer, invasion of spinal cord parenchyma, and encasement of vascular structure stand as exceptions to this rule.

2. Incidence, location, and subtypes

SM count for 25–46% of the intradural-extramedullary lesions, second to spinal schwannomas, which is the most frequent entity of this location [10]. SM favor females [4, 6, 11, 12], its incidence is significantly higher in Caucasians and Asian Pacific islanders than in Afro-Americans and Native Americans [13].

Despite being described at every age [14, 15], the highest incidence is in the fifth and sixth decade age group [4, 6, 7, 11]. Below the age of 18, predilection for female sex is not present. This feature, matched with a peak of incidence during peri-menopausal period, is consistent with the widely described and recognized neoplastic cells responsitivity to female sex hormones, similar to what happens for intracranial meningiomas [11, 12]. The exact incidence of SM is not known even though is estimated about 0.5–2 cases per 100,000 persons per year [3].

The relatively higher incidence in the thoracic spine is also noted in current literature compared to the other biomechanically active segments [6–8, 16]. The dural attachment is most frequently found in the anterior/anterolateral dura. Our series (**Figure 1** and **Table 1**) confirms these data [1, 2, 6, 7].

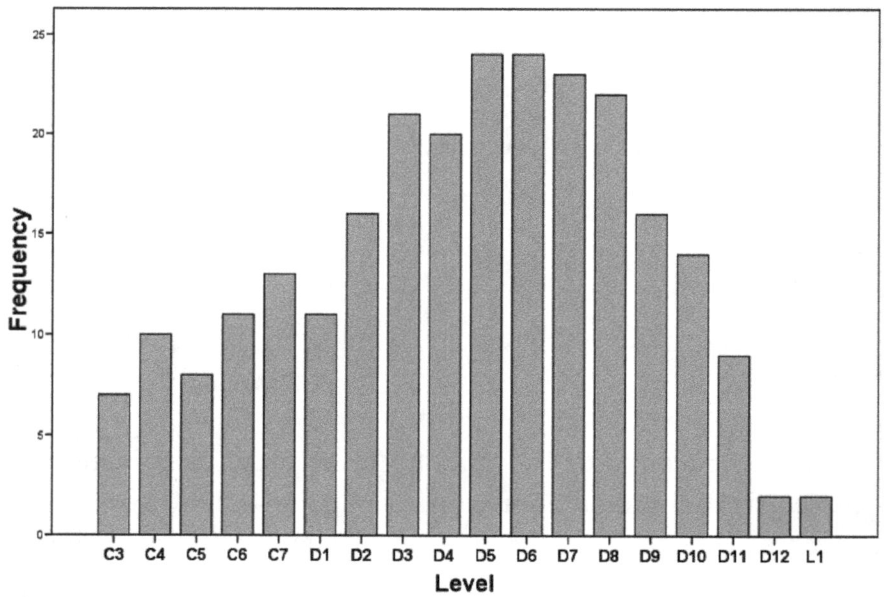

Figure 1. Incidence of spinal meningiomas in our cohort according to sagittal topography.

Total no. of patients	224
Lost to follow-up	15
Incomplete report (clinical and surgical)	22
Lesion involving CVJ	14
Residual cohort	173
Sex	
Woman	138 (79.8%)
Men	35 (20.2%)
Age	55.6 ± 13.1 years
Clinical presentation	
Pain	57 (32.9%)
Motor or gait disorders	55 (31.8%)
Paresthesias	53 (30.6%)
Sensory deficit	8 (4.6%)
Mean duration of preoperative symptoms	20.01 ± 18.86 months (range, 0–120 months)
Axial topography	
Posterior	11 (6.4%)
Posterolateral	42 (24.3%)
Anterolateral	73 (42.2%)
Anterior	15 (8.7%)
Lateral	32 (18.5%)
Simpson grade of resection	
I	52 pts (30%)
II	119 pts (68.8%)
III	2 pts (1.2%)
Neurological status at follow-up	
Improved	150 (86.7%)
Stable	11 (6.4%)
Worsened	12 (6.9%)
Sagittal topography according to biomechanical levels of the spine	
Subaxial cervical	14.2%
Cervicothoracic Junction	9.5%
Thoracic spine	75.5%
Thoracolumbar Junction	0.8%
Complications	
Total complication rate	7 (4.04%)
CSF leakage	3 (1.73%)
Spinal epidural hematoma	2 (1.15%)
Syringomyelia	1 (0.58%)
Adverse reaction to dural sealant	1 (0.58%)
WHO grading of the lesions	
I	170 pts (98.3%)
II	2 pts (1.15%)
III	1 pt (0.58%)

Table 1. Details of the final cohort.

SM histological subtypes are the same as their intracranial counterpart. The percentage of atypical/anaplastic SM is significantly lower than intracranial meningiomas [12]. In our series, WHO Grade I (**Table 1**) was the most represented subgroup of lesions in our cohort (98.3% of the lesions). These data are similar to other series [4, 6, 11, 12].

A higher incidence of SM is also well documented in patients suffering from neurofibromatosis. When a SM is detected in early life, it should raise suspicion of neurofibromatosis, especially in patients below the fourth decade and with extrathoracic sagittal location [12].

3. Diagnosis

3.1. Symptoms and physical findings

Literature recognize pain as the typical symptom at clinical onset of SM [6, 7, 17]. Pain can be axial, radicural, or radiating to upper or lower limbs, depending on the location of the tumor; it is commonly associated with paresthesias, hot and cold sensations, and sensory disturbances, followed by gait instability evolving in an obvious motor deficit, which is usually late due to the typical growth slowness of this lesions [2]. Sphincter impairment is a late finding and involves from 15 to 40% of the patients [18].

In our cohort, the most common disturbance at clinical onset was pain in 32.9% of cases (57 patients), followed by motor and gait disorder in 31.8% of cases, (55 patients); less frequently we observed paresthesias (30.6%, 53 patients), and occasionally a pure sensory disturbance was detectable (4.6%, 8 patients). Only 18.5% of patients complained a single disturbance at onset. The second disturbance in order of appearance was a motor disorder (61 patients, 35.3%) and occasionally a sphincter disturbance (10 patients, 5.8%). The average duration of symptoms was 20.01±18.86 months (range, 0–120 months) (**Table 1**).

Pain was described as axial (cervical or thoracic; 30 patients; 17.34%), radicular (radiating to corresponding dermatome; 5 patients; 2.89%), or radiating to distant dermatomes (e.g. thoracic cord meningiomas with pain radiating to lower limbs; 22 patients; 12.71%). A total of 21 patients (12.13%) were retrospectively estimated to suffer from a pure radiculopathy, 37 from a pure myelopathy (21.38%), and 115 from myeloradiculopathy (66.47%).

3.2. Radiology

Standard X-ray plain film is of limited value, it may demonstrate pedicle or soma erosion, abnormalities in the normal spine curvatures [18]. X-ray standard myelography may outline a contrast block at the level of the extradural lesion, but it has been disused in the common everyday clinical practice. Spine contrast-enhanced CT scans provide detailed information about bony anatomy; it finds a contemporary huge value while investigating extensively calcified lesions or in defining the detailed anatomy of recurrent SM [6, 17].

Since its introduction (at our Institution in 1991), a preoperative magnetic resonance imaging (MRI) scans have become the gold standard in defining this pathology. T1w, T2w, T1w gadolinium-enhanced sequences are routinely performed to investigate anatomical details of the lesions (**Figure 2A, B,** E, and **F**). Gadolinium-enhanced MRI imaging demonstrated an homogeneously enhanced mass delocating spinal cord parenchyma and nerve roots, intra-extradural extension of the lesion, and dural tail; it may not sufficiently help the differential diagnosis between spinal schwannomas and meningiomas [14].

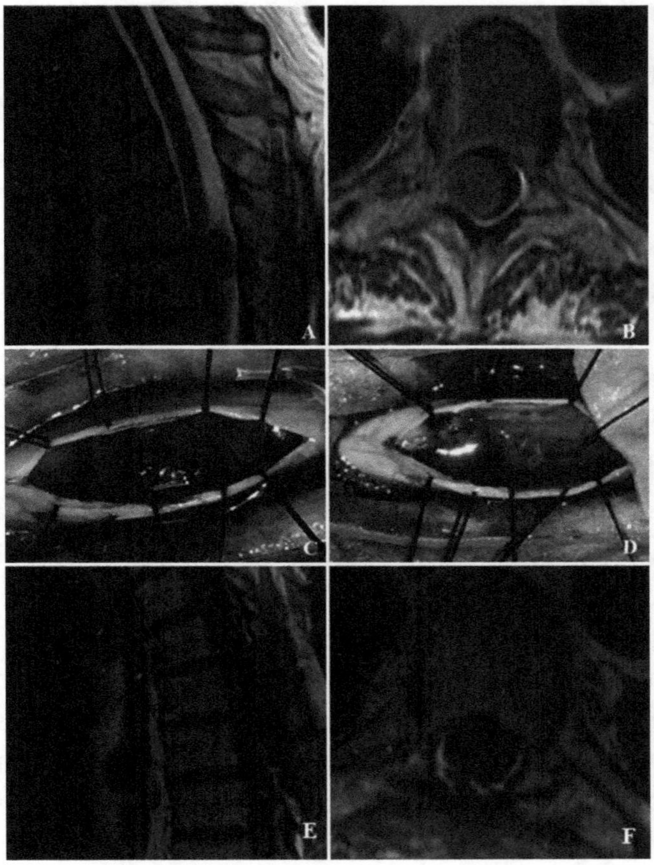

Figure 2. A. Sagittal T2w and B. Axial T1w gadolinium enhanced images of a thoracic spinal meningioma causing spinal cord dislocation. C. Intraoperative pre- and D. post- total resection of the lesion. Dura mater was extensively coagulated with no remnant of the disease, realizing a Simpson Grade of Resection II. E. Sagittal and F. Axial T1w gadolinium enhanced postoperative MRI demonstrating complete resection of the tumor and spinal cord decompression.

4. Surgical treatment—technical standards, pitfalls, and advances

Standard prone position is commonly used to approach a SM. Mayfield clamp may prove useful in cases of high subaxial cervical SM. A preoperative radioscopic localization of the involved levels is routinely carried out. After a standard midline skin incision and hypodermal tissues sharp dissection, fascia is incised in a standard midline fashion, and subperiostal exposure of laminae and articular processes is performed. A standard laminotomy (or hemilaminectomy) exposes the dural sac. In case of thoracic spine anterior/anterolateral axially located lesion, a costo-trasversectomy to enlarge surgical corridor can be performed. Midline temporary 4 or 5-0 silk tack-up sutures lead to a safer midline dural opening. Under magnification of the operative microscope, a microsurgical lesionectomy is performed (**Figure 2C** and **D**). Regardless of the potential infiltrative pattern or encasement of spinal vascular structures and nerve roots, a CUSA debulking is made to avoid any traction on the spinal cord.

Total removal is the target in all posteriorly located lesions, dural attachment must be removed, and a duraplasty completes the procedure. For anterior/anterolateral lesions, macroscopically complete excision is always associated with generous coagulation of the dural attachment.

Experience and literature have led us to strongly prefer laminotomy over laminectomy to perform a standard posterior midline approach for the evidence-based risk of iatrogenic postoperative instability. In order to clarify the difference between laminectomy and laminotomy, we use the term "laminotomy" to describe a "partial laminectomy" sparing of the medial facet of the articular process.

The reported incidence of postoperative instability in cervical spine is as high as 56% in more than four-level laminectomies and 11% in less than four level [19], whereas in thoracolumbar spine, instability appears in 25% of patients receiving more than two-level laminectomies [20]. Postoperative deformity is reported in 9.4% of patients receiving laminectomy compared to 3% of patients receiving laminotomy [21].

In most cases, a standard posterior approach allows surgeon to work in an adequate surgical corridor to achieve complete excision even for anterior/anterolateral lesions. In our experience, standard posterior approach is the gold standard in huge number of cases. However, intraextradural lesion with infiltration of the vertebral body, massively calcified lesions, anterior/anterolateral lesions, or recurrent tumors with spinal cord invasion stand as notable exceptions to this rule. In these cases, lateral or anterior approaches, with generous arthrectomy, pedicle resection, and partial/total vertebrectomy, performed to gain an optimal attachment control and safer spinal cord manipulation may be required [8, 16, 22, 23].

5. Neurological and functional outcome and complications

SM are slowly growing lesion, typically benign. Usually, they carry a fair neurological and functional prognosis [1, 6–9]. However, cases of anteriorly located or calcified lesions, recurrences, and cases in which there is violation of the arachnoidal layer, invasion of spinal cord parenchyma, and encasement of vascular structure stand as exceptions to this rule.

For this reason, one of the major efforts in SM surgery research and literature has historically been to preoperatively identify cases with a worse functional and neurological prognosis.

With the same aforementioned purpose, we critically reviewed our entire cohort of patients operated on for SM excision through a detailed retrospective analysis. Functional and neurological data about the outcome of each patient were recoded with Frankel [24] and McCormick [25] scales.

Frankel scale is a functional evaluation scale, initially conceived for spinal cord injury (SCI) but capable of assessing residual function "below" the level of a lesion. It is extremely easy and extremely sensitive with respect to coarse variations of the spinal cord function. McCormick scale, designed for intramedullary neoplasms, provides information about spinal cord function in relation to the quality of life and patient's independence (e.g. walking ability and the degree of impairment in the upper limbs). In our cohort, these scales appear to be strongly associated (Pearson's bivariate correlation p 0.01; r= −0.820 McCormick Pre-Frankel, Frankel −0.934 McCormick at Follow-Up), validating each other.

The scales are reported in **Table 2**.

	Frankel scale
A	Complete neurological injury—no motor or sensory function below the level of the injury
B	Preserved sensation only—no motor function below the level of the injury
C	Preserved motor nonfunctional—some motor function observed below the level of the injury
D	Preserved motor function—useful motor function below the level of the injury
E	Normal motor—no clinically detected abnormality in motor or sensory function with normal sphincter function; abnormal reflexes and subjective sensory abnormalities may be present
	McCormick scale
1	Intact neurologically, normal ambulation, and minimal dysesthesia
2	Mild motor or sensory deficit and functional independence
3	Moderate deficit, limitation of function, and independent w/external aid
4	Severe motor or sensory deficit, limited function, and dependent
5	Paraplegia or quadriplegia, even w/flickering movement

Table 2. Frankel and McCormick scales.

The preoperative Frankel functional classes most represented in our cohort were classes A, B, and C (respectively 15, 9, and 91 patients, amounting to 66.5% of the total). These classes reflect a deeper neurological impairment. Preoperative McCormick grade III, IV, and V was recorded, respectively, in 76, 36, and 18 patients (75.1% of the sample), whereas in the postoperative period, A, B, and C and III, IV, and IV classes were represented by 28.3% (49 patients) and 28.6% (53 patients).

The number of patients who experienced a significant improvement at follow-up amounted to 150 (86.7%), 11 were stable (6.4%) and the remaining 12 worsened (6.9%). In this cohort, the worst functional preoperative status showed a clear tendency to more modest improvements both on Frankel and McCormick scales (Pearson's bivariate correlation, both p 0.01, r = 0.511 and 0.618).

In our sample, a long duration of preoperative symptoms and severe preoperative impairment are related to worse outcomes; this result is similar to other reports [8, 26]. The author (A.R.) has previously reported a clear possibility of recovery even in patients harboring deep functional preoperative impairment [26], outlining that age (under 60) and duration of preoperative impairment stand as the most important predictors of neurological recovery.

Anteriorly located lesions imply the most difficult setting in SM surgery [4, 7, 8, 12]. Consistent with the literature [7, 8], in our series, anterior/anterolateral lesions were identified as a subgroup with worse outcome compared to different axial topographies. Purely anterior lesions with arachnoidal adhesions to spinal cord and vascular encasement lead to an increased risk of spinal cord traction and surgical damage.

Some authors report massive calcification of the lesion as a predictor of neurological postoperative deterioration [6, 8]. In our series, only three patients harbored massively calcified spinal meningiomas, and thus this feature failed to reach statistical significance to confirm these findings.

Recurrence of SM in our sample was predictive of worse outcome. Our recurrence rate was 2.3% (4/173 cases). In the current literature, this rate varies between 1.3 and 13% [2, 4, 6, 9, 14, 18, 27, 28]. Obviously, WHO grading of the lesions is correlated with the probability of local relapses. In recurrent SM surgery, arachnoidal scarring caused by the first procedure can make tumor debulking harder and, despite the regular use of intraoperative neuromonitoring and CUSA, can lead to a worse outcome. In our cohort, patients harboring recurrent lesions were 4, a total of just two patients underwent a second SM excision surgery, and, although underrepresented compared to the entire sample (2 of 4 patients on 173 patients of the entire cohort), showed a statistical association with worse outcomes. Therefore, whenever feasible, our experience suggests, according to Literature, that first surgery should always be as aggressive as possible [7, 23].

No postoperative death was recorded in our sample. Mortality rate in SM surgery is usually extremely low, ranging between 0.8 and 2% in series reported after 1999 [6–8].

6. Complications

In SM surgery, complications can be coarsely divided in two subgroups: neurological postoperative worsening and surgical complications causing neurological impairment. Among the last subgroup, most common surgical complications include spinal epidural hematoma, CSF leakage with or without deep or superficial infections, syringomyelia, and iatrogenic instability [2, 6, 7, 19–21].

The first subgroup was extensively discussed in the previous paragraph as well as concerns about iatrogenic instability are described in surgical treatment section.

Surgical complications counted for a total of 7/173 cases (4.04% of patients). A total of four patients (two postoperative spinal epidural hematoma, one syringomyelia, and one adverse reaction to dural sealant) required a revision surgery. The remaining underwent conservative treatments (three patients with CSF leakage resolved with lumbar drainage).

Lumbar drainage is reserved for the management of at least 4–5 days of persistent wound CSF leakage. In this series, three patients suffered from wound CSF leakage and were treated conservatively by bedrest and lumbar drainage positioning. These complications were completely resolved in 5–7 days and did not require a surgical revision. Lumbar drainage use for CSF leakages treatment is hugely validated by experience and literature [29, 30].

No case of deep or superficial infection was recorded in our series. According to contemporary Literature, at present, deep and superficial infections are exceptional complications [7, 17].

7. Simpson grade of resection and recurrences

In the spinal compartment, recurring lesions are less common than meningiomas rising within the intracranial compartment (10–26%) [4]. Mirimanoff et al. [28] showed that the long-term follow-up of patients operated on for spinal meningioma removal can indicate up to 13% of recurrence at 10 years. However, the main limitation of this study is the small size of the cohort investigated (18 patients). Nakamura et al. [23] reported a recurrence rate as high as 30% at 12-year follow-up for patients who received a Simpson grade II resection. Setzer et al. [16] reported a stratification of recurrence probability by WHO histological grading: 1.4% for grade I, 50% for grade II, and 100% for grade III and IV, in 43.5 ± 24.8 months of follow-up.

As previously mentioned, recurrence of SM in our sample was predictive of worse outcome. Our recurrence rate was 2.3% (4/173 cases). In the current literature, this rate varies between 1.3 and 13% [2, 4, 6, 9, 14, 18, 27, 28].

Simpson grade I was obtained in 52 patients (30%). In all these cases, dural attachment, mainly posterior or posterolateral, was removed and a duraplasty with eterologous dural patch was performed. The rationale for this procedure is that literature analysis reveals a difference in terms of recurrence probability for Simpson grade I and II [2, 18, 23], and these data are confirmed in our series. In case of duraplasty, dural sealant was routinely used, since its use is substantially supported by literature [31].

Our routine postoperative SM follow-up protocol consists of a minimum 4 years of clinical and radiological follow-up reserved for patients with Simpson grade of resection I and WHO grade I lesions. Simpson grade of resection > I and WHO grade > I patients underwent a closer clinical and radiological follow-up. Such a follow-up protocol appears justified in relation to the natural history of SM, an extremely slowly growing lesion, which favors fifth/sixth decade. Some recurrences may be ignored because they never reach clinical significance in the lifespan of the patient. Our policy toward recurrent lesions is to reoperate only on those with MRI-demonstrated progressive regrowth tendency, because, according to literature and experience, operating a recurrent SM is often technically challenging [7, 8, 32, 33].

8. Conclusions

Spinal meningiomas are common primary spinal tumors, in most cases benign and with a good surgical prognosis. However, specific location, infiltration of spinal cord, vascular encasement, or spinal root involvement can bring on to a less favorable prognosis. We can adfirm that the negative prognostic factors in our study were: anterior or anterolateral axial location, protracted symptoms before diagnosis, WHO Grade > I, Simpson grade II and III resection, sphincter involvement, and worse functional grade at onset.

Author details

Antonino Raco[1], Alessandro Pesce[1*] and Massimo Miscusi[2]

*Address all correspondence to: ale_pesce83@yahoo.it

1 "Sapienza" University, Rome, Italy

2 "ICOT" Hospital, Latina – "Sapienza" Univesity, Rome, Italy

References

[1] Bret P, Lecuire J, Lapras C, Deruty R, Dechaume JP, Assaad A. Intraspinal meningiomas. A series of 60 cases. Neurochirurgie. 1976; 22:5–22.

[2] Solero CL, Fornari M, Giombini S, Lasio G, Oliveri G, Cimino C, Pluchino F. Spinal meningiomas: review of 174 operated cases. Neurosurgery. 1989; 25:153–160.

[3] Westwick HJ, Shamji MF. Effects of sex on the incidence and prognosis of spinal meningiomas: a Surveillance, Epidemiology, and End Results study. J Neurosurg Spine. 2015; 29:1-6.

[4] Maiuri F, De Caro ML, de Divitiis O, Vergara P, Mariniello G. Spinal meningiomas: Age-related features, Clin Neurol Neurosurg. 2011; 113(1):34–38.

[5] Cushing H, Eisenhardt L. Meningiomas: Their Classification, Regional Behavior, Life History, and Surgical End Results. Springfield, IL, Charles C Thomas, 1938.

[6] Sandalcioglu EI, Hunold A, Muller O, Bassiouni H, Stolke D, Asgari S. Spinal meningiomas: Critical review of 131 surgically treated patients. Eur Spine J. 2008; 17:1035–1041.

[7] Klekamp J, Samii M. Surgical results for spinal meningiomas. Surg Neurol.1999; 52(6): 552–562.

[8] Westwick HJ, Yuh SJ, Shamji MF. Complication avoidance in the resection of spinal meningiomas. World Neurosurg. 2015; 83(4):627-634.

[9] Roux FX, Nataf F, Pinaudeau M, Borne G, Devaux B, Meder JF. Intraspinal meningiomas: review of 54 cases with discussion of poor prognosis factors and modern therapeutic management. Surg Neurol. 1996; 46(5):458–463.

[10] Albanese V, Platania N. Spinal intradural extramedullary tumors. J Neurosurg Sci. 2002; 16:18–24.

[11] Yoon SH, Chung CK, Jahng TA. Surgical outcome of spinal canal meningiomas, J Kor Neurosurg Soc. 2007; 42(4):300-304.

[12] Saracenia C, Harropb J. Spinal meningioma: Chronicles of contemporary neurosurgical diagnosis and management. Clin Neurol Neurosurg. 2009; 111(3):221–226.

[13] Kshettry VR, Hsieh JK, Ostrom QT, Kruchko C, Benzel EC, Barnholtz-Sloan JS. Descriptive epidemiology of spinal meningiomas in the United States. Spine (Phila Pa 1976). 2015; 40(15):E886-E889.

[14] Cohen-Gadol AA, Zikel OM, Koch CA, Scheithauer BW, Krauss WE. Spinal meningiomas in patients younger than 50 years of age: a 21-year experience. J Neurosurg. 2003; 98(3 Suppl):258–263.

[15] Fortuna A, Nolletti A, Nardi P, Caruso R. Spinal neurinomas and meningiomas in children. Acta Neurochir (Wien). 1981. 55(3-4), 329-341.

[16] Setzer M, Vatter H, Marquardt G, Seifert V, Vrionis FD. Management of spinal meningiomas: surgical results and a review of the literature. Neurosurg Focus. 2007; 23(4):E14.

[17] Kleklamp J, Samii M. "Extramedullary Tumors" in Surgery of Spinal Tumors. 1st ed. Springer-Verlag Berlin Heidelberg. 2007. p. 248-260.

[18] Levy WJ Jr, Bay J, Dohn D. Spinal cord meningioma. J Neurosurg. 1982; 57(6):804–812

[19] Katsumi Y, Honma T, Nakamura T: Analysis of cervical instability resulting from laminectomies for removal of spinal cord tumor. Spine (Phila Pa 1976). 1989; 14(11): 1171-1176.

[20] Papagelopoulos PJ, Peterson HA, Ebersold MJ, Emmanuel PR, Choudhury SN, Quast LM. Spinal column deformity and instability after lumbar or thoracolumbar laminectomy for intraspinal tumors in children and young adults. Spine (Phila Pa 1976). 1997; 22(4):442-451.

[21] McGirt MJ, Garces-Ambrossi GL, Parker SL, et al. Short-term progressive spinal deformity following laminoplasty versus laminectomy for resection of intradural spinal tumors: analysis of 238 patients. Neurosurgery. 2010; 66(5):1005-1012.

[22] Arima H, Takami T, Yamagata T, et al. Surgical management of spinal meningiomas: A retrospective case analysis based on preoperative surgical grade. Surg Neurol Int. 2014; 5(Suppl 7): S333–S338.

[23] Nakamura M, Tsuji O, Fujiyoshi K, et al. Long-term surgical outcomes of spinal meningiomas. Spine (Phila Pa 1976). 2012; 37(10):E617-E623.

[24] Frankel HL, Hancock DO, Hyslop G, et al. The value of postural reduction in the initial management of closed injuries of the spine with paraplegia and tetraplegia. Paraplegia. 1969; 7(3):179-192.

[25] McCormick PC, Stein BM: Intramedullary tumors in adults. Neurosurg Clin N Am. 1990;1(3):609-630.

[26] Ciappetta P, Domenicucci M, Raco A. Spinal meningiomas: prognosis and recovery factors in 22 cases with severe motor deficits. Acta Neurol Scand. 1988; 77(1):27-30.

[27] Schick U, Marquaedt G, Lorenz R. Recurrence of benign spinal neoplasm. Neurosurg Rev. 2001; 24(1):20-25.

[28] Mirimanoff RO, Dosoretz DE, Linggood RM, Ojemann RG, Martuza RL. Meningioma: analysis of recurrence and progression following neurosurgical resection. J Neurosurg 1985; 62:18–24.

[29] Khan M. Rihn J, Steele G. et al. Postoperative management protocol for incidental dural tears during degenerative lumbar spine surgery: A review of 3,183 consecutive degenerative lumbar cases. Spine (Phila Pa 1976). 2006; 31(22): 2609-2613

[30] Shapiro SA, Scully T. Closed continuous drainage of cerebrospinal fluid via a lumbar subarachnoid catheter for treatment or prevention of cranial/spinal cerebrospinal fluid fistula. Neurosurgery 1992; 30(2):241-245.

[31] Weinstein JS, Liu KC, Delashaw JB Jr, et al. The safety and effectiveness of a dural sealant system for use with nonautologous duraplasty materials. J Neurosurg. 2010;112(2):428-433

[32] Caroli E, Acqui M, Roperto R, Ferrante L, D'Andrea G. Spinal en plaque meningiomas: a contemporary experience. Neurosurgery 2004; 55:1275–1279.

[33] Gezen F, Kahraman S, Canakci Z, Beduk A. Review of 36 cases of spinal cord meningioma. Spine (Phila Pa 1976). 2000; 25:727-731.

Permissions

All chapters in this book were first published in ISDPD, by InTech Open; hereby published with permission under the Creative Commons Attribution License or equivalent. Every chapter published in this book has been scrutinized by our experts. Their significance has been extensively debated. The topics covered herein carry significant findings which will fuel the growth of the discipline. They may even be implemented as practical applications or may be referred to as a beginning point for another development.

The contributors of this book come from diverse backgrounds, making this book a truly international effort. This book will bring forth new frontiers with its revolutionizing research information and detailed analysis of the nascent developments around the world.

We would like to thank all the contributing authors for lending their expertise to make the book truly unique. They have played a crucial role in the development of this book. Without their invaluable contributions this book wouldn't have been possible. They have made vital efforts to compile up to date information on the varied aspects of this subject to make this book a valuable addition to the collection of many professionals and students.

This book was conceptualized with the vision of imparting up-to-date information and advanced data in this field. To ensure the same, a matchless editorial board was set up. Every individual on the board went through rigorous rounds of assessment to prove their worth. After which they invested a large part of their time researching and compiling the most relevant data for our readers.

The editorial board has been involved in producing this book since its inception. They have spent rigorous hours researching and exploring the diverse topics which have resulted in the successful publishing of this book. They have passed on their knowledge of decades through this book. To expedite this challenging task, the publisher supported the team at every step. A small team of assistant editors was also appointed to further simplify the editing procedure and attain best results for the readers.

Apart from the editorial board, the designing team has also invested a significant amount of their time in understanding the subject and creating the most relevant covers. They scrutinized every image to scout for the most suitable representation of the subject and create an appropriate cover for the book.

The publishing team has been an ardent support to the editorial, designing and production team. Their endless efforts to recruit the best for this project, has resulted in the accomplishment of this book. They are a veteran in the field of academics and their pool of knowledge is as vast as their experience in printing. Their expertise and guidance has proved useful at every step. Their uncompromising quality standards have made this book an exceptional effort. Their encouragement from time to time has been an inspiration for everyone.

The publisher and the editorial board hope that this book will prove to be a valuable piece of knowledge for researchers, students, practitioners and scholars across the globe.

List of Contributors

Paul S. Sung and Pamela Danial
Department of Physical Therapy, Central Michigan University, MI, USA

Irene Paterniti, Emanuela Esposito and Salvatore Cuzzocrea
Department of Chemical, Biological, Pharmaceutical and Environmental Sciences, University of Messina, Messina, Italy

Andrej Cupar
Faculty of Mechanical Engineering, Institute of Structures and Design, University of Maribor, Maribor, Slovenia

Zoran Stjepanovič and Andreja Rudolf
Faculty of Mechanical Engineering, Institute of Engineering Materials and Design, University of Maribor, Maribor, Slovenia

Simona Jevšnik
Inlas, Slovenske Konjice, Slovenia

Rija Erveš
Faculty of Civil Engineering, University of Maribor, Maribor, Slovenia

Josette Bettany-Saltikov
School of Health and Social Care, Teesside University, Victoria Road, Middlesbrough, UK

Gokulakannan Kandasamy
School of Social Sciences Business and Law, Teesside University, Middleborough, UK

Dariusz Czaprowski
Department of Physiotherapy, Józef Rusiecki University College, Olsztyn, Poland
Center of Body Posture, Olsztyn, Poland

Lukasz Stolinski
Spine Disorders and Pediatric Orthopedic Department, University of Medical Sciences, Poznan, Poland

Susan Henning, Lisa C. Mangino and Jean Massé
Advance Physical Therapy, Chapel Hill, NC, USA

Luiz Cláudio Lacerda Rodrigues
Santa Marcelina Medical School, São Paulo, Brazil
Oswaldo Cruz German Hospital, Rua Treze de Maio, São Paulo - SP, Brazil

Shu-Yan Ng
Wanchai Chiropractic Clinic, Wanchai, Hong Kong

Wing-Yan Chan, Tsz-Ki Ho and Yin-Ling Ng
Spine Technology Ltd, Wanchai, Hong Kong

Grant I. Wood
Align Clinic, San Mateo, California, USA

Manuel Rigo
Institute Elena Salvá, Barcelona, Spain

Moreno D'Amico
G. D'Annunzio University, Chieti, Italy
Bioengineering and Biomedicine Company Srl, San Giovanni Teatino, Chieti, Italy

Edyta Kinel
Department of Rheumatology and Rehabilitation, Clinic of Rehabilitation, University of Medical Sciences, Poznan, Poland

Gabriele D'Amico and Piero Roncoletta
Bioengineering and Biomedicine Company Srl, San Giovanni Teatino, Chieti, Italy

Prachi Bakarania, Hagit Berdishevsky and Kelly Grimes
Columbia University Medical Center, New York, NY, USA

John Tunney
East Coast Orthotics & Prosthetics, New York, NY, USA

Yizhar Floman and Michael A. Millgram
Israel Spine Center, Assuta Hospital Tel Aviv, Israel

Bauer Sabine
Institute for Medical Engineering and Information Processing, University Koblenz-Landau, Koblenz, Germany

Paulus Dietrich
Institute for Computer Science, University Koblenz-Landau, Koblenz, Germany

Antonino Raco and Alessandro Pesce
"Sapienza" University, Rome, Italy

Massimo Miscusi
"ICOT" Hospital, Latina – "Sapienza" Univesity, Rome, Italy

Index

www.ingramcontent.com/pod-product-compliance
Lightning Source LLC
LaVergne TN
LVHW081038210926
848485LV00004B/1056